*JOURNAL OF PROSTHODONTICS
ON COMPLETE AND
REMOVABLE DENTURES*

JOURNAL OF PROSTHODONTICS ON COMPLETE AND REMOVABLE DENTURES

Edited by

JONATHAN P. WIENS, DDS, MSD, FACP

JENNIFER WIENS PRIEBE, DDS, MS, FACP

DONALD A. CURTIS, DMD, FACP

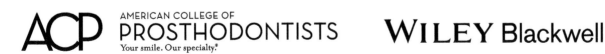

AMERICAN COLLEGE OF
PROSTHODONTISTS
Your smile. Our specialty.®

WILEY Blackwell

Registered Office
John Wiley & Sons, Inc., 111 River Street, Hoboken, NJ 07030, USA

Editorial Office
111 River Street, Hoboken, NJ 07030, USA

For details of our global editorial offices, customer services, and more information about Wiley products visit us at www.wiley.com.

Wiley also publishes its books in a variety of electronic formats and by print-on-demand. Some content that appears in standard print versions of this book may not be available in other formats.

Library of Congress Cataloging-in-Publication Data

Names: Wiens, Jonathan P. (Jonathan Peter), 1948– editor. | Priebe, Jennifer
 Wiens, 1975– editor. | Curtis, Donald A., 1954– editor. | American College
 of Prosthodontists, issuing body.
Title: Journal of prosthodontics on complete and removable dentures / edited
 by Jonathan P. Wiens, Jennifer Wiens Priebe, Donald A. Curtis.
Other titles: Complete and removable dentures | Journal of Prosthodontics.
Description: Hoboken, NJ : Wiley, 2018. | Includes bibliographical references
 and index. |
Identifiers: LCCN 2017051208 (print) | LCCN 2017052066 (ebook) | ISBN
 9781119442639 (pdf) | ISBN 9781119442646 (epub) | ISBN 9781119442622
 (cloth)
Subjects: | MESH: Denture, Complete | Mouth, Edentulous | Technology,
 Dental—methods | Collected Works
Classification: LCC RK656 (ebook) | LCC RK656 (print) | NLM WU 5 | DDC
 617.6/92—dc23
LC record available at https://lccn.loc.gov/2017051208

Cover images: (Main image) Courtesy of Dr. Sreenivas Koka;
　　　　　　　(Top inset) Courtesy of Charles J. Goodacre;
　　　　　　　(Bottom insert) Courtesy of Jonathan P. Wiens
Cover design by Wiley

Set in 10/12 pt TimesLTStd-Roman by Thomson Digital, Noida, India

Printed in the United States of America

10 9 8 7 6 5 4 3 2 1

CONTENTS

PREFACE

Textbooks on removable complete dentures have historically included an emphasis on technical procedures and materials sciences as they apply to the rehabilitation of the edentulous patient. However, in this compilation of 30 articles from the *Journal of Prosthodontics*, we have also selected articles that provide insight to the functional, psychosocial, nutritional, and comorbid factors that influence our ability to improve outcomes for the edentulous patient. This is relevant, as the total number of patients in the United States needing dentures has been increasing and because the edentulous state is interconnected to a patient's general well being.

This textbook started with the review of over 2,000 *Journal of Prosthodontics* articles related to removable complete dentures. The authors established a ranking that resulted in the 30 most impactful articles.* We divided the 30 articles into five thematic parts: Part I; Edentulism and Comorbidities, Part II; Oral Health, Biofilms, and Denture Stomatitis, Part III; Treatment Innovations, Part IV; Functional Parameters and Assessment, and Part V; Esthetic Considerations. Of the 30 articles selected, the article by Felton, Cooper, Duqum, et al on "Evidence-based guidelines for the care and maintenance of complete dentures" is featured on the book cover.

We encourage you to review this textbook with the idea of advancing your understanding of removable complete dentures. In addition to the above-selected articles, we suggest readers consider searching additional valuable literature on removable complete dentures that is available in the *Journal* online. Valuable information can be found by searching for removable complete dentures and keywords such as education, parameters of care, materials testing, occlusion, treatment methods, patient acceptance, satisfaction, adaptability, maxillofacial prosthetics, laboratory, CAD/CAM digital dentures, anatomy, and preprosthetic surgery.

The editors appreciate the opportunity to provide this textbook on removable complete dentures and hope that you will find value in reading the selected articles.

JONATHAN P. WIENS, DDS, MSD, FACP
JENNIFER L. PRIEBE, DDS, MS, FACP
DONALD A. CURTIS, DMD, FACP

---

*All author affiliations and addresses were correct at the time of their original publication.

PART I

EDENTULISM AND COMORBIDITIES

1

EVIDENCE-BASED GUIDELINES FOR THE CARE AND MAINTENANCE OF COMPLETE DENTURES: A PUBLICATION OF THE AMERICAN COLLEGE OF PROSTHODONTISTS

David Felton, DDS, MS, FACP,[1] Lyndon Cooper, DDS, PHD, FACP,[2] Ibrahim Duqum, BDS, MS,[3] Glenn Minsley, DMD,[4] Albert Guckes, DDS, MS,[4] Steven Haug, DDS, MSD, FACP,[5] Patricia Meredith, DDS, MS,[6] Caryn Solie, RDH,[7] David Avery, AAS, CDT,[8] and Nancy Deal Chandler, MA, RHIA, CAE[9]

[1]Professor, Department of Prosthodontics, School of Dentistry, University of North Carolina Chapel Hill, Chapel Hill, NC
[2]Stallings Distinguished Professor and the Chair, Department of Prosthodontics, School of Dentistry, University of North Carolina Chapel Hill, Chapel Hill, NC
[3]Clinical Assistant Professor, Department of Prosthodontics, School of Dentistry, University of North Carolina Chapel Hill, Chapel Hill, NC
[4]Associate Professor, Department of Prosthodontics, School of Dentistry, University of North Carolina Chapel Hill, Chapel Hill, NC
[5]Professor, Restorative Dentistry, School of Dentistry, Indiana University, Indianapolis, IN
[6]Clinical Associate Professor, Department of Oral Pathology, Radiology and Medicine, School of Dentistry, University of Iowa, Iowa City, IA
[7]Dental Hygienist, Spanish Springs Family Dental, Sparks, NV
[8]Director of Training and Education, Drake Precision Dental Laboratory, Charlotte, NC
[9]Executive Director, American College of Prosthodontists, Chicago, IL

Keywords
Dentures; edentulism; biofilm; adhesives; denture cleansers; denture relining; denture rebasing; denture repair; denture wear; stomatitis.

Correspondence
David Felton, Department of Prosthodontics, School of Dentistry, University of North Carolina Chapel Hill, 330 Brauer Hall, CB #7450, Chapel Hill, NC 27599-7450.
E-mail: dave_felton@dentistry.unc.edu

guidelines in collaboration with the Academy of General Dentistry, the American Dental Association Council on Scientific Affairs, the American Dental Hygienists' Association, the National Association of Dental Laboratories, and GlaxoSmithKline Consumer Healthcare.

Funding for the guidelines development project and for this special supplement was provided by GlaxoSmithKline Consumer Healthcare.

Published in *Journal of Prosthodontics* 2011; Vol. 20, Suppl 1, pp. S1–S12

doi: 10.1111/j.1532-849X.2010.00683.x

ABSTRACT

The current rates of edentulism have been estimated to be between 7% and 69% of the adult population internationally. In the United States, while the incidence of edentulism continues to decline, rapid population growth coupled with current economic conditions suggest that edentulism and conventional denture use will continue at current or higher numbers. Unfortunately, evidence-based guidelines for the care and maintenance of removable complete denture prostheses do not exist. In 2009, the American College of Prosthodontists (ACP) formed a task force to establish evidence-based guidelines for the care and maintenance of complete dentures. The task force comprised members of the ACP, the Academy of General Dentistry, American Dental Association (ADA) Council on Scientific Affairs, the American Dental Hygienists' Association, the National Association of Dental Laboratories, and representatives from GlaxoSmithKline Consumer Healthcare. The review process included the assessment of over 300 abstracts and selection of over 100 articles meeting inclusion criteria of this review. The task force reviewed synopses of the literature and formulated 15 evidence-based guidelines for denture care and maintenance. These guidelines were reviewed by clinical experts from the participating organizations and were published in February 2011 issue of *The Journal of the American Dental Association* for widespread distribution to the dental community. These guidelines reflect the views of the task force.

It is estimated that between 7% and 69% of adult populations internationally are affected with complete edentulism, which is defined as the loss of all permanent teeth.[1] Additionally, 26% of the U.S. population between the ages of 65 and 74 years are edentulous, and low income and education levels have the highest correlation with tooth loss.[2–4] While the incidence of complete edentulism in the United States continues to decline (approximately 6% between 1988 and 2000,[5] continued growth in the population strongly suggests that edentulism rates will remain constant or increase over the next few decades.[6] However, with the increasing need and expected demand for complete denture services, there are few published guidelines on the daily and long-term care and maintenance of complete denture prostheses.

METHODS

In 2009, the American College of Prosthodontists (ACP) formed a task force to develop contemporary, evidence-based guidelines for the care and maintenance of complete dentures. This task force comprised individuals representing the ACP, the Council on Scientific Affairs of the American Dental Association, the Academy of General Dentistry, the American Dental Hygienists' Association, the National Association of Dental Laboratories, and representatives from GlaxoSmithKline Consumer Healthcare.

A literature search was conducted by task force members using PubMed, EMBASE, known prosthodontic references and materials obtained from the U.S. Centers for Disease Control and Prevention. Search words and MEDLINE Medical Subject Headings for the search included the terms "complete dentures," "edentulism" and various combinations of those terms and the following: "biofilm," "adhesives," "cleansers," "cleaning," "relines," "rebases," "repairs," "nocturnal (or continuous) wear," "stomatitis," and "maintenance." Abstracts of the following types of articles were reviewed: Cochrane Reviews, systematic reviews, general literature reviews, meta-analyses, randomized controlled trials, prospective clinical trials, cross-sectional studies, retrospective cohort studies and any in vitro studies that introduced novel approaches to evaluation of the topic. Over 300 abstracts were reviewed, and set inclusion and exclusion criteria allowed the identification of 150 manuscripts, which were reviewed by members of the ACP. Inclusion criteria included:

- clinical trials involving more than 10 participants;
- clinical trials of more than 7 days' duration;
- crossover trials with or without a washout period.

The ACP task force members reviewed the abstracts and excluded from further assessment those studies that did not meet the inclusion criteria. The same task force members printed and reviewed full-text articles and collated all data from the manuscripts on manuscript review matrixes. The reviewers summarized data for discussion by the entire task force. Over 120 manuscripts were included in this review. After the reviewing task force members conducted a careful analysis of the manuscripts, they provided summaries to all task force members for review, and a meeting was held at the School of Dentistry, University of North Carolina Chapel Hill, in May 2010 to develop the guidelines. After the meeting and multiple conference calls, the document that follows was developed and agreed upon by the task force members.

This document provides the practicing clinician with the evidence-based guidelines for the care and maintenance of complete dentures. In the main portion of the document, the guidelines are reported in bold type followed immediately by the evidentiary documentation. This document has been distributed to the communities of interest for review and input, and subsequently this document has been developed for distribution.

GUIDELINES FOR THE CARE AND MAINTENANCE OF DENTURES

Based on the best available evidence, the following are guidelines for the care and maintenance of dentures:

1. **Careful daily removal of the bacterial biofilm present in the oral cavity and on complete dentures is of paramount importance to minimize denture stomatitis and to help contribute to good oral and general health.**

2. **To reduce levels of biofilm and potentially harmful bacteria and fungi, patients who wear dentures should do the following:**

   (a) **Dentures should be cleaned daily by soaking and brushing with an effective, nonabrasive denture cleanser.**

   (b) **Denture cleansers should ONLY be used to clean dentures outside of the mouth.**

   (c) **Dentures should always be thoroughly rinsed after soaking and brushing with denture-cleansing solutions prior to reinsertion into the oral cavity. Always follow the product usage instructions.**

3. **Although the evidence is weak, dentures should be cleaned annually by a dentist or dental professional using ultrasonic cleansers to minimize biofilm accumulation over time.**

4. **Dentures should never be placed in boiling water.**

5. **Dentures should not be soaked in sodium hypochlorite bleach, or in products containing sodium hypochlorite, for periods that exceed 10 minutes. Placement of dentures in sodium hypochlorite solutions for periods longer than 10 minutes may damage dentures.**

6. **Dentures should be stored immersed in water after cleaning, when not replaced in the oral cavity, to avoid warping.**

7. **Denture adhesives, when properly used, can improve the retention and stability of dentures and help seal out the accumulation of food particles beneath the dentures, even in well-fitting dentures.**

8. **In a quality-of-life study[88] patient ratings showed that denture adhesives may improve the denture wearer's perceptions in retention, stability, and quality of life; however, there is insufficient evidence that adhesives improve masticatory function.**

9. **Evidence regarding the effects of denture adhesives on the oral tissues when used for periods longer than 6 months is lacking. Thus, extended use of denture adhesives should not be considered without periodic assessment of denture quality and health of the supporting tissues by a dentist, prosthodontist, or dental professional.**

10. **Improper use of zinc-containing denture adhesives may have adverse systemic effects. Therefore, as a precautionary measure, zinc-containing denture adhesives should be avoided.**

11. **Denture adhesive should only be used in sufficient quantities (three or four pea-sized dollops) on each denture to provide sufficient added retention and stability to the prostheses.**

12. **Denture adhesives should be completely removed from the prosthesis and the oral cavity on a daily basis.**

13. **If increasing amounts of adhesives are required to achieve the same level of denture retention, the patient should see a dentist or dental professional to evaluate the fit and stability of the dentures.**

14. **While existing studies provide conflicting results, it is not recommended that dentures should be worn continuously (24 hours per day) in an effort to reduce or minimize denture stomatitis.**

15. **Patients who wear dentures should be checked annually by the dentist, prosthodontist, or dental professional for maintenance of optimum denture fit and function, for evaluation for oral lesions and bone loss, and for assessment of oral health status.**

EDENTULISM: ITS RELATIONSHIP TO ORAL AND SYSTEMIC HEALTH

The oral health of the completely edentulous patient is a significant factor related to the quality of life, nutrition, social interactions and general systemic health of denture-wearing patients (for a review, see Felton[7]). While often not life-threatening, the presence of oral biofilm on complete dentures has been associated with denture stomatitis, as well as with more serious systemic conditions, especially in the dependent elderly. Published reports regarding the relationship between oral health and systemic diseases in the edentulous, the partially edentulous and the dentate patient are increasing.

Oral bacteria have been implicated in bacterial endocarditis,[8–10] aspiration pneumonia,[11–20] chronic obstructive pulmonary disease,[21] generalized infections of the respiratory tract[22] and other systemic diseases.[23,24] Excellent reviews of the pathogenic potential of denture plaque have been published.[25,26]

A 2008 report by Ishikawa and colleagues[27] indicated that weekly professional cleaning of complete dentures (brushing, cleaning of dentures with denture brush, ultrasonic irrigation of denture with denture cleanser, swabbing of oral tissues with a sponge brush) significantly decreased multiple oral bacterial strains when compared with the daily chemical disinfection methods, and suggested this to be a viable strategy for reducing aspiration pneumonia in the dependent elderly. Clearly, evidence is mounting regarding the relationship between proper complete denture hygiene and overall systemic health.

DENTURE BIOFILMS

Dentures accumulate plaque, stain and calculus similar to the natural dentition. Failure to properly clean the accumulated biofilm from the dentures is associated with an increased incidence of localized denture stomatitis[28–30] in addition to the more serious systemic diseases noted earlier. Denture plaque is a complex aggregate of oral bacteria, fungi and other organisms; it is estimated to contain more than 10^{11} organisms per milligram (wet weight)[24] involving more than 30 different species.[31] While there is general consensus that the composition of denture plaque is similar to that of plaque in the dentate patient,[32] the biomass may vary between individuals and between sites in the oral cavity and sites on the dentures.

It has also been determined that dental biofilms accumulate more readily on rough denture surfaces than on smooth ones. In an in vitro study by Charman and colleagues,[33] denture acrylic resin samples were prepared to four different degrees of surface roughness, after which *Streptococcus oralis* was cultured on the samples. Specific areas of the acrylic resin were observed by using microscopy over eight incubation time points (inoculation period of 5 hours). Surface roughness varied from highly polished roughness average (Ra) value of 0.07 microns, to brushing with a mechanical brushing machine (Oral-B soft toothbrush) with baking soda (Ra value of 0.29 μm), to brushing with the same machine using silica toothpaste (Ra value of 0.38 μm), to sanding with silicon carbide paper (Ra value of 1.14 μm). The study demonstrated that there was increased coverage of the denture with *Streptococcus* bacteria as the surface roughness increased, and that heat-processed denture base acrylic was less likely to grow organisms than were cold-cured resin bases. The study may have a significant effect on the efficacy of denture cleaning, general denture hygiene and biofilm reformation of various cleaning regimens, and the results indicate that nonabrasive cleansers may offer a more appropriate regimen. Care should be taken not to scratch the surface of processed denture bases or acrylic prosthetic denture teeth; however, one needs to understand that the intaglio surface of the denture base, that surface in contact with the oral tissues, is never polished.

DENTURE STOMATITIS

Careful daily removal of the bacterial biofilm present in the oral cavity and on complete dentures is of paramount importance to minimize denture stomatitis and to help contribute to good oral and general health.

Denture stomatitis is a common occurrence in denture wearers, resulting in an area of erythema beneath the denture. Its etiology is multifactorial, and it may be associated with both local and systemic factors.[34] For a review on the topic, see Loewy.[35] As many as 67% of existing denture wearers are thought to have *Candida*-associated denture stomatitis.[36] The role of *Candida albicans* in the pathogenesis of denture stomatitis has been well investigated, and multiple strains of *Candida* have been found to populate the denture base, as well as the oral tissues.[30]

Recently, Campos et al[37] collected samples from both the oral tissues and corresponding regions on the intaglio surfaces of the dentures in patients who were healthy (had no inflammation), and from patients with denture stomatitis. They identified 82 bacterial species in healthy patients and those with denture stomatitis, including three types of *Candida* sp. However, 26 bacterial phylotypes were found only in the healthy denture wearers (with a strong representation of *Streptococcus* sp), while 32 phylotypes were exclusively found in those patients with denture stomatitis. The stomatitis group was represented by *Streptococcus* sp (23%), *Atopobium* sp (16%), and *Prevotella* sp (11%). *C. albicans* was identified as the primary fungal species in the stomatitis group, while there was a greater diversity of three *Candida* sp found in the healthy population (*C. albicans*, 22%; *Candida glabrata*, 54%; *Candida tropicalis*, 24%). The authors concluded that there appear to be distinct biofilms present in healthy subjects and in those with denture stomatitis. Denture stomatitis is a disease that is chronic and multifactorial, and it tends to compromise the edentulous patient's quality of life. Eradicating this disease requires treatment of both the oral tissues and the removable prostheses.

DENTURE CLEANING

To reduce levels of biofilm and potentially harmful bacteria and fungi, patients who wear dentures should do the following:

- **Dentures should be cleaned daily by soaking and brushing with an effective, nonabrasive denture cleanser.**
- **Denture cleansers should ONLY be used to clean dentures outside of the mouth.**
- **Dentures should always be thoroughly rinsed after soaking and brushing with denture-cleansing solutions prior to reinsertion into the oral cavity. Always follow the product usage instructions.**

Although the evidence is weak, dentures should be cleaned annually by a dentist or dental professional using ultrasonic cleansers to minimize biofilm accumulation over time.

Dentures should never be placed in boiling water.

Dentures should not be soaked in sodium hypochlorite bleach, or in products containing sodium hypochlorite, for periods that exceed 10 minutes. Placement of dentures in sodium hypochlorite solutions for periods longer than 10 minutes may damage dentures.

Dentures should be stored immersed in water after cleaning, when not replaced in the oral cavity, to avoid warping.

Because of the defined relationship of biofilm to stomatitis, dentists and healthcare providers must carefully instruct the edentulous patient in the proper methods for cleaning and maintaining dentures. An important unanswered question is what defines a "clean" removable denture.

The characteristics of an ideal denture cleanser should include the following

- It should, at a minimum, demonstrate antibiofilm activity to remove biofilm and stains and should be antibacterial and antifungal to minimize the level of biofilm and potentially harmful pathogens in the biofilm below clinically relevant levels; however, this acceptable level has yet to be defined.
- It should be nontoxic
- It should be compatible with denture materials, and should not modify (roughen) or degrade the surface of the acrylic resin denture base or prosthetic teeth.
- It should be short acting (≤ 8 hours).
- It should be easy to use for the patient or caregiver.
- It should have an acceptable (or no) taste.
- It should be cost effective.

Three literature reviews on denture cleansers were identified by the task force. Abelson's[38] review focused on the literature published between 1936 and 1983. The Abelson review described the nature of denture plaque and its role in oral disease. Additionally, Abelson reviewed the development of denture cleansers, their mechanism of cleansing and their efficacy. The Abelson review suggested that the use of abrasive pastes may be the most efficacious method of denture cleansing, that hypochlorite solutions were highly effective but potentially damaging to prostheses, and that new standards for evaluating denture cleansers were needed.

A second review by Nikawa et al[39] focused on the literature published between 1979 and 1995. This review covered more than 20 articles that evaluated the efficacy of denture cleansers and determined that the results obtained were highly dependent on the methods used to evaluate the selected cleansing methods. Nikawa et al,[39] like Abelson,[38] called for the development of a standardized method for evaluation of denture cleansers.

Third, a Cochrane Review on interventions for cleaning dentures was recently published by de Souza et al.[40] After careful comparison of the six clinical trials in this Cochrane Review[41–46] the authors suggested that there was no evidence that any denture-cleaning method is more beneficial than others for the health of the denture-bearing tissues or has a higher level of patient satisfaction or preference than that of others.

Brushing with denture creams and pastes: Three in vivo studies considered the efficacy of denture paste in biofilm removal. Dills et al[41] suggested that brushing with a denture paste was inferior to use of an effervescent cleaner or to use of the same cleaner followed by paste brushing. Panzeri et al[42] demonstrated that brushing with two types of pastes (one antibacterial and one with a fluorosurfactant) reduced the biofilm mass when compared with brushing with water; however, brushing with either paste had no impact on *Candida* sp colonization. Finally, Barnabé et al[43] compared brushing the dentures with coconut soap followed by soaking in sodium hypochlorite (NaOCl) (10 minutes) to brushing with soap and soaking in water. This cross-sectional study indicated that both treatments reduced the levels of denture stomatitis, but that neither treatment reduced the levels of *Candida* sp cultured from the prostheses. Thus, *Candida* sp appears to be resistant to mechanical debridement from the denture base. Other methods of denture cleansing appear superior to this method, and the abrasiveness of denture pastes is of concern.

Soaking and brushing with commercially available denture cleansers (effervescent tablets): Commercially available denture cleansers use various active agents—including hypochlorites, peroxides, enzymes, acids and oral mouth rinses—to remove biofilm from dentures. Each of these immersion cleansers has a different mode of action and a different rate of efficacy for removal of adherent denture biofilms. While the denture-cleaning methods tested were capable of reducing the biomass present on dentures over the various time courses evaluated, none of the in vivo trials reviewed demonstrated that any of the methods used was bactericidal.[44–48] In vitro studies, however, have demonstrated that NaOCl was superior to all other types of commercially available denture cleansers.[49–55] In addition, the emergence of methicillin-resistant *Staphylococcus aureus* (MRSA), a major pathogen in the immuno-compromised patient, has become a major issue in hospitalized patients, as MRSAs increase mortality rates significantly. An in vitro investigation by Lee and colleagues[57] indicated that NaOCl was capable of killing MRSA. Neither of the commercially available denture cleansers used in this trial was bactericidal against the pathogens tested, but both reduced the biomass levels.

Ultrasonic cleaning: Ultrasonic cleaning of dentures occurs frequently in both the dental office and the dental laboratory. The mode of action of ultrasonic devices is unique in that they produce ultrasonic sound waves (20 to 120 kHz), which create microscopic cavities (bubbles) that grow and implode. This implosion creates voids that result in localized areas of suction. Materials adhering to the denture are loosened and removed by this action. This action is commonly known as "cavitation." Two representative types of solutions that are commercially available for use in the ultrasonic cleaner are BioSonic Enzymatic (Coltène/Whaledent, Cuyahoga Falls, OH), which contains nonionic detergents, protease enzymes and 400 parts per million isopropyl alcohol, and Ultra-Kleen (Sterilex, Hunt Valley, MD), which requires the mixing of two solutions that results in the formation of an alkaline-peroxide cleanser. Interestingly, while ultrasonic cleaning demonstrated remarkably improved kill rates of bacteria, neither of these two solutions tested were completely bactericidal.[57,58] The literature review indicated that the use of other commercially available denture cleansers in conjunction with ultrasonic cleaning in the dental office has not been investigated.

Precautions associated with use of denture cleansers: In 2008 the U.S. Food and Drug Administration[59] (FDA) issued a requirement for manufacturers of denture cleansers to revise their labeling regarding contents, and to consider alternatives to the types of ingredients present in this class of products. This action was in response to 73 severe reactions, including at least one death, linked to denture cleansers. The specifically identified ingredient, persulfate, is known to cause allergic reactions. Persulfates are used in denture cleansers as part of the cleaning and bleaching process. Symptoms of the reaction to persulfates include

- irritation of the tissues;
- tissue damage;
- rash;

- hives;
- gum tenderness;
- breathing problems;
- low blood pressure.

The FDA noted that other reactions may be the result of misuse of the product by patients. The requirement specifically involves labeling revisions to ensure that denture wearers understand that these products are for use only when the dentures are outside the mouth. Symptoms related to misuse of the denture cleansers can include:

- damage to the esophagus;
- abdominal pain;
- burns;
- breathing problems;
- low blood pressure;
- seizures;
- bleaching of tissues;
- internal bleeding;
- vomiting.

Alternative denture cleansing methods: Currently, there are few techniques that sterilize complete dentures following intraoral use. Microwave irradiation of dentures immersed in sterile water at 650 Watts for three minutes sterilizes dentures without causing surface degradation of the prosthesis. However, the long-term effects of this technique have not been investigated.[60–63] Additionally, boiling of a denture base has been shown to deform the base, rendering it unusable. All other forms of denture cleansing appear to reduce the bacterial and fungal biofilm, but are disinfecting the prosthesis only. Of the immersion products available, NaOCl may be the most effective product available, but only when used properly (10-minute soaking). Soaking dentures for extended periods of time (i.e., overnight) in NaOCl may degrade the acrylic resin components, causing color changes (lightening), and therefore should be avoided. Additionally, once cleaned, dentures should remain immersed in water to prevent over drying of the base, with resultant warping of the prosthesis.

DENTURE CARE AND MANAGEMENT

Denture adhesives, when properly used, can improve the retention and stability of dentures and help seal out the accumulation of food particles beneath the dentures, even in well-fitting dentures.

In a quality-of-life study,[88] patient ratings showed that denture adhesives may improve the denture wearer's perceptions of retention, stability and quality of life;

however, there is insufficient evidence that adhesives improve masticatory function.

Evidence regarding the effects of denture adhesives on the oral tissues when used for periods longer than 6 months is lacking. Thus, extended use of denture adhesives should not be considered without periodic assessment of denture quality and health of the supporting tissues by a dentist, prosthodontist or dental professional.

Improper use of zinc-containing denture adhesives may have adverse systemic effects. Therefore, as a precautionary measure, zinc-containing denture adhesives should be avoided.

Denture adhesive should only be used in sufficient quantities (three or four pea-sized dollops) on each denture to provide sufficient added retention and stability to the prostheses.

Denture adhesives should be completely removed from the prosthesis and the oral cavity on a daily basis.

If increasing amounts of adhesives are required to achieve the same level of denture retention, the patient should see a dentist or dental professional to evaluate the fit and stability of the dentures.

While existing studies provide conflicting results, it is not recommended that dentures should be worn continuously (24 hours per day) in an effort to reduce or minimize denture stomatitis.

Patients who wear dentures should be checked annually by the dentist, prosthodontist, or dental professional for maintenance of optimum denture fit and function, for evaluation for oral lesions and bone loss, and for assessment of oral health status.

Use of denture adhesives: Complete dentures are retained in the oral cavity through a complex interaction of factors that include close adaptation of the intaglio surface of the prosthesis to the underlying tissues, appropriate peripheral extension of the denture borders, the presence of a thin film of saliva of acceptable viscosity between the prosthesis and the tissues, and atmospheric pressure. Following tooth removal and denture placement, significant resorption of the residual ridges typically occurs over the first 3 to 12 months. The resorption usually continues at a lower level throughout the life of the patient.[64,66] As bone is lost, the adaptation of the denture to the bearing tissues is compromised, resulting in ill-fitting dentures with compromised retention that decrease the wearer's chewing ability. Denture wearers may have conditions that significantly affect retention and stability of their oral prostheses. In addition to hard- and soft-tissue changes over time, these patients often experience problems with diminished neuromuscular control, reduced bite force, and alterations in the quantity and quality of saliva due to age or medications. Several methods have been developed to enhance both fit and retention of aging prostheses. These methods include denture adhesives, prosthesis relining, rebasing and the use of endosseous dental implants. Denture adhesives are widely available in formulations of creams, powders, pads/wafers, strips, or liquids.

Advantages of using denture adhesives: Twenty clinical trials were identified and reviewed that focused on the use of denture adhesives relative to their effect on denture retention, stability, movement, bite force, ability to chew test foods, food occlusion or patient satisfaction. Most of these studies were of short duration (same-day evaluation). Some trials randomly allocated patients to various experimental groups (depending on numbers of adhesives investigated), and most investigated effects on the maxillary denture only. Some did not have a control group, and many were crossover in design (comparing dentures without adhesives to the same prosthesis with adhesive).

In a study of 146 denture-wearing patients in a dental school in Adelaide, South Australia, Coates[67] found that 52.0% of the patients surveyed saw no need for using denture adhesives, as they managed their dentures well, 20.5% did not know denture adhesives existed, and 32.9% had used denture adhesives in the past, but only 6.9% of those previously using adhesives continued to use them on a regular basis. Instruction regarding denture adhesives and their proper use is important.

Despite limitations, several studies yielded results indicating that denture adhesives improved retention and stability of both ill-fitting and well-fitting dentures.[68–78] Some studies measured the adhesive-related improvement in retention and stability[78–81] and showed more improvement in old or ill-fitting dentures than in new prostheses. However, Grasso and colleagues[76,82] reported no difference in improvement between well-fitting and poorly fitting prostheses.

Regarding mastication, the use of denture adhesives has been reported to significantly improve the bite force a denture patient is able to exert compared with using no adhesives.[79,82–85] Rendell and colleagues[86] further evaluated chewing rates in denture wearers using a multichannel magnetometer tracking device and found that the mean chewing rates increased after application of denture adhesive.[70] Ghani and Picton[74] used subjective measures to evaluate whether adhesives improved chewing ability, comfort, retention and patient confidence in denture wearers.

Functional changes associated with denture adhesive application is time dependent. Rendell et al[85,86] found that chewing improved immediately after applying the adhesive and continued to increase after two and four hours. While many studies indicate that adhesives are effective for up to eight hours, one trial by Kapur et al[76] indicated that the mandibular denture, in spite of showing initial improvements in retention, underwent significant loss of retention following chewing of test foods and imbibing of taste solutions. The duration of effectiveness of adhesive retention is variable and often product dependent.

Improvements in oral health-related quality of life (OHR-QOL): The condition of complete edentulism and the use of complete dentures have been shown to have a negative impact on the patient's QOL.[87] The effect of denture adhesives on OHR-QOL have recently been reported in a longitudinal study of 14 denture-wearing patients conducted by Nicholas et al.[88] These patients were selected from 143 denture-wearing patients because of their low QOL scores following denture insertion. In this 6-month prospective trial, patients had their QOL assessed at the time of denture insertion and 3 months following insertion. At the 3 month time point, the patients were provided with denture adhesives, and they were assessed again at 6 months following denture placement (3 months after adhesive introduction). They were assessed by means of a Geriatric Oral Health Assessment Index questionnaire,[89] which assesses their OHR-QOL. The results indicated that, while the denture adhesive may have improved the participants' ability to manage conventional dentures and enhance their QOL, no improvement in masticatory performance was found. Thus, while many studies have reported improvements in denture retention and stability with adhesive use, there is limited evidence at this time to suggest that OHR-QOL is improved by using denture adhesives.

Precautions when using denture adhesives: *Cytotoxic effects*. Several articles have evaluated the potential cytotoxic effects of denture adhesives. Two studies were in vitro studies, including studies for evaluating the irritation and cytotoxic potential of commercially available adhesives (creams, powders, and pads). Al et al[90] demonstrated that only one of six adhesive types evaluated induced severe cytotoxic reactions. The authors did, however, raise concerns that adhesives may contribute to mucosal inflammation in denture wearers. Dahl[91] investigated the mucosal irritation induced in vitro by 27 different dental adhesive products. He found that most adhesives damaged the blood vessels of the test apparatus, indicating potential irritant effects on the mucous membranes.

Two in vitro studies revealed both bacterial and fungal contaminants in denture adhesives. Gates et al[92] tested four brands of adhesives and suggested that microwave irradiation of the adhesives for 10 minutes in their original containers may reduce the contaminants. However, in their study, the irradiation had no effect on five of the 24 containers of adhesives tested. The authors recommended caution when prescribing adhesives to the immune compromised patient cohort. Eckstrand and colleagues[93] evaluated 19 commercially available adhesives for microbial contamination and formaldehyde content. Using the agar overlay technique, the authors found that all of the materials tested caused severe cytologic effects. Formaldehyde was found in substantial amounts in four products and in minor amounts in two other products.

In vivo trials have found few negative effects attributed to adhesive use. In a cross-sectional study of 12 maxillary-complete-denture wearers, Kim and colleagues[94] collected samples from the patients' saliva and dentures to evaluate total viable counts of *Candida* sp 2 weeks prior to use of adhesives and after 2 weeks of adhesive use. The authors found no statistical difference between test (adhesive use) and control (nonadhesive use) relative to *Candida* sp counts either in the saliva or on the maxillary denture. They indicated that patient compliance and home care may have played a role in the lack of differences between the groups.

In a similar assessment of 24 denture-wearing patients, Oliveira and colleagues[95] compared the number of colony-forming units (CFUs) and *Candida* sp in saliva samples collected at denture placement and at 7-day and 14-day intervals from patients using an adhesive denture strip. Twelve patients (test group) using the adhesive tape were compared with 12 nonadhesive-wearing patients. There was no statistical difference between the groups at the 2-week analysis. However, neither of these trials evaluated the extended use of adhesives in denture wearers.

Finally, Al et al[90] suggested that since denture adhesives are commonly used throughout the day, denture adhesives may contribute to mucosal inflammation in denture wearers. However, as there are no longitudinal trials of continual use of denture adhesives, the effects of long-term use of adhesives on oral tissues is currently unknown.

Toxicity of zinc-containing adhesives: The most serious of the chronic and excessive use of denture adhesives reported to date is potential neurotoxicity related to the presence of zinc as a component of the adhesive. Zinc is an essential mineral normally found in some foods or used as a dietary supplement. It is involved in numerous aspects of cellular metabolism.[96]

The daily recommended allowances for zinc are 8 mg for women and 11 mg for men, respectively. Acute overdose can lead to nausea, vomiting, loss of appetite, cramps, diarrhea and headaches. Tolerable upper limits of zinc have been recommended at 40 mg per day[95]. Unfortunately, material safety data sheets for denture adhesives do not list the specific amounts of zinc contained by the adhesives. Case-series studies by Nations et al[97] of four patients, and by Hedera et al[98] of 11 patients, identified patients experiencing progressive neurological symptoms (myelopolyneuropathy) following extended chronic overuse of zinc-containing adhesives. This misuse of the adhesives by the patients resulted in hypocupremia and hyperzincemia with resultant neurological symptoms. However, no attempt was made in either study to assess whether the existing dentures exhibited acceptable fit, retention, occlusion and stability, or whether the patients affected were correctly using the zinc-containing adhesives. Both sets of authors identified denture adhesives as the sole source of the neurologic disease. Since these were published, at least one manufacturer has voluntarily removed all of its zinc-containing adhesives from the market as a precautionary measure and replaced them with zinc-free products.

Application and removal of adhesives from the intaglio surface of dentures: There are no studies reported to our knowledge that have evaluated the patient's ability to effectively place denture adhesives on the intaglio surface of the denture. However, three studies have evaluated the patient's ability to effectively remove the adhesive.

Sato[68] compared the ability of edentulous patients to remove an experimental gel and commercially available cream adhesive from both the intaglio surface of the denture and the maxillary soft tissues. The authors colored the adhesive with 0.4% indigo carmine to allow identification of the adhesive by the patient to facilitate its removal, and also evaluated the patient's ability to remove the adhesive from the maxillary soft tissues using a standardized five-stage method. Each stage involved the use of an undetermined mouth rinse, followed by application of cotton gauze or rinsing with hot water (70 °C) for two minutes; each technique was repeated five times by each patient. The authors found that repeating the process five times did not remove the cream adhesive, while a single stage completely removed the experimental gel adhesive.

A second study, by Uysal et al,[71] of 32 denture-wearing patients evaluated four adhesives in several categories (retention, function, cleansibility, etc.) on newly relined dentures. All adhesives were applied by the investigators, and patients were instructed to use the denture with adhesive for 24 hours. Patients were instructed to clean the dentures with their individual habitual cleaning method, which was not specified. Patients' perceptions were tallied. Although 20% to 30% of patients using each of the four adhesives reported that removal of the adhesive from their oral cavity and denture base was difficult to very difficult, no attempt to assess the degree of cleaning was performed by the authors.

A third study[73] similarly compared the perceptions of 32 patients regarding 10 different factors related to three commercially available adhesives and one formulated by a pharmacy (tragacanth powder). After application of one of the four adhesives and use for 1 day, the patients were interviewed regarding their opinions about the adhesive used. Unfortunately, there was no effort made to verify the patient's ability to successfully clean the tissues or the intaglio surface of the dentures; rather, only the patient's perceptions were collected.

Only the Sato[68] study adequately evaluated the patient's ability to successfully remove the adhesive from the tissues and denture base. Finally, there have been no long-term studies to investigate the potential effects of adhesive buildup on hard or soft oral tissues, if the patient fails to remove the adhesive completely.

Correct application of denture adhesives: The following clinical technique has been advocated by several manufacturers of denture adhesives for proper application to the denture base:

- Clean and dry the intaglio (tissue side) surface of the dentures.

- For the maxillary denture, apply three or four pea-sized increments of denture creams to the anterior ridge, midline of the palate, and posterior border.
- For the mandibular denture, apply three pea-sized increments of denture cream to several areas of the edentulous ridge.
- If using powder adhesive (instead of cream as noted above), wet the base with water, apply a thin film of powder to the entire tissue-contacting surface and shake off any excess.
- If using pad adhesives, place the correct size onto the denture and cut off any excess that extends beyond the denture border with sharp scissors.
- Seat the dentures independently; hold each firmly in place for 5 to 10 seconds.
- Remove any excess material that expresses into the cheek or tongue space.
- Bite firmly to spread the adhesive and remove any additional excess that expresses into the cheek or tongue spaces.

Residual ridge resorption: Multiple factors may lead to bone loss beneath complete dentures. Bone loss is associated with changes that affect the support and adaptation of complete dentures. Loss of alveolar bone, or residual ridge resorption (RRR), is multifactorial in nature. Factors that have been implicated in RRR include local and systemic effectors of bone resorption that include asthma (due to the use of corticosteroid inhalants),[99,100] fluoride consumption, hormone replacement therapy,[101] prior use of removable partial dentures prior to denture therapy,[102] poor oral hygiene,[103] and continuous wearing of dentures.[102,103] In a cross-sectional cohort study of 185 elderly patients in Finland, Xie and Ainamo[100] found that 67% of subjects studied wore their dentures day and night. Acceptable denture quality, as viewed by the examiners, was found to exist in only 10% of the mandibular prostheses and 36% of the maxillary prostheses. Mucosal lesions were found in 16% of the mandibles and 35% of the maxillae. Flabby ridges (suggestive of bone loss) were observed in 24% of the maxillae. The authors found that residual ridge reduction was significantly related to denture quality in both arches, and to prior use of a removable partial denture (odds ratio [OR] = 2.4). There has been one clinical study in humans that demonstrated that leaving dentures out at night, when compared with continual wearing of dentures, resulted in less bone loss beneath the denture bases.[104] However, other studies, including those by Bergman et al[105] and Kalk and de Baat,[106] have failed to corroborate these findings. The Kalk and de Baat study, a cross-sectional study of 92 patients, found a direct correlation between the number of years a patient was edentulous and resorption of the edentulous ridges, and with the number of previous dentures used by the patient. However, the authors could not find a significant correlation between bone loss and wearing dentures 24 hours a day.

Mucosal lesions and denture stomatitis: In a cross-sectional study of 889 elderly patients in Chile, Espinoza et al[107] found that 574 (nearly 65%) were completely edentulous. Of the entire group of patients examined, 53% of the patients had one or more oral mucosal lesions, the most frequent being denture stomatitis (22.3% of all patients, and 34.0% of all denture wearers). The OR for having oral mucosal lesions was 3.26 for the denture-wearing population when compared with the dentate population. Nocturnal wearing of dentures was associated with an increased likelihood of developing oral lesions (OR = 2.25).

Shulman et al[108] used data from the Third National Health and Nutrition Examination Survey (NHANES III) to explore the risk factors associated with denture stomatitis in the United States. Of 3,450 denture-wearing adults, they found that 27.9% displayed denture stomatitis. The prevalence of developing denture stomatitis was associated with continuous wearing of both the maxillary (OR = 6.20) and mandibular (OR = 5.21) prostheses, as well as with low vitamin A levels and cigarette smoking.

The connection between *Candida* sp and denture stomatitis has been known for decades. Studies by Emami et al[109] and Jeganathan et al[110] have demonstrated the direct relationship between the presence of *C. albicans* and other oral microorganisms and nocturnal denture wear. In Jeganthan et al's[110] study of 75 denture patients, the continuous wearing of dentures resulted in 61% of patients' developing denture stomatitis, compared with 18% of those who did not wear their dentures at night.

In a study of 68 denture-wearing patients from two university clinics, Barbeau and colleagues[111] investigated the relationship between denture stomatitis and *C. albicans*. Risk factors were determined for the patients on the basis of the findings. The investigators concluded that nocturnal wear of dentures and smoking was associated with extensive inflammation of the denture-bearing tissues. Unlike in most studies, the authors could not find a correlation between various *Candida* sp and stomatitis.

Arendorf and Walker,[112] in a matched cross-sectional study of 60 dentate and 60 denture-wearing patients, found that *C. albicans* and related denture stomatitis were found more frequently in patients who wore dentures continually than in those who removed them while sleeping. Similar findings were reported in a short-term evaluation of 24 patients by Compagnoni et al.[113]

The use of nystatin and other antifungal agents has been recommended as part of the treatment regimen to combat *Candida*-related denture stomatitis. A longitudinal controlled trial by Bergendal[114] evaluated the treatment regimen of 48 patients with denture stomatitis compared with 27 patients with healthy mucosa (control group). Treatment

of the stomatitis group included fabrication of new dentures, surgical and nystatin treatment, oral hygiene instruction and nutritional counseling. All patients were reassessed after 1 year. The authors found that the use of nystatin did not affect the healing of palatal erythema evaluated 1 year later. Additionally, the nocturnal use of dentures was directly associated with continual presence of denture stomatitis.

Peltola et al[115] examined 42 edentulous patients who had been treated with new complete dentures by dental students in Finland 30 months previously. The authors determined that the frequency of cleaning dentures was not correlated statistically with the condition of the oral mucosa, and those patients who wore their dentures day and night did not have any more stomatitis or hyperplastic changes than those who took them out at night. Finally, a review by MacEntee[116] documented several studies that demonstrated the ill effects of wearing dentures longer than 5 years. The ill effects were primarily related to the presence of soft-tissue lesions.

Relines, rebase of dentures and denture recall interval: The Glossary of Prosthodontic Terms, eighth edition,[117] defines reline as "the procedures used to resurface the tissue side of a denture with new base material, thus producing an accurate adaptation to the denture foundation area." Similarly, the term "rebase" is defined as "the laboratory process of replacing the entire denture base material on an existing prosthesis." While these procedures are seemingly similar, the reline procedure is most often used when factors other than loss of bone or soft-tissue support has changed for the patient (i.e., the vertical dimension, occlusion, phonetics and functionality of the dentures are acceptable), and these changes are compensated for by the addition of new acrylic resin to the intaglio surface of the denture. In those instances in which these other factors have apparently been compromised, the rebase procedure is used. This procedure can effect marked changes in denture architecture that influence vertical dimension, phonetics and associated function. The reorientation of teeth to the denture-bearing surface by means of the rebase procedure provides these potential benefits and at the same time provides a pristine intaglio surface opposing the mucosa.

Unfortunately, there are no published clinical guidelines to assist the clinician in determining how frequently to reline or rebase the dentures. A study by Marchini and colleagues[118] evaluated 236 complete-denture wearers in a Brazilian university dental clinic. They found that only 44% of the patients had sought treatment following completion of the dentures, and that this was at 10 years post completion. Another 23% of the patients had visited their dentist between 6 and 10 years following completion of denture therapy. Additionally, 78% of the patients indicated that they had received no instruction regarding denture cleaning, and 92% indicated that they had not been instructed to return for routine recall appointments. Denture stomatitis was found in 42% of the patients, although nearly 90% of those affected reported no symptoms. Finally, the authors found a positive relationship between the lack of oral hygiene instructions and the incidence of denture stomatitis. Family income and periodicity of recalls were also directly related to hygiene levels and incidence of stomatitis.

In the Peltola et al[115] study noted in the section earlier, the authors found that the retention of the maxillary denture was "moderate to poor" in 41% of the patients, and that the retention of the mandibular prosthesis was "moderate to poor" in 76% of the patients. The frequency of cleaning of the prostheses did not correlate with the necessity for relining procedures. The overall improvement of denture renewal (in this case, remaking of the prostheses), and improvements in quality and fit of the new dentures was found to have a positive effect on the patients' satisfaction with their prostheses, and on improved health of the denture-bearing tissues.

A finite element study of bone resorption beneath a maxillary complete denture was conducted by Maeda and Wood[119] simulating a poorly fitting denture and a newly rebased denture. The authors postulated, on the basis of their loading study, that RRR in the maxillary arch may be associated with compressive strains developed in the alveolar bone. Rebasing the denture accentuated the stresses, unless the position of the occlusal loads was carefully located (over the lingual cusps of maxillary posterior teeth, not the facial cusps). The authors recommend carefully adjusting the occlusion following rebasing procedures to provide lingual cusp contacts and balanced occlusion in protrusive and lateral excursions.

Recently, a Cochrane Review was conducted by Sutton et al[120] to investigate the effectiveness of denture occlusal schemes in improving patient satisfaction and, thus, in improving the success of the dentures. The authors could only find a single crossover clinical trial of 30 patients that compared a lingualized occlusal scheme with zero-degree teeth that met their inclusion criteria. The authors of this crossover trial[121] did find a statistically significant difference in favor of the lingualized occlusal scheme (OR = 10). However, the Cochrane Review suggested that the evidence was too weak to suggest that cusped posterior teeth were superior to flat-plane prosthetic teeth.

There are no studies to our knowledge that have evaluated appropriate recall intervals for the completely edentulous patient, and few references to what constitutes an appropriate recall interval in published textbooks. Because patient-specific and time-dependent changes of the denture-bearing tissues occur, all clinicians should periodically evaluate each denture wearer for RRR, changes in vertical dimension of occlusion, phonetics, integrity of the denture bases and prosthetic tooth wear, as well as for other biological reasons, including general systemic health, health of the oral soft tissues, oral cancer screening and blood pressure screenings.

FUTURE RESEARCH NEEDS

The ACP Task Force acknowledges that there are significant gaps in the literature related to complete denture care and maintenance. While primarily higher levels of evidence were sought in the search strategy, the task force did not attempt to categorize the reference materials on the basis of the strength of the evidence. Additionally, on the basis of the current level of evidence, the task force recommends that future clinical and laboratory research focus on the following areas:

1. Further exploration of effective cleaning methods will improve the quality of denture use, that is, microwave cleaning. This includes the long-term clinical evaluation and improvement of specific denture-cleaning components for safety, efficacy and ease of use.
2. The impact of denture hygiene on oral and general health requires additional investigation.
3. Proper identification of the inflammatory process in denture stomatitis could enable clinicians to prescribe proper treatments for this condition.
4. The long-term effects (longer than 6 months) of denture adhesive use on oral tissue health need to be determined. Additionally, methods for enhancing the removal of adhesives from the tissue-contacting surface of dentures and oral soft tissues should be developed.

DISCLOSURE

Funding for the guidelines development project was provided by GlaxoSmithKline Consumer Healthcare. The authors declare no conflicts of interest.

ACKNOWLEDGMENT

The authors thank Dr. Zvi Loewy, DDS, PhD, Vice President, Dental Care Future Team; Dr. Frank Gonser, DDS, PhD, MBA, Director, Medical Affairs, Dental Care Future Team; Sonya Greco, MT, MBA, Senior Manager of Professional Relations, US GlaxoSmithKline; and Grace Chu, RPh, MBA, Director, Medical Marketing, Dental Care Future Team, all of Glaxo-SmithKline Consumer Healthcare, for their support.

REFERENCES

1. Petersen PE, Bourgeois D, Bratthall D, et al: Oral health information systems—towards measuring progress in oral health promotion and disease prevention. *Bull World Health Organ* 2005;83:686–693.

2. Healthy People 2010. Volume II, Section 21: Oral Health. "www.healthypeople.gov/Document/HTML/Volume2/21Oral.htm". Accessed November 21, 2010.

3. National Center for Health Statistics. Healthy People 2000 Review 1998–99. Hyattsville, MD: U.S. Department of Health and Human Services, Public Health Service, Centers for Disease Control and Prevention, National Center for Health Statistics; 1999.

4. Burt BA, Eklund SA, Ismail AI: *Dentistry, Dental Practice, and the Community* (ed 5). Philadelphia, Saunders, 1999, pp. 205–206.

5. Beltran-Aguilar ED, Barker LK, Canto MT, et al: Surveillance for dental caries, dental sealants, tooth retention, edentulism, and enamel fluorosis—United States, 1988–1994 and 1999–2002. *MMWR Surveill Summ* 2005;54:1–43.

6. Douglass CW, Shih A, Ostry L: Will there be a need for complete dentures in the United States in 2020? *J Prosthet Dent* 2002;87:5–8.

7. Felton DA: Edentulism and comorbid factors. *J Prosthodont* 2009;18:88–96.

8. Berbari E, Cockerill FR 3rd, Steckelberg JM: Infective endocaditis due to unusual or fastidious microorganisms. *Mayo Clin Proc* 1997;72:532–542.

9. Li X, Kolltveit KM, Tronstad L, et al: Systemic diseases caused by oral infection. *Clin Microbiol Rev* 2000;13:547–558.

10. Drangsholt MT: A new causal model of dental diseases associated with endocarditis. *Ann Periodont* 1998;3:184–196.

11. Abe S, Ishihara K, Adachi M, et al: Oral hygiene evaluation for effective oral care in preventing pneumonia in dentate elderly. *Arch Gerontol Geriatr* 2006;43:53–64.

12. Sumi Y, Miura H, Sunakawa M, et al: Colonization of denture plaque by respiratory pathogens in dependent elderly. *Gerodontology* 2002;19:25–29.

13. Sumi Y, Miura H, Michiwaki Y, et al: Colonization of dental plaque by respiratory pathogens in dependent elderly. *Arch Gerontol Geriatr* 2007;44:119–124.

14. Sumi Y, Kagami H, Ohtsuka Y, et al: High correlation between the bacterial species in denture plaque and pharyngeal microflora. *Gerodontology* 2003;20:84–87.

15. Raghavendran K, Mylotte JM, Scannapieco FA: Nursing home-associated pneumonia, hospital-acquired pneumonia and ventilator-associated pneumonia: the contribution of dental biofilms and periodontal inflammation. *Peridontol 2000* 2007;44:164–177.

16. Yoon MN, Steele CM: The oral care imperative: the link between oral hygiene and aspiration pneumonia. *Top Geriatr Rehabil* 2007;23:280–288.

17. Imsand M, Janssens J-P, Auckenthaler R, Mojo et al: Bronchopneumonia and oral health in hospitalized older patients: a pilot study. *Gerondontology* 2002;19:66–72.

18. Green SL: Anaerobic pleuro-pulmonary infections. *Postgrad Med* 1979;65:62–74.

19. Rossi T, Peltonen R, Laine J, et al: Eradication of the long-term carriage of methicillin-resistant *Staphylococcus aureus* in patients wearing dentures: a follow-up of 10 patients. *J Hosp Infect* 1996;34:311–320.

20. Johanson WG Jr, Pierce AK, Stanford JP, et al: Nosocomial infections with gram-negative bacilli: the significance of colonization of the respiratory tract. *Ann Intern Med* 1972;77:701–706.

21. Scannapieco FA: Pneumonia in nonambulatory patients: the role of oral bacteria and oral hygiene (published correction appears in JADA 2008;139[3]:252). JADA 2006;137(10 Suppl):21S–25S.

22. Mojon P, Budtz-Jorgensen E, Michel JP, et al: Oral health and history of respiratory tract infection in frail institutionalised elders. *Gerodontology* 1997;14:9–16.

23. Senpuku H, Sogame A, Inoshita E, et al: Systemic diseases in association with microbial species in oral biofilm from elderly requiring care. *Gerontology* 2003;49:301–309.

24. Nikawa H, Hamada T, Yamamoto T: Denture plaque: past and recent concerns. *J Dent* 1998;26:299–304.

25. Coulthwaite L, Verran J: Potential pathogenic aspects of denture plaque. *Br J Biomed Sci* 2007;64:180–189.

26. Verran J, Maryan CJ: Retention of *Candida albicans* on acrylic resin and silicone of different surface topography. *J Prosthet Dent* 1997;77:535–539.

27. Ishikawa A, Yoneyama T, Hirota K, et al: Professional oral health care reduces the number of oropharyngeal bacteria. *J Dent Res* 2008;87:594–598.

28. Zissis A, Yannikakis S, Harrison A: Comparison of denture stomatitis prevalence in two population groups. *Int J Prosthodont* 2006;19:621–625.

29. Ramage G, Tomsett K, Wickes BL, et al: Denture stomatitis: a role for *Candida* biofilms. *Oral Surg Oral Med Oral Pathol Oral Radiol Endod* 2004;98:53–59.

30. Coco BJ, Bagg J, Cross LJ, et al: Mixed *Candida albicans* and *Candida glabrata* populations associated with the pathogenesis of denture stomatitis. *Oral Microbiol Immunol* 2008;23:377–383.

31. Aas JA, Paster BJ, Stokes LN, et al: Defining the normal bacterial flora of the oral cavity. *J Clin Micorbiol* 2005;43:5721–5732.

32. Theilade E, Budtz-Jorgensen E, Theilade J: Predominant cultivable microflora of plaque on removable dentures in patients with healthy oral mucosa. *Arch Oral Biol* 1983;28:675–680.

33. Charman KM, Fernandez P, Loewy Z, et al: Attachment of *Streptococcus oralis* on acrylic substrates of varying roughness. *Lett Appl Microbiol* 2009;48:472–477.

34. Wilson J: The aetiology, diagnosis and management of denture stomatitis. *Br Dent J* 1998;185:380–384.

35. Loewy Z: Epidemiology and etiology of denture stomatitis. *J Prosthodont.* In press.

36. Arendorf TM, Walker DM: Denture stomatitis: a review. *J Oral Rehabil* 1987;14:217–227.

37. Campos MS, Marchini L, Bernardes LA, et al: Biofilm microbial communities of denture stomatitis. *Oral Microbiol Immunol* 2008;23:419–424.

38. Abelson DC: Denture plaque and denture cleansers: review of the literature. *Gerodontics* 1985;1:202–206.

39. Nikawa H, Hamada T, Yamashiro H, et al: A review of in vitro and in vivo methods to evaluate the efficacy of denture cleansers. *Int J Prosthodont* 1999;12:153–159.

40. de Souza RF, de Freitas Oliveira Paranhos H, Lovato da Silva CH, et al: Interventions for cleaning dentures in adults. *Cochrane Database Syst Rev* 2009;(4):CD007395.

41. Dills SS, Olshan AM, Goldner S, et al: Comparison of the antimicrobial capability of an abrasive paste and chemical-soak denture cleaners. *J Prosthet Dent* 1988;60:467–470.

42. Panzeri H, Lara EH, Paranhos Hde F, et al: In vitro and clinical evaluation of specific dentifrices for complete denture hygiene. *Gerodontology* 2009;26:26–33.

43. Barnabé W, de Mendonca Neto T, Pimenta FC, et al: Efficacy of sodium hypochlorite and coconut soap used as disinfecting agents in the reduction of denture stomatitis, Streptococcus mutans and Candida albicans. *J Oral Rehabil* 2004;31:453–459.

44. Gornitsky M, Paradisl I, Landaverde G, et al: A clinical and microbiological evaluation of denture cleansers for geriatric patients in long-term care institutions. *J Can Dent Assoc* 2002;68:39–45.

45. Sheen SR, Harrison A: Assessment of plaque prevention on dentures using an experimental cleanser. *J Prosthet Dent* 2000;84:594–601.

46. Mima EG, Pavarina AC, Neppelenbroek KH, et al: Effect of different exposure times on microwave irradiation on the disinfection of a hard chairside reline resin. *J Prosthodont* 2008;17:312–317.

47. Nalbant AD, Kalkanci A, Filiz B, et al: Effectiveness of denture cleaning agents against the colonization of Candida spp and the in vitro detection of the adherence of these yeast cells to denture acrylic surfaces. *Yonsei Med J* 2008;49:647–654.

48. DePaola LG, Minah GE, Elias SA, et al: Clinical and microbial evaluation of treatment regimens to reduce denture stomatitis. *Int J Prosthodont* 1990;3:369–374.

49. da Silva FC, Kimpara ET, Mancini MN, et al: Effectiveness of six different disinfectants on removing five microbial species and effects on the topographic characteristics of acrylic resin. *J Prosthodont* 2008;17:627–633.

50. Devine DA, Percival RS, Wood DJ, et al: Inhibition of biofilms associated with dentures and toothbrushes by tetra-sodium EDTA. *J Appl Microbiol* 2007;103:2516–2524.

51. Ferreira MA, Pereira-Cenci T, Rodrigues de Vasconcelos LM, et al: Efficacy of denture cleansers on denture liners contaminated with *Candida* species. *Clin Oral Invest* 2009;13:237–242.

52. Hong G, Murata H, Li YA, et al: Influence of denture cleansers on the color stability of three types of denture base acrylic resins. *J Prosthet Dent* 2009;101:205–213.

53. Paranhos HF, Silva-Lovato CH, de Souza RF, et al: Effect of three methods for cleaning dentures on biofilms formed in vitro on acrylic resin. *J Prosthodont* 2009;18:427–431.

54. Nguyen CT, Masri R, Driscoll CF, et al: The effect of denture cleansing solutions on the retention of pink Locator attachments: an in vitro study. *J Prosthodont* 2010;19:226–230.

55. Maeda Y, Kenny F, Coulter WA, et al: Bactericidal activity of denture-cleaning formulations against planktonic health care-associated and community-associated methicillin-resistant *Staphylococcus aureus*. *Am J Infect Control* 2007;35:619–622.

56. Lee D, Howlett J, Pratten J, et al: Susceptibility of MSRA biofilms to denture-cleansing agents. *FEMS Microbiol Lett* 2009;291:241–246.

57. Muqbil I, Burke FJ, Miller CH, et al: Antimicrobial activity of ultrasonic cleaners. *J Hosp Infect* 2005;60:249–255.

58. Sheen SR, Harrison A: Assessment of plaque prevention on dentures using an experimental cleanser. *J Prosthet Dent* 2000;84:594–601.

59. U.S. Food and Drug Administration. U.S. Food and Drug Administration Alert. FDA public Health Notification: Denture Cleanser Allergic Reactions and Misuse. February 14, 2008. www.fda.gov/MedicalDevices/Safety/AlertsandNotices/PatientAlerts/ucm064558.htm. Accessed November 21, 2010.

60. Ribeiro DG, Pavarina AC, Dovigo LN, et al: Denture disinfection by microwave irradiation: a randomized clinical study. *J Dent* 2009;37:666–672.

61. Mima EG, Pavarina AC, Neppelenbroek KH, et al: Effect of different exposure times on microwave irradiation on the disinfection of a hard chairside reline resin. *J Prosthodont* 2008;17:312–317.

62. Campanha NH, Pavarina AC, Vergani CE, et al: Effect of microwave sterilization and water storage on the Vickers hardness of acrylic resin denture teeth. *J Prosthet Dent* 2005;93:483–487.

63. Pavarina AC, Neppelenbroek KH, Guinesi AS, et al: Effect of microwave disinfection on the flexural strength of hard chairside reline resins. *J Dent* 2005;33:741–748.

64. Atwood DA: Bone loss of edentulous alveolar ridges. *J Periodontol* 1974;50(4 spec no): 11–21.

65. Atwood D, Coy WA: Clinical, cephalometric, and densitometric study of reduction of residual ridges. *J Prosthet Dent* 1971;26:280–295.

66. Tallgren A: The continuing reduction of the residual alveolar ridges in complete denture wearers: a mixed-longitudinal study covering 25 years. *J Prosthet Dent* 1972;27:120–132.

67. Coates AJ: Usage of denture adhesives. *J Dent* 2000;28:137–140.

68. Sato Y, Kaiba Y, Hayakawa I: Evaluation of denture retention and ease of removal from oral mucosa on a new gel-type denture adhesive. *Nihon Hotetsu Shika Gakkai Zasshi* 2008;52:175–182.

69. Pradies G, Sanz I, Evans O, et al: Clinical study comparing the efficacy of two denture adhesives in complete denture patients. *Int J Prosthodont* 2009;22:361–367.

70. Kulak Y, Ozcan M, Arikan A: Subjective assessment by patients of the efficiency of two denture adhesive pastes. *J Prosthodont* 2005;14:248–252.

71. Uysal H, Altay OT, Alparslan N, et al: Comparison of four different denture cushion adhesives: a subjective study. *J Oral Rehabil* 1998;25:209–213.

72. Kelsey CC, Lang BR, Wang RF: Examining patients' responses about the effectiveness of five denture adhesive pastes. *JADA* 1997;128:1532–1538.

73. Berg E: A clinical comparison of four denture adhesives. *Int J Prosthodont* 1991;4:449–456.

74. Ghani F, Picton DC: Some clinical investigations on retention forces of maxillary complete dentures with the use of denture fixatives. *J Oral Rehabil* 1994;21:631–640.

75. Lang A, Garcia T, Bohnenkamp DM, et al: Effects of denture adhesive on retention of mandibular complete dentures (abstract 0308). *J Dent Res* 2007;86(spec issue research A).

76. Kapur KK. A clinical evaluation of denture adhesives. *J Prosthet Dent* 1967;18:550–558.

77. Grasso JE: Denture adhesives. *Dent Clin North Am* 2004;48: 721–733.

78. Chew CL, Boone ME, Swartz ML, et al: Denture adhesives: their effects on denture retention and stability. *J Dent* 1985;13:152–159.

79. de Baat C, van't Hof M, van Zeghbroeck L, et al: An international multicenter study on the effectiveness of a denture adhesive in maxillary dentures using disposable gnathometers. *Clin Oral Investig* 2007;11:237–243.

80. Hasegawa S, Sekita T, Hayakawa I: Effect of denture adhesive on stability of complete dentures and the masticatory function. *J Med Dent Sci* 2003;50:239–247.

81. Zhao K, Cheng XR, Chao YL, et al: Laboratory evaluation of a new denture adhesive. *Dent Mater* 2004;20:419–424.

82. Grasso JE. Denture adhesives: changing attitudes. *JADA* 1996;127(1):90–96.

83. Psillakis JJ, Wright RF, Grbic JT, et al: In practice evaluation of a denture adhesive using a gnathometer. *J Prosthodont* 2004;13:244–250.

84. Ozcan M, Kulak Y, de Baat C, et al: The effect of a new denture adhesive on bite force until denture dislodgement. *J Prosthodont* 2005;14:122–126.

85. Cheng XR, Zhao K, Han GL: In vitro cytotoxicity evaluation of denture adhesive. *Chin J Dent Res* 2000;3:59–62.

86. Rendell JK, Gay T, Grasso JE, et al: The effect of denture adhesive on mandibular movement during chewing. *JADA* 2000;131:981–986.

87. Veyrune JL, Tubert-Jeannin S, Dutheil C, et al: Impact of new prostheses on the oral health related quality of life of edentulous patients. *Gerodontology* 2005;22:3–9.

88. Nicolas E, Veyrune JL, Lassauzay C: A six-month assessment of oral health-related quality of life of complete denture wearers using denture adhesive: a pilot study. *J Prosthodont* 2010;19: 443–448.

89. Atchison KA, Dolan TA: Development of the Geriatric Oral Health Assessment Index. *J Dent Educ* 1990;54:680–687.

90. Al RH, Dahl JE, Morisbak E, et al: Irritation and cytotoxic potential of denture adhesives. *Gerodontology* 2005;22: 177–183.

91. Dahl JE: Potential of dental adhesives to induce mucosal irritation evaluated by the HET-CAM method. *Acta Odontol Scand* 2007;65:275–283.

92. Gates WD, Goldschmidt M, Kramer D: Microbial contamination in four commercially available denture adhesives. *J Prosthet Dent* 1994;71:154–158.

93. Ekstrand K, Hensten-Pettersen A, Kullmann A: Denture adhesives: cytotoxicity, microbial contamination, and formaldehyde content. *J Prosthet Dent* 1993;69:314–317.

94. Kim E, Driscoll CF, Minah GE: The effect of a denture adhesive on the colonization of Candida species in vivo. *J Prosthodont* 2003;12:187–191.

95. Oliveira MC, Oliveira VM, Vieira AC, et al: In vivo assessment of the effect of an adhesive for complete dentures on colonisation of *Candida* species. *Gerodontology* 2009 Sep 22. [Epub ahead of print].

96. National Institutes of Health, Office of Dietary Supplements. Dietary Supplement FactSheet: Zinc. "http://ods.od. nih.gov/FactSheets/Zinc.asp". Accessed November 22, 2010.

97. Nations SP, Boyer PJ, Love LA, et al: Denture cream: an unusual source of excess zinc, leading to hypocupremia and neurologic disease. *Neurology* 2008;71:639–643.

98. Hedera P, Peltier A, Fink JK, et al: Myelopolyneuropathy and pancytopenia due to copper deficiency and high zinc levels of unknown origin II: the denture cream is a primary source of excessive zinc. *Neurotoxicology* 2009;30:996–999.

99. Xie Q, Narhi TO, Nevalainen JM, et al: Oral status and prosthetic factors related to residual ridge resorption in elderly subjects. *Acta Odontol Scand* 1997;55:306–313.

100. Xie Q, Ainamo A: Association of edentulousness with systemic factors in elderly people living at home. *Community Dent Oral Epidemiol* 1999;27:202–209.

101. Klemetti E, Kroger H, Lassila L: Fluoridated drinking water, estrogen therapy and residual ridge resorption. *J Oral Rehabil* 1997;24:47–51.

102. Adams LP, Wilding RJ: A photogrammetric method for monitoring changes in the residual alveolar ridge form. *J Oral Rehabil* 1985;12:443–450.

103. Penhall B: Preventive measures to control further bone loss and soft tissue damage in denture wearing. *Aust Dent J* 1980;25:319–324.

104. Carlsson GE, Ragnarson N, Astrand P: Changes in height of the alveolar process in edentulous segments. II: a longitudinal clinical and radiographic study over 5 years of full upper denture patients with residual lower anteriors. *Sven Tandlak Tidskr* 1969;62:125–136.

105. Bergman B, Carlsson GE, Ericson S: Effect of differences in habitual use of complete dentures on underlying tissues. *Scand J Dent Res* 1971;79:449–460.

106. Kalk W, de Baat C: Some factors connected with alveolar bone resorption. *J Dent* 1989;17:162–165.

107. Espinoza I, Rojas R, Aranda W, et al: Prevalence of oral mucosal lesions in elderly people in Santiago, Chile. *J Oral Pathol Med* 2003;32:571–575.

108. Shulman JD, Rivera-Hidalgo F, Beach MM: Risk factors associated with denture stomatitis in the United States. *J Oral Pathol Med* 2005;34:340–346.

109. Emami E, de Grandmont P, Rompré PH, et al: Favoring trauma as an etiological factor in denture stomatitis. *J Dent Res* 2008;87:440–444.

110. Jeganathan S, Payne JA, Thean HP: Denture stomatitis in an elderly edentulous Asian population. *J Oral Rehabil* 1997;24:468–472.

111. Barbeau J, Seguin J, Goulet JP, et al: Reassessing the presence of *Candida albicans* in denture-related stomatitis. *Oral Surg Oral Med Oral Pathol Oral Radiol Endod* 2003;95: 51–59.

112. Arendorf TM, Walker DM: Oral candidal populations in health and disease. *Br Dent J* 1979;147:267–272.

113. Compagnoni MA, Souza RF, Marra J, et al: Relationship between *Candida* and nocturnal denture wear: quantitative study. *J Oral Rehabil* 2007;34:600–605.

114. Bergendal T: Status and treatment of denture stomatitis patients: a 1-year follow-up study. *Scand J Dent Res* 1982;90: 227–238.

115. Peltola MK, Raustia AM, Salonen MA: Effect of complete denture renewal on oral health: a survey of 42 patients. *J Oral Rehabil* 1997;24:419–425.

116. MacEntee MI: The prevalence of edentulism and diseases related to dentures: a literature review. *J Oral Rehabil* 1985;12:195–207.

117. Academy of Prosthodontics; Academy of Prosthodontics Foundation. The Glossary of Prosthodontic Terms (ed 8). St. Louis, Mosby, 2005, pp. 67–68.

118. Marchini L, Tamashiro E, Nascimento DF, et al: Self-reported denture hygiene of a sample of edentulous attendees at a university dental clinic and the relationship to the condition of the oral tissues. *Gerodontology* 2004;21:226–228.

119. Maeda Y, Wood WW: Finite element method simulation of bone resorption beneath a complete denture. *J Dent Res* 1989;68:1370–1373.

120. Sutton AF, Glenny AM, McCord JF: Interventions for replacing missing teeth: denture chewing surface designs in edentulous people. *Cochrane Database Syst Rev* 2005;(1):CD004941.

121. Clough HE, Knodle JM, Leeper SH, et al: A comparison of lingualized occlusion and monoplane occlusion in complete dentures. *J Prosthet Dent* 1983;50:176–179.

2

CLASSIFICATION SYSTEM FOR COMPLETE EDENTULISM

Thomas J. McGarry, DDS, FACP,[1] Arthur Nimmo, DDS, FACP,[2] James F. Skiba, DDS,[3] Robert H. Ahlstrom, DDS, MS,[4] Christopher R. Smith, DDS,[5] and Jack H. Koumjian, DDS, MSD, FACP[6]

[1] Private practice, Oklahoma City, OK
[2] Professor and Director of Implant Dentistry, Department of Restorative Dentistry, University of Detroit Mercy School of Dentistry, Detroit, MI
[3] Private practice, Montclair, NJ
[4] Private practice, Reno, NV
[5] Private practice, San Antonio, TX
[6] Clinical Professor, Department of Restorative Dentistry, UCSF School of Dentistry and Private Practice, Palo Alto, CA

Keywords

Complete dentures; diagnosis; treatment planning; prosthodontics; dental education; graduate dental education; outcomes assessment; quality assurance; treatment outcomes

Correspondence

Thomas J. McGarry, DDS, 4320 McAuley Boulevard, Oklahoma City, OK 73120

Presented at the Annual Session of the American College of Prosthodontists in Orlando, FL, November 5, 1997.

Funded by The American College of Prosthodontists.

Accepted January 21, 1999

Published in *Journal of Prosthodontics* 1999; Vol. 8, Issue 1, pp. 27–39

ABSTRACT

The American College of Prosthodontists has developed a classification system for complete edentulism based on diagnostic findings. These guidelines may help practitioners determine appropriate treatments for their patients. Four categories are defined, ranging from Class I to Class IV, with Class I representing an uncomplicated clinical situation and a Class IV patient representing the most complex and higher-risk situation. Each class is differentiated by specific diagnostic criteria. This system is designed for use by dental professionals who are involved in the diagnosis of patients requiring treatment for complete edentulism. Potential benefits of the system include: 1) better patient care, 2) improved professional communication, 3) more appropriate insurance reimbursement, 4) a better screening tool to assist dental school admission clinics, and 5) standardized criteria for outcomes assessment.

Completely edentulous patients exhibit a broad range of physical variations and health concerns. Classifying all edentulous patients as a single diagnostic group is insensitive to the multiple levels of physical variation and the differing treatment procedures required to restore function and comfort. A graduated classification of complete edentulism has been developed that describes varying levels of loss of denture-supporting structures.

This article defines complete edentulism as follows: the physical state of the jaw(s) following removal of all erupted teeth and the condition of the supporting structures available for reconstructive or replacement therapies. The condition of edentulism, for the purpose of this article, is divided into four levels according to specific diagnostic criteria.

The absence of organized diagnostic criteria for complete edentulism has been a long-standing impediment to effective care for patients. Recognition of the diverse nature, scope, and degree of complete edentulism, although thoroughly described in the dental literature, has not been organized to efficiently guide dental educators, general dentists, prosthodontists, and third-party payers in providing the appropriate treatment for each patient. A system for facilitating patient identification is needed to improve patient treatment outcomes.

The American College of Prosthodontists (ACP) recognized its responsibility to the public and the profession to correct this dilemma. The Subcommittee on Prosthodontic Classification was formed in 1995 and charged with developing classification systems for prosthodontic patients. Timely implementation of this system will benefit patients, clinicians, and educators. The classification system for complete edentulism is presented in the following sections.

DEVELOPMENT OF THE CLASSIFICATION SYSTEM

A classification system has been successfully used to assess periodontal status for more than 20 years.[1] Recently, the American Association of Endodontists devised an evaluation system for determining endodontic risk factors.[2] These factors serve as guidelines to determine when patients with advanced treatment needs should be referred for consultation with a specialist. The classification system for complete edentulism will establish separate diagnostic entities for four levels of edentulism, ranked according to degree of difficulty of treatment.

A review of the prosthodontic literature was used to identify the many variables associated with complete edentulism. A questionnaire was then constructed to categorize the 89 variables identified. The questionnaire that was circulated within the subcommittee asked for comments and literature citations to support inclusion of a variable into a diagnostic system. The data collected via this questionnaire were formatted into a new survey instrument that differentiated variables into four subclasses:

1. Physical findings;
2. Prosthetic history;
3. Pharmaceutical history;
4. Systemic disease evaluation.

The variables in these four subclasses of variables were further evaluated to determine their importance in relation to:

- Educational requirement: What additional clinical skill or knowledge is necessary to manage this variable?
- Clinical responsibility: Is this variable most significant to the patient, practitioner, or the dental laboratory technician?
- Clinical technique modification: Will this variable require a change in conventional five-step technique, and could this variable have a significant effect on patient satisfaction?
- Clinical and laboratory time requirement: Will this variable require additional time by the practitioner, clinical staff, and/or the dental laboratory technician?
- Overall clinical significance: Will this variable require advanced education to manage?

The subcommittee established a ranking of individual variables. Subsequently, a classification system was developed based on the most objective variables. The survey was sent to a cross-sectional sample of 10% of the ACP fellows and members and to representatives of prosthodontic organizations. A five-step scoring grid was included that asked if the classification would be one of the following: very helpful, helpful, not helpful and had minor flaws, or had major flaws. Of the 250 drafts sent out, 56 were returned. When the results were tallied, 73.4% of responses expressed the view that the classification would be very helpful or helpful. Nine percent said the system would not be helpful. Minor flaws were identified by 15.6% of the respondents, and 1.7% stated that the system had major flaws; however, no consistent flaws were identified in the comments. The additional information gained from this survey and initial draft comments was incorporated into a definitive document.

SYSTEM APPLICATIONS

This system, when combined with the appropriate Parameter of Care,[3] will establish a basis for diagnosis and treatment procedures. In addition, patients will be provided with treatment justifications for third-party payers to ensure that the patient is able to receive appropriate prosthodontic care, should referral to a specialist be necessary.

The classification system will be of value to dental faculty responsible for screening new edentulous patients. Dental educators will need to determine which classes of complete edentulism can be treated within their predoctoral clinical program.[4] Patients diagnosed at more advanced levels should be referred to graduate prosthodontics programs or to a practicing prosthodontist.

Data gathered and organized using this system will enable the dental educator, general dentist, or prosthodontist to review clinical outcomes on evidence-based diagnostic criteria. By identifying the advanced patient before treatment and making the appropriate referral, when indicated, the incidence of retreatment should decrease.

The classification system will be subject to monitoring and revision as new diagnostic and treatment information becomes available in the literature. The experiences gained in its application in practice will enable the provider to determine which treatment procedures would be most appropriate for a patient with a specific diagnosis.

With the premise that complete edentulism has differing degrees of severity, the committee sought to identify and group the most significant diagnostic criteria. The following criteria should help in applying the guidelines in a consistent manner.

A SYSTEMATIC REVIEW OF DIAGNOSTIC CRITERIA FOR THE EDENTULOUS PATIENT

The diagnostic criteria are organized by their objective nature and not in their rank of significance. Because of variations in adaptive responses, certain criteria are more significant than others.[5] However, objective criteria will allow for the most accurate application of the classification system and measurement of its efficacy. Objectivity also will provide reliable outcome data and mechanisms for review by third-party payers and peer-review panels. The diagnostic criteria used in the classification system are listed in the worksheet (Table 1).

Bone Height: Mandible Only

The identification and measurement of residual bone height is the most easily quantified objective criterion for the mandibular edentulous ridge.[6-9] In addition, it represents a measurement of the chronic debilitation associated with complete edentulism in the mandible. Despite the lack of a known etiology, it has been established that the loss of denture-supporting structures does occur.[6,8] Atwood's description in 1971 of alveolar bone loss is still applicable today: "Chronic progressive, irreversible and disabling process probably of multifactoral origin. At the present time, the importance of various cofactors is unknown." The continued decrease in bone volume affects: 1) denture-bearing area; 2) tissues

remaining for reconstruction; 3) facial muscle support/attachment; 4) total facial height[9]; and 5) ridge morphology.

The results of a radiographic survey of residual bone height measurement are affected by the variation in the radiographic techniques and magnification of panoramic machines of different manufacturers. To minimize variability in radiographic techniques, the measurement should be made on the radiograph at that portion of the mandible of the *least* vertical height. The values assigned to each of the four types listed below are averages that historically have been used in relation to preprosthetic surgical procedures. A measurement is made and the patient is classified as follows:

- Type I (most favorable): residual bone height of 21 mm or greater measured at the least vertical height of the mandible (Fig 1);
- Type II: residual bone height of 16 to 20 mm measured at the least vertical height of the mandible (Fig 2);
- Type III: residual alveolar bone height of 11 to 15 mm measured at the least vertical height of the mandible (Fig 3);
- Type IV: residual vertical bone height of 10 mm or less measured at the least vertical height of the mandible (Fig 4).

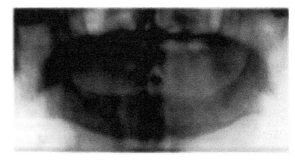

FIGURE 1   Radiograph with residual bone height of 21 mm or greater measured at the least vertical height of the mandible (Type I).

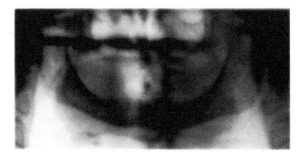

FIGURE 2   Radiograph with residual bone height of 16 to 20 mm measured at the least vertical height of the mandible (Type II).

TABLE 1   Checklist for Classification of Complete Edentulism

	Class I	Class II	Class III	Class IV
Bone Height-Mandibular				
21 mm or greater				
16–20 mm				
11–15 mm				
10 mm or less				
Residual Ridge Morphology-Maxilla				
Type A - resists vertical & horizontal, hamular notch, no tori				
Type B - no buccal vest., poor hamular notch, no tori				
Type C - no ant vest, min support, mobile ant. ridge				
Type D - no ant/post vest, tori, redundant tissue				
Muscle Attachments-Mandibular				
Type A - adequate attached mucosa				
Type B - no b attach mucosa (22–27), +mentalis m				
Type C - no ant b&l vest (22–27), +genio & mentalis m				
Type D - att mucosa only in post				
Type E - no att mucosa, cheek/lip moves tongue				
Maxillomandibular Relationships				
Class I				
Class II				
Class III				
Conditions requiring Preprosthetic Surgery				
Minor soft tissue procedures				
Minor hard tissue procedures				
Implants – simple				
Implants with bone graft – complex				
Correction of dentofacial deformities				
Hard tissue augmentation				
Major soft tissue revisions				
Limited Interarch Space				
18–20 mm				
Surgical correction needed				
Tongue Anatomy				
Large (occludes interdental space)				
Hyperactive – with retracted position				
Modifiers				
Oral manifestations of systemic disease				
mild				
moderate				
severe				
Psychosocial				
moderate				
major				
TMD symptoms				
Hx of paresthesia or dysesthesia				
Maxillofacial defects				
Ataxia				
Refractory Patient				

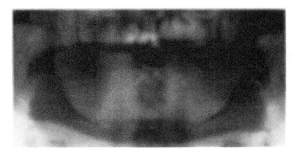

FIGURE 3   Radiograph with residual bone height of 11 to 15 mm measured at the least vertical height of the mandible (Type III).

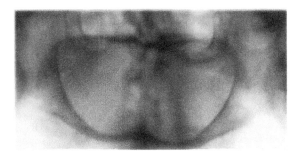

FIGURE 4   Radiograph with residual bone height of 10 mm or less measured at the least vertical height of the mandible (Type IV).

Residual Ridge Morphology: Maxilla Only

Residual ridge *morphology* is the most objective criterion for the maxilla, because measurement of the maxillary residual bone *height* by radiography is not reliable.[11] The classification system continues on a logical progression, describing the effects of residual ridge morphology and the influence of musculature on a maxillary denture.[12]

Type A (most favorable) (Fig 5)
- Anterior labial and posterior buccal vestibular depth that resists vertical and horizontal movement of the denture base.

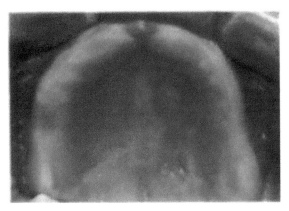

FIGURE 5   Type A maxillary residual ridge.

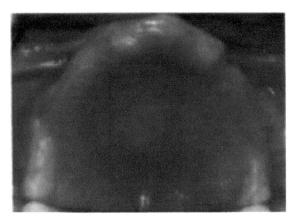

FIGURE 6   Type **B** maxillary residual ridge.

- Palatal morphology resists vertical and horizontal movement of the denture base.
- Sufficient tuberosity definition to resist vertical and horizontal movement of the denture base.
- Flamular notch is well defined to establish the posterior extension of the denture base.
- Absence of tori or exostoses.

Type B (Fig 6)
- Loss of posterior buccal vestibule.
- Palatal vault morphology resists vertical and horizontal movement of the denture base.
- Tuberosity and hamular notch are poorly defined, compromising delineation of the posterior extension of the denture base.
- Maxillary palatal tori and/or lateral exostoses are rounded and do not affect the posterior extension of the denture base.

Type C (Fig 7)
- Loss of anterior labial vestibule.
- Palatal vault morphology offers minimal resistance to vertical and horizontal movement of the denture base.

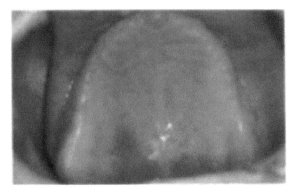

FIGURE 7   Type C maxillary residual ridge.

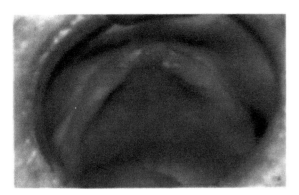

FIGURE 8   Type D maxillary residual ridge.

- Maxillary palatal tori and/or lateral exostoses with bony undercuts that do not affect the posterior extension of the denture base.
- Hyperplastic, mobile anterior ridge offers minimum support and stability of the denture base.[13,14]
- Reduction of the post malar space by the coronoid process during mandibular opening and/or excursive movements.

Type D (Fig 8)
- Loss of anterior labial and posterior buccal vestibules.
- Palatal vault morphology does not resist vertical or horizontal movement of the denture base.
- Maxillary palatal tori and/or lateral exostoses[15] (rounded or undercut) that interfere with the posterior border of the denture.
- Hyperplastic, redundant anterior ridge.
- Prominent anterior nasal spine.

Muscle Attachments: Mandible Only

The effects of muscle attachment and location are most important to the function of a mandibular denture.[9,16–18] These characteristics are difficult to quantify. The classification system follows a logical progression to describe the effects of muscular influence on a mandibular denture. The clinician examines the patient and selects the category that is most descriptive of the mandibular muscle attachments.

Type A (most favorable) (Fig 9)
- Attached mucosal base without undue muscular impingement during normal function in all regions.

Type B (Fig 10)
- Attached mucosal base in all regions except labial vestibule.
- Mentalis muscle attachment near crest of alveolar ridge.

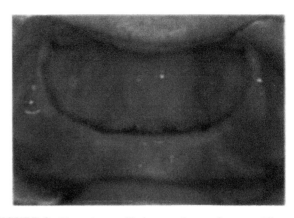

FIGURE 9   Type A mandibular muscle attachments. All vestibules are adequate.

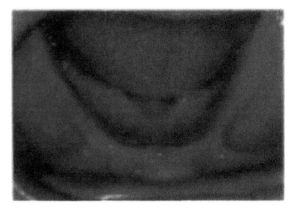

FIGURE 10   Type B mandibular muscle attachments. Loss of anterior labial vestibule.

Type C (Fig 11)
- Attached mucosal base in all regions except anterior buccal and lingual vestibules—canine to canine.
- Genioglossus and mentalis muscle attachments near crest of alveolar ridge.[15]

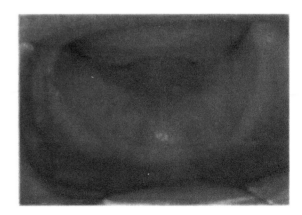

FIGURE 11   Type C mandibular muscle attachments. Loss of anterior labial and lingual vestibules.

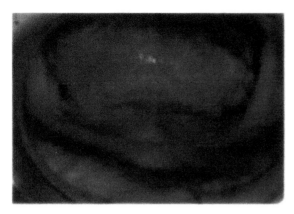

FIGURE 12   Type D mandibular muscle attachments. Only the posterior lingual vestibule remains.

Type D (Fig 12)
- Attached mucosal base only in the posterior lingual region.
- Mucosal base in all other regions is detached.

Type E (Fig 13)
- No attached mucosa in any region.

Maxillomandibular Relationship

The classification of the maxillomandibular relationship characterizes the position of the artificial teeth in relation to the residual ridge and/or to opposing dentition. Examine the patient and assign a class as follows:

- Class I (most favorable): Maxillomandibular relation allows tooth position that has normal articulation with the teeth supported by the residual ridge.
- Class II: Maxillomandibular relation requires tooth position outside the normal ridge relation to attain

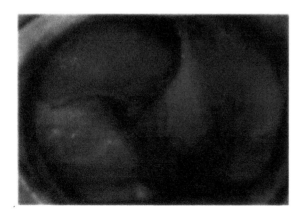

FIGURE 13   Type E mandibular muscle attachments. No discernible vestibular anatomy remains.

esthetics, phonetics, and articulation (eg, anterior or posterior tooth position is not supported by the residual ridge; anterior vertical and/or horizontal overlap exceeds the principles of fully balanced articulation).
- Class III: Maxillomandibular relation requires tooth position outside the normal ridge relation to attain esthetics, phonetics, and articulation (ie crossbitc—anterior or posterior tooth position is not supported by the residual ridge).

Integration of Diagnostic Findings

The previous four subclassifications are important determinants in the overall diagnostic classification of complete edentulism. In addition, variables that can be expected to contribute to increased treatment difficulty are distributed across all classifications according to their significance.

Classification System for Complete Edentulism

Class I (Fig 14 A–H)

This classification level characterizes the stage of edentulism that is most apt to be successfully treated with complete dentures using conventional prosthodontic techniques.[6] All four of the diagnostic criteria are favorable.

- Residual bone height of 21 mm or greater measured at the least vertical height of the mandible on a panoramic radiograph.
- Residual ridge morphology resists horizontal and vertical movement of the denture base; Type A maxilla.
- Location of muscle attachments that arc conducive to denture base stability and retention; Type A or B mandible.
- Class I maxillomandibular relationship.

Class II (Fig 15 A–H)

This classification level distinguishes itself by the continued physical degradation of the denturesupporting anatomy, and, in addition, is characterized by the early onset of systemic disease interactions, patient management, and/or lifestyle considerations.

- Residual bone height of 16 to 20 mm measured at the least vertical height of the mandible on a panoramic radiograph.
- Residual ridge, morphology that resists horizontal and vertical movement of the denture base; Type A or B maxilla.

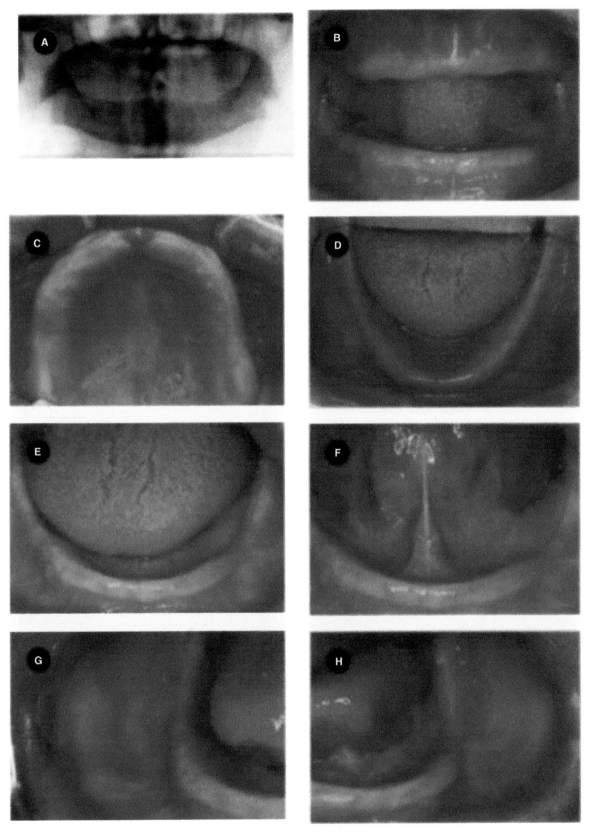

FIGURE 14   Class I patient. (*A*) Panoramic radiograph. (*B*) Facial view at the approximate occlusal vertical dimension. (*C*) Occlusal view: maxillary arch. (*D*) Occlusal view: mandibular arch. (*E*) Facial view: tongue in resting position. (*F*) Facial view: tongue elevated. (*G*) Lateral view of mandible: patient right. (*H*) Lateral view of mandible: patient left.

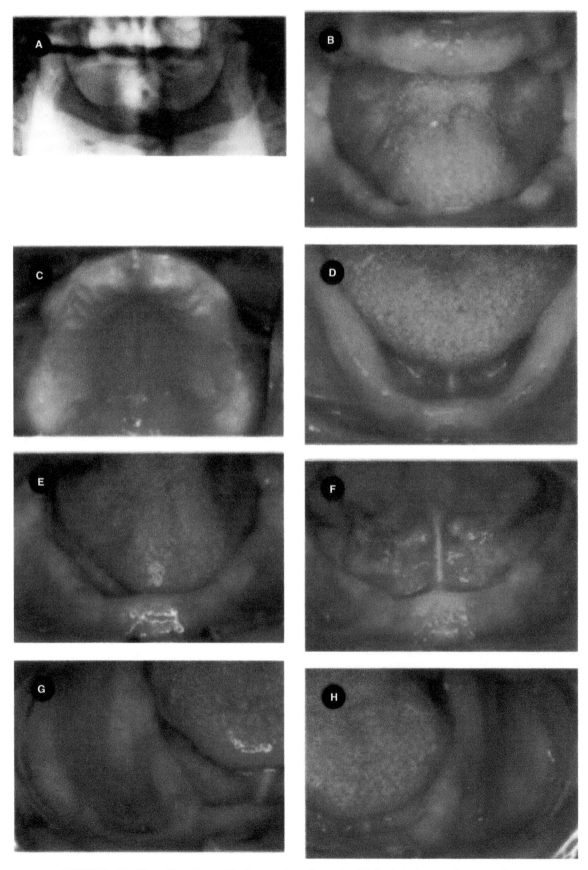

FIGURE 15 Class II patient. (*A*) Panoramic radiograph. (*B*) Facial view at the approximate occlusal vertical dimension. (*C*) Occlusal view: maxillary arch. (*D*) Occlusal view: mandibular arch. (*E*) Facial view: tongue in resting position. (*F*) Facial view: tongue elevated. (*G*) Lateral view of mandible: patient right. (*H*) Lateral view of mandible: patient left.

- Location of muscle attachments with limited influence on denture base stability and retention; Type A or B mandible.
- Class I maxillomandibular relationship.
- Minor modifiers, psychosocial considerations, mild systemic disease with oral manifestations[6]

Class III (Fig 16 A–H)

This classification level is characterized by the need for surgical revision of supporting structures to allow for adequate prosthodontic function. Additional factors now play a significant role in treatment outcomes.

- Residual alveolar bone height of 11 to 15 mm measured at the least vertical height of the mandible on a panoramic radiograph.
- Residual ridge morphology has minimum influence to resist horizontal or vertical movement of the denture base; Type C maxilla.
- Location of muscle attachments with moderate influence on denture base stability and retention; Type C mandible.
- Class I, II, or III maxillomandibular relationship.
- Conditions requiring preprosthetic surgery[13]:
  1. minor soft tissue procedures;
  2. minor hard tissue procedures including alveoloplasty[18];
  3. simple implant placement, no augmentation required;
  4. multiple extractions leading to complete edentulism for immediate denture placement.
- Limited interarch space (18–20 mm).
- Moderate psychosocial considerations[19,20] and/or moderate oral manifestations of systemic diseases or conditions such as xerostomia.[21]
- TMD symptoms present.[14]
- Large tongue (occludes interdental space)[22] with or without hyperactivity.
- Hyperactive gag reflex.[23,24]

Class IV (Fig 17)

This classification level depicts the most debilitated edentulous condition. Surgical reconstruction is almost always indicated but cannot always be accomplished because of the patient's health, preferences, dental history, and financial considerations. When surgical revision is not an option, prosthodontic techniques of a specialized nature must be used to achieve an adequate treatment outcome.

- Residual vertical bone height of 10 mm or less measured at the least vertical height of the mandible on a panoramic radiograph.
- Residual ridge offers no resistance to horizontal or vertical movement; Type D maxilla.
- Muscle attachment location that can be expected to have significant influence on denture base stability and retention; Type D or E mandible.
- Class I, II, or III maxillomandibular relationships.
- Major conditions requiring preprosthetic surgery:
  1. complex implant placement,[25] augmentation required;
  2. surgical correction of dentofacial deformities;
  3. hard tissue augmentation required;
  4. major soft tissue revision required, ie, vestibular extensions with or without soft tissue grafting.
- History of paresthesia or dysesthesia.
- Insufficient interarch space with surgical correction required.
- Acquired or congenital maxillofacial defects.
- Severe oral manifestation of systemic disease or conditions such as sequelae from oncological treatment.
- Maxillo-mandibular ataxia (incoordination).
- Hyperactivity of tongue that can be associated with a retracted tongue position and/or its associated morphology.
- Hyperactive gag reflex managed with medication.
- Refractory patient (a patient who presents with chronic complaints following appropriate therapy). These patients may continue to have difficulty achieving their treatment expectations despite the thoroughness or frequency of the treatments provided.
- Psychosocial conditions warranting professional intervention.

GUIDELINES FOR USE OF THE COMPLETE EDENTULISM CLASSIFICATION SYSTEM

In those instances when a patient's diagnostic criteria are mixed between two or more classes, *any single criterion of a more complex class* places the patient into the more complex class. The analysis of diagnostic factors is facilitated with the use of a worksheet (Table 1).

Use of this system is indicated for pretreatment evaluation and classification of patients. Reevaluation of classification status should be considered following preprosthetic surgery. Retrospective analysis on a posttreatment basis may alter a patient's classification.

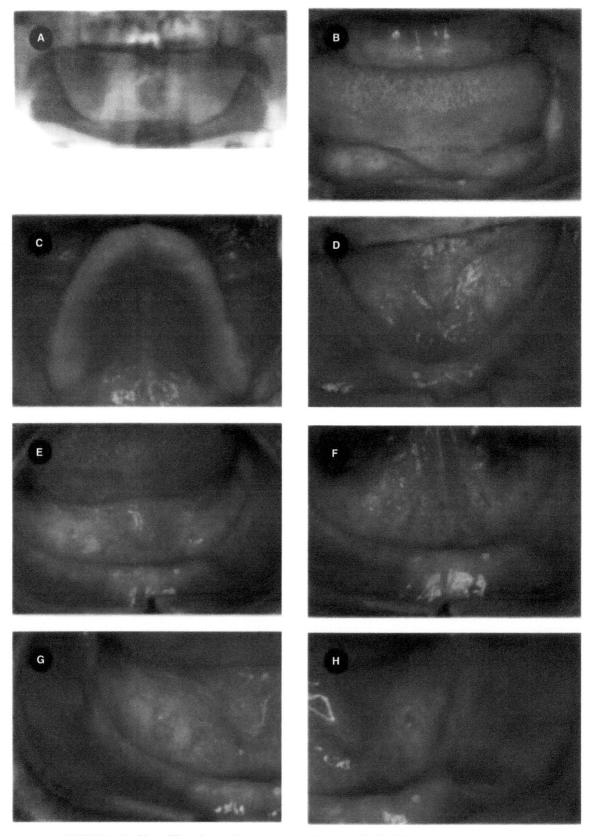

FIGURE 16   Class III patient. (*A*) Panoramic radiograph. (*B*) Facial view at the approximate occlusal vertical dimension. (*C*) Occlusal view: maxillary arch. (*D*) Occlusal view: mandibular arch. (*E*) Facial view: tongue in resting position. (*F*) Facial view: tongue elevated. (*G*) Lateral view of mandible: patient right. (*H*) Lateral view of mandible: patient left.

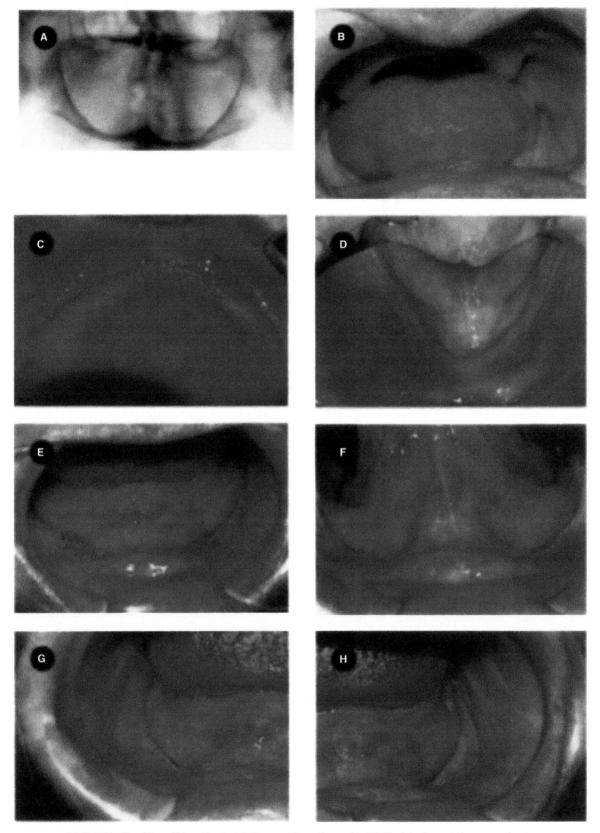

FIGURE 17 Class IV patient. (*A*) Panoramic radiograph. (*B*) Facial view at the approximate occlusal vertical dimension. (*C*) Occlusal view: maxillary arch. (*D*) Occlusal view: mandibular arch. (*E*) Facial view: tongue in resting position. (*F*) Facial view: tongue elevated. (*G*) Lateral view of mandible: patient right. (*H*) Lateral view of mandible: patient left.

CLOSING STATEMENT

The classification system for complete edentulism is based on the most objective criteria available to facilitate uniform utilization of the system. With such standardization, communication will be improved among dental professionals and third parties. This classification system will help to identify those patients most likely to require treatment by a specialist or by a practitioner with additional training and experience in advanced techniques. This system should also be valuable to research protocols as different treatment procedures are evaluated.

ACKNOWLEDGMENT

The authors thank Dr. Nancy Arbree and Ms. Betty Freeman for their assistance in the preparation of this manuscript. The authors also wish to recognize Dr. Kent Cohenour, Oral and Maxillofacial Surgeon, for his contribution to the original concept of a classification for complete edentulism.

REFERENCES

1. Genco RJ: Classification and Clinical Radiographic Features of Periodontal Disease, in Robert J. Genco, Henry M. Goldman, D. Walter Cohen (eds): *Contemporary Periodontics* (ed 6). St. Louis, MO, CV Mosby, 1990, p 65.

2. American Association of Endodontists. *Evaluating endodontic treatment risk factors.* Spring/Summer 1997. AAE, Chicago, IL.

3. Parameters of Care for The American College of Prosthodontists. *J Prosthod* 1996;5:3–71.

4. Nimmo A, Woolsey GD, Arbree NS, et al: Defining predoctoral prosthodontic curriculum: A workshop sponsored by The American College of Prosthodontists and the Prosthodontic Forum. *J Prosthod* 1998;7:30–34.

5. Zarb GA: Biomechanics of the edentulous state, in Zarb GA, Bolender CL, Carlsson GE (eds): *Prosthodontic Treatment for Edentulous Patients* (ed 11). St. Louis, MO, Mosby-Year Book, 1997, p 15.

6. Atwood DA: Some clinical factors related to rate of resorption of residual ridges. *J Prosthet Dent* 1962;12:441.

7. Ortman HR: Factors of bone resorption of the residual ridge. *J Prosthet Dent* 1962;12:429–440.

8. Tallgren A: The continuing reduction of the residual alveolar ridges in complete denture wearers: A mixed-longitudinal study covering 25 years. *J Prosthet Dent* 1972;27:120–132.

9. Davis DM: Developing an analogue/substitute for the mandibular denture-bearing area, in Zarb, Bolender, Carlsson (eds). *Prosthodontic Treatment for Edentulous Patients* (ed 11) St. Louis, MO. Mosby-Year Book, Inc, 1997, pp 162–173.

10. Zarb GA: Biomechanics of the edentulous state, in Zarb, Bolender, Carlsson (eds): *Prosthodontic Treatment for Edentulous Patients* (ed 11) St. Louis, MO, Mosby-Year Book, 1997, pp 23–24.

11. Davis DM: Developing an analogue/substitute for the maxillary denture-bearing area, in Zarb, Bolender, Carlsson (eds). *Prosthodontic Treatment for Edentulous Patients, 11th edition,* St. Louis, MO, Mosby-Year Book, 1997, pp 141–149.

12. Kolb HR: Variable denture-limiting structures of the edentulous mouth. Part I. Maxillary border areas. *J Prosthet Dent* 1966;16:194–201.

13. Hilierup S: Preprosthetic surgery in the elderly. *J Prosthet Dent* 1994;72:551–558.

14. Carlsson GE: Clinical morbidity and sequelae of treatment with complete dentures. *J Prosthet Dent* 1998;79:20.

15. Kazanjian VH: Surgery as an aid to more efficient service with prosthetic dentures. *J Am Dent Assoc* 1935;22:566–581.

16. DeVan MM: Basic principles in impression making. *J Prosthet Dent* 1952;2:26–35.

17. Tilton GE: The denture periphery. *J Prosthet Dent* 1952;2:290–306.

18. Kolb HR: Variable denture-limiting structures of the edentulous mouth. Part II. Mandibular border areas. *J Prosthet Dent* 1966;16:202–212.

19. van Waas MA: The influence of psychologic factors on patient satisfaction with complete dentures. *J Prosthet Dent* 1990;63:545–548.

20. Vervoorn JM, Duinkerke ASH, Luteijn F, et al: Relative importance of psychologic factors in denture satisfaction. *Commun Dent Oral Epidemiol* 1991;19:45–47.

21. Pendleton EC: The anatomy of the maxilla from the point of view of full denture prosthesis. *J Am Dent Assoc* 1932;19:543–572.

22. Rinaldi P, Sharry J: Tongue force and fatigue in adults. *J Prosthet Dent* 1963;13:857.

23. Borkin DW: Impression technique for patients that gag. *J Prosthet Dent* 1958;9:386–387.

24. Krol AJ: A new approach to the gagging problem. *J Prosthet Dent* 1963;13:611–616.

25. Carlson B, Carlsson GE: Prosthodontic complications in osseointegrated dental implant treatment. *Int J Oral Maxillofac Implants* 1994;9:90–94.

26. Jacob R: Maxillofacial prosthodontics for the edentulous patient, in Zarb, Bolender, Carlsson (eds). *Prosthodontic Treatment for Edentulous Patients* (ed 11) St. Louis, MO, Mosby-Year Book, 1997, pp 469–490.

3

COMPLETE EDENTULISM AND COMORBID DISEASES: AN UPDATE

DAVID A. FELTON, DDS, MS, FACP[1]

Department of Restorative Dentistry, West Virginia University School of Dentistry, Morgantown, WV

Keywords

Complete edentulism; comorbid disease; malnutrition; obesity; rheumatoid arthritis; cardiovascular disease; pneumonia; COPD; cancer; dementia; mortality

Correspondence

David A. Felton, Department of Restorative Dentistry, West Virginia University School of Dentistry, Robert C. Byrd Health Sciences Center, 1 Medical Center Drive, Morgantown, WV 26506. E-mail: dafelton@hsc.wvu.edu

This manuscript was presented at the 2015 Annual Session of the Academy of Prosthodontics in Austin, TX, April 28-May 2, 2015.

The author denies any conflict of interest.

Accepted June 17, 2015

Published in *Journal of Prosthodontics* 2016; Vol. 25, pp. 5–20

doi: 10.1111/jopr.12350

ABSTRACT

The relationship between complete edentulism, which is the terminal outcome of a multifactorial oral disease process and other comorbid diseases, was first reported in 2009. Although the relationship between edentulism and a multitude of systemic diseases was reported, none of the publications studied could determine causality of tooth loss on the incidence of any comorbid disease. Since that publication, there has been a renewed interest in this relationship, and a plethora of new articles have been published. This article will provide an update on articles published since 2008 on the relationship between edentulism and comorbid diseases, and will include the relationship between complete edentulism and such comorbid conditions as malnutrition, obesity, cardiovascular disease, rheumatoid arthritis, pulmonary diseases (including chronic obstructive pulmonary disease), cancer, and even mortality.

As prosthodontists and dentists, we have been treating the clinical condition of complete edentulism for over a millennium. Unfortunately, treatment of the edentulous patient may have in many academic institutions focused on the technical aspects of removable prostheses rather than the clinical rationale for treatment and long-term outcomes. According to World Health Organization (WHO) criteria, the completely edentulous patient meets WHO criteria for being: (1) physically impaired, (2) disabled, and (3) handicapped.[1–3]

Consider the patient shown in Figure 1, a 23-year-old male with a history of chronic soft drink consumption, who presented in pain for dental treatment. Rather than attempting to salvage some remaining mandibular anterior teeth to retain a removable partial dental prosthesis, the patient was edentulated and allowed to heal. He underwent two additional surgeries before denture fabrication; the first surgery was required due to the failure to recognize and remove lateral bony exostoses that impeded successful prosthesis insertion, and a second surgery was required to remove 5 to 7 mm of alveolar bone due to a lack of adequate interarch space. Finally, complete denture prostheses were inserted on healed alveolar ridges. Given that the average life expectancy in the

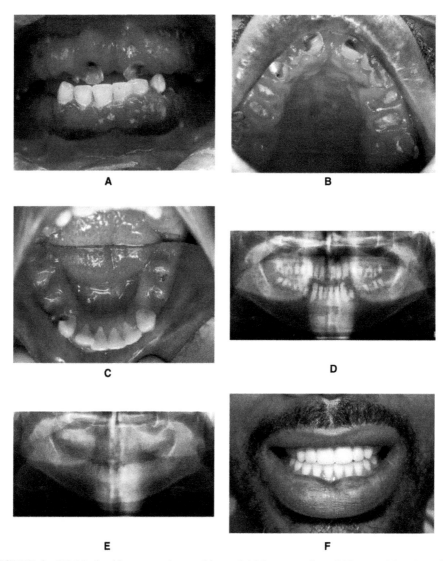

FIGURE 1 (A) Maximal intercuspation position at initial presentation of 23-year-old male patient exhibiting significant loss of tooth structure and dental caries. (B) Occlusal view of maxillary arch at initial presentation. (C) Occlusal view of mandibular dental arch at initial presentation. (D) Initial panoramic film denoting multiple carious lesions, periapical abscesses, and significant vertical bone height. (E) Panoramic film following tooth extraction, but before alveolar surgery to provide adequate interarch space for removable complete denture prostheses. (F) Definitive prostheses inserted at established occlusal vertical dimension. Note significant amount of tooth display.

United States is 78.8 years, what does this 23-year-old edentulous patient have to look forward to over the next 55 years, and how might edentulation at this early age impact his overall systemic health?

Incidence of Complete Edentulism in the United States And globally

Over a decade ago, Douglas et al[4] suggested that complete edentulism in the United States was not declining, and may, in fact, be on the rise. The authors suggested that the apparent decline in edentulism of approximately 10% per decade will be more than offset by the increase in the population growth of adults over the age of 55. They suggested that the completely edentulous population in the United States would increase from 33.6 to 37.9 million by 2020, due to population growth and increased life expectancies for the elderly.

Slade et al[5] evaluated edentulism trends in the United States. They investigated population trends in U.S. adults >15 years of age using five national cross-sectional health surveys (1957 to 1958, 1971 to 1975, 1988 to 1998, 1999 to 2002, and 2009 to 2012). These surveys included 155,524 individuals. The authors found that the prevalence of edentulism declined from 18.9% at the 1957 to 1958 cohort to 4.9% in the most recent age cohort. They reported the rate of edentulism in the United States in 2010 at 12.2 million. As might be expected, edentulism was a rare condition in high-income households, and states with higher levels of poverty experienced higher levels of edentulism. Slade et al projected that the rate of decline would slow to 2.6% by 2050; however, they also concluded that rate of decline in edentulism may be offset by population growth and aging. Wu et al[6] reported similar findings. They evaluated social stratification and tooth retention in 11,812 adults 50+ years of age between 1988 and 2004, using NHANES surveys. During this time, the rate of edentulism declined from 24.6% to 17.4%. In addition, the mean number of missing teeth declined from 8.19 to 6.5. Wu et al concluded that tooth loss and edentulism were directly related to race, lower income, and lower education levels. Given these data, it appears that the need for complete denture education must be continued for the next four or five decades in the United States.

Globally, complete edentulism also appears to be on the decline. Kassebaum et al[7] studied the effects of 291 diseases and their 1160 sequelae occurring between 1990 and 2010 globally. A total of 68 studies were selected and included 285,746 people in 26 countries ages 12 and older. A meta-analysis was conducted of the data. The results indicated that the global incidence of complete edentulism decreased from 4.4% to 4.1% between 1990 and 2010. Clearly, dentistry and prosthodontics have made an impact on tooth loss and complete edentulism; however, although a decline has been observed, we have not eliminated complete edentulism

or the need for complete denture education, at least in the United States.

Tooth Loss and Comorbid Disease

The relationship between tooth loss and other systemic comorbid conditions is, at best, multifactorial (Fig 2). What, then, is a comorbid condition? Comorbidity is one or more diseases (or disorders) that exist in addition to the primary disorder or disease for a given patient (in this case, complete edentulism). The combined relationship between the primary condition and the comorbidity can have profound impacts on the individual's overall health. In medicine, the Charlson Comorbidity Index[8] is the most widely used validated method for quantifying the effects of multiple diseases on a patient. It predicts the 1-year mortality rates for individuals with multiple systemic diseases. Of 22 possible conditions the Index uses, oral health is not one of the possible disease entities.

In an evaluation of the relationship between complete edentulism and other systemic comorbid conditions, Felton[9] reported on a multitude of studies indicating that completely edentulous patients had a greater risk of developing coronary artery plaque formation, and for having certain cancers. In addition, edentulous patients had a greater incidence of asthma (OR = 10.52) and diabetes. In addition, one study found a direct relationship between the number of remaining teeth and the incidence of dementia.[10] Unfortunately, none of the studies reviewed could confirm whether the relationship between complete edentulism and these comorbid conditions was causal (i.e., a direct cause and effect relationship) or casual.

The purpose of this report, then, is to provide an updated review of the current literature on the relationship between tooth loss, complete edentulism, and comorbid disease conditions.

METHODS

To further investigate this relationship, the National Library of Medicine's PubMed web site was used to search the literature using the following parameters:

(1) Articles published since 2008
(2) Patient cohorts studied had to have a minimum of 50 patients, and a control group for comparison.
(3) MESH terms included complete edentulism, dentures, and tooth loss in combination with the following comorbidities: nutrition, cancer, cardiovascular disease, cognition or dementia, diabetes, mortality, respiratory or chronic obstructive pulmonary disease (COPD), and rheumatoid arthritis (RA).
(4) Some portion of the investigated patient cohort had to be completely edentulous

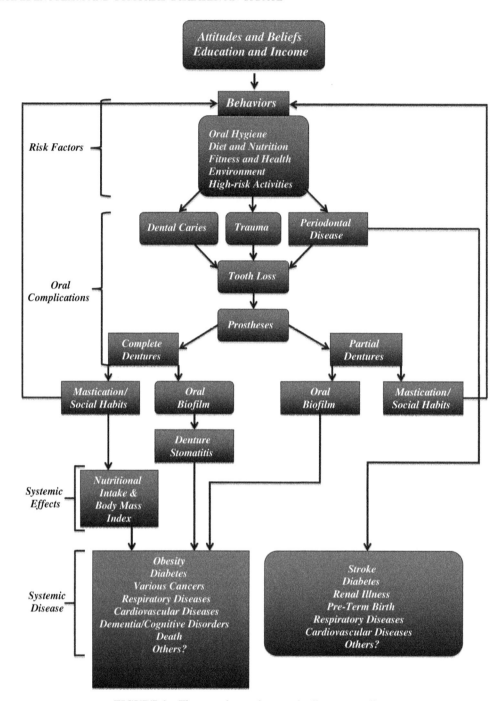

FIGURE 2 The complex oral-systemic disease paradigm.

(5) Abstracts were reviewed, and articles printed and reviewed to determine if they met the inclusion criteria by a single author.

RESULTS

A total of 225 abstracts of potential articles published since the 2009 report were reviewed, resulting in 95 full-text articles for review. Of these, 48 were found to meet the inclusion criteria. These were subdivided into categories evaluating edentulism and its relationship to the following comorbid conditions:

(1) Impact on nutrition and obesity
(2) Cardiovascular diseases
(3) Diabetes
(4) RA
(5) Respiratory diseases, including COPD

(6) Cancer

(7) Cognitive disorders

(8) Mortality

Tables 1–10 present some of the pertinent data from the 2009 paper highlighted at the start of the table in bold/italic type, and the more recent data in standard type. In addition, some discussion is required to distinguish between the use of "Odds ratio" and "Hazard ratio," which are reported from many of the manuscripts. As used here, "Odds ratio" is obtained from the use of logistic regression analysis, and relates to the ratio of proportions. In other words, an odds ratio of 2.3 implies that one patient cohort is at a 2.3-time greater risk for developing a systemic comorbidity than a different patient cohort (i.e., edentulous vs. dentate). "Hazard ratio" is obtained from a Cox regression (i.e., survival analysis) statistical evaluation (i.e., the number of new cases

of a "disease" occurring per population cohort, per unit time). The hazard ratio is the relative risk of the disease comorbidity occurring based on a comparison of event rates during a given time period.

DISCUSSION

Complete Edentulism, Nutrition, Malnutrition, and Obesity

Malnutrition and obesity are the two general aspects of nutrition that have been studied related to tooth loss and denture wear.

Nutrition and Malnutrition (Table 1) In our previous report, Nowjack-Ramer and Sheiham,[11] Sahyoun et al,[12] and Slade et al[13] reported that tooth loss negatively

TABLE 1   Edentulism, nutrition, and malnutrition

Author	N	Study type	Age (years)	Measured	Outcome	Risk, If reported, as OR/HR
Nowjack-Ramer and Sheiham 2007[11]	*6985*	*Cross-sectional*		*Tooth loss, dietary intake*	*Reduced dentition had reduced intake of fruits and vegetables*	
Sahyoun et al 2003[12]	*5958*	*Cross-sectional*	*50+*	*Healthy eating index (HEI) and tooth loss*	*<4 pairs of posterior teeth resulted = malnutrition. Edentulous = malnutrition*	
Slade 1996[13]	*1160*	*Cross-sectional*	*60+*	*Chewing ability, #remaining teeth*	*58% of denture wearers reported difficulty chewing*	
Saarela et al 2014[19]	1475	Cross-sectional		Nutritional status	Edentulism without a prosthesis = malnutrition	
De Marchi et al 2008[15]	471	Cross-sectional	60 to 92	Malnutrition	26% at risk for malnutrition; one to eight teeth protective against malnutrition	OR = 3.26 with 1 denture
Lancker et al 201 2[14]	10,916	Systematic review	60 to 89.6	Malnutrition	Association exists between oral health and malnutrition	
loannldou et al 2014[15]	2749	Cross-sectional NHANES III	>60	Protein and caloric Intake	Tooth loss = decreased Intake of vital nutrients	OR = 1.42 for each 5 teeth lost
De Marchi et al 2011[16]	471	Cross-sectional	60 to 89	Fruit, vegetable Intake	44% were edentulous 49% did not consume recommended F-V	
Han & Klm 2014[17]	1168	Cross-sectional KNHANES	75.1 (mean)	Nutritional Intake	With dentures: 1 2.8% malnourished; without dentures: 20%	OR = 1.89

TABLE 2   Edentulism and obesity

Author	N	Study type	Age (years)	Measured	Outcome	Risk, if reported, as OR/HR
Sheiham et al 2002[20]	*629*	*Cross-sectional*	*65+*	*# remaining teeth, body mass index (BMI)*	*<21 teeth, or edentulous increased risk of obesity*	*OR = 3.0*
De Marchi et al 2012[21]	471	Cross-sectional	60 to 92	Central obesity	Obesity if <8 teeth. Tooth loss associated with obesity	OR = 3.28
Do Nascimento et al 2013[22]	900	Cross-sectional	72.7 (mean)	Obesity	Not wearing dentures = increased obesity	OR = 2.88

TABLE 3   **Edentulism and cardiovascular disease**

Author	N	Study type	Age (years)	Measured	Outcome	Risk, if reported, as OR/HR
Taguchi et al 2004[24]	*67*	*Cross-sectional*	*44 to 68*	*Tooth loss, hypertension*	*Tooth loss = increased risk of hypertension*	*OR = 3.59*
Desvarieux et al 2003[25]	*711*	*Cross-sectional*	*57 to 75*	*Tooth loss, periodontal health*	*Tooth loss = increased incidence of carotid artery plaques*	
Schwahn et al 2004[26]	*2738*	*Cross-sectional*	*20 to 59*	*Tooth loss, plasma fibrinogen*	*Periodisease, tooth loss associated with inflammation*	*OR = 1.88*
Medina-Solis et al 2014[27]	13,966	Cross-sectional	50.9	Tooth loss, angina pectoris	10.2% were edentulous 2.3% had angina. Edentulism correlated with age, more in younger age group	OR = 12.93
Polzer et al 2012[28]	108 to 41,407	Systematic review-meta analysis	18 to 85	Tooth loss, circulatory mortality	Circulatory mortality linked to tooth loss. All-cause mortality linked	

TABLE 4   **Edentulism and diabetes**

Author	N	Study type	Age (years)	Measured	Outcome	Risk, if reported, as OR/HR
Cleary and Hutton 1995[29]	*370*	*Cross-sectional*	*50 to 95*	*Health, #teeth, non-insulin diabetes*	*Edentulous = higher risk of developing non-insulin dependent diabetes mellitus*	*OR = 4.06*
Medina-Solis et al 2006[30]	*14,000*	*Cross-sectional*	*18 to 90*	*#teeth, health status*	*30.6% edentulous above 65 years. Edentulism increased risk of diabetes*	*OR = 1.82*
Azogui-Levi and Dray-Spira 2012[31]	19,231 (1111 with diabetes mellitus)	Cross-sectional	35+	± diabetes and dental problems	Diabetes = dental problems. Diabetes = removable prostheses	OR = 1.47 OR = 2.17
Patel et al 2013[32]	2508	Cross-sectional	50+	#teeth and diabetes	Edentulism = 28% diabetic v 14% (nondiabetic)	OR = 2.25

TABLE 5   **Edentulism and rheumatoid arthritis**

Author	N	Study type	Age (years)	Measured	Outcome	Risk, if reported, as OR/HR
De Pablo et al 2008[34]	4461	Cross-sectional	60+	#remaining teeth, perio disease, edentulism	RA patients = higher incidence of perio, more missing teeth, greater risk of edentulism	OR = 1.82 for perio disease OR = 2.27 if edentulous
Demmer et al 2011[35]	9702	Cross-sectional	25 to 74	#remaining teeth, perio disease, edentulism	Perio disease and >5 missing teeth = higher incidence of RA (but not statistically significant). Edentulous = greater risk of RA	OR = 1.92 if edentulous

TABLE 6   Edentulism and respiratory diseases

Author	N	Study type	Age (years)	Measured	Outcome	Risk, if reported, as OR/HR
Xie et al 1997, 1999[38,39]	*293*	*Cross-sectional*	*75+*	*Tooth loss, smoking, asthma*	*Asthma more likely in edentulous, increased ridge resorption*	*OR = 10.52 OR = 6.0*
Sjögren et al 2008[40]	3545	Systematic review	Elderly	Oral health, respiratory tract infections	Good oral hygiene reduces RTI and reduced resp. mortality	Risk reduction of 6.8% to 11.7%
Iinuma et al 2015[41]	524	Prospective for 36 months	85+ years	Denture wear and pneumonia	Nocturnal denture = pneumonia 22% death rate	OR = 2.3 for pneumonia
Pryzbylowska et al 2014[42]	53 COPD pts.	in vivo	62 to 88	Cultured dentures for COPD biofilm	90% COPD pts had pathogenic bact. Yeast in 75%	
Ortega et al 2014[43]	65	Observe-transverse	Mean 79.7	Dysphagia	40% edentulous 16% aspiration +	

TABLE 7   Edentulism and COPD

Author	N	Study type	Age (years)	Measured	Outcome	Risk, if reported, as OR/HR
Barros et al 2013[44]	11,387	Prospective cohort over 5 years	45 to 64	Inflammatory biomarkers & COPD	Edentulous at higher risk for COPD incr IL-6 = COPD biofilm on dentures	OR = 2.37 for gold type 1,2
Offenbacher et al 2012[45]	13,465 (2084 edent)	Cross-sectional	45 to 64	COPD in edentulous	28.3% of edentulous had COPD v 19.6%dentate	OR = 1.3 (GOLD 2) OR = 2.5 (GOLD 3)

TABLE 8   Edentulism and cancer

Author	N	Study type	Age (years)	Measured	Outcome	Risk, if reported, as OR/HR
Hiraki et al 2008[46]	*5240*	*Cross-sectional*		*Tooth loss, various cancer types*	*Edentulism = increased cancer of: lung esophagus bladder*	*OR = 1.54 OR = 2.36 OR = 2.85*
Ansai et al 2013[47]	656	Prospective for 12 years	80 years at baseline	Oral exam, cause of death	Tooth loss = cancer death 17 cancer deaths	HR = 1.03
Shakeri et al 2013[48]	922	Case-controlled study	40 to 75	Oral exam	8 or fewer teeth, or edentulous, at higher risk for cancer	OR = 1.6 for both
Zeng et al 2013[49]	6282 6873 cont.	Meta-analysis	18 to 89	Tooth loss, head/ neck cancer incidence	Loss of 15 teeth incr risk. Loss of 20 teeth incr risk	OR = 1.72 OR = 1.89

influenced nutritional intake, and that edentulous patients were at greater risk for malnutrition than the dentate or partially dentate cohort. In a systematic review, Lancker et al[14] found a direct correlation between poor oral health and malnutrition. Ioannidou et al[15] found that tooth loss was related to a decreased intake of vital nutrients, and that the risk was 1.42 times greater for each five teeth lost. De Marchi et al[16] reported that the edentulous patient cohort did not consume the recommended amount of fruits and vegetables. Han and Kim[17] reported that in the denture-wearing cohort, 12.8% were malnourished while using dentures, whereas 20% experienced malnutrition if dentures were not used. De Marchi et al[18] found that the edentulous patient was 3.26 times more likely to suffer from malnutrition (OR = 3.26

TABLE 9   Edentulism and cognitive impairment

Author	N	Study type	Age (years)	Measured	Outcome	Risk, if reported, as OR/HR
Stein et al 2007[10]	*144*	*Prospect for 40 years*		*Memory impairment tooth loss, brain histology*	*22% had one or more copies of Alzheimer's gene. # missing teeth = incr dementia incidence*	
Okamoto et al 2014[50]	2335	Prospect for 5 years		Memory impairment and tooth loss	Fewer teeth + decreased cognition 10.3% declined edent was worse	OR = 1.02 in dentate 2.39 in edent
Eshkoor et al 2014[51]	1210 with dementia	National cross-sectional		Oral health, physical and cognitive impairment	Falls incr 17% Falls decreased for wearing dentures	OR = 1.58 (funct decline) OR = 0.66
Kisely et al 2011[52]	27,843 cont.	Meta-analysis		Oral health, dementia	Edentulism increased risk of dementia	OR = 3.4
Naorungroj et al 2014[53]	5878	Cross-sectional over 6 years	45 to 64	Cognitive function, oral health	Edentulism 18.2%. Cognitive change in 6 years greater in edent	
Naorungroj et al 2014[53]	558	Cross-sectional over 8 years	52 to 75	Oral health, cognitive function	13.8% edentulous. Greater cognitive decline in edent (NS)	
Paganini-Hill et al 2012[54]	5468		52 to 105	Cognitive function, oral health	Greater risk for dementia if NOT wearing dentures	HR = 1.91
Tsakos et al 2015[55]	3166	Longitudinal	60+	Cognitive function, oral health	Edent recalled 0.88 fewer words, at slower rate; edent = cognitive decline	
Zenthofer et al 2014[56]	94	Cross-sectional	Mean 82.9	OHRQoL index, oral health	No teeth = lower ORHQoL scores 39.4% edent	

TABLE 10   Edentulism and mortality

Author	N	Study type	Age (years)	Measured	Outcome	Risk, if reported, as OR/HR
Brown 2009[57]	41 K	Cross-sectional, 16-year follow-up	18+	Cause of death, edentulism	12.3% edent (46% over age 75). Risk of death 10% with teeth, 19% if edentulous	OR = 1.5
Holm-Pedersen et al 2008[58]	573	Cross-sectional at 5 to 20 years	70	Disability, oral assessment	40% edentulous; edentulous = higher risk of mortality	OR = 3.79 OR = 2.67 if 9 = teeth
Osterberg et al 2008[59]	1803	Cross-sectional over 20 years	70	Cause of death, oral health	Dentures = highest mortality	HR = 0.98
Ansai et al 2013[60]	656	Prospect over 12 years	80+	Cause of death, oral exam	Tooth loss = cancer deaths; survival lowest in edentulous	HR = 1.03
Janket et al 2013[61]	256, 250 cont	Cross-sectional, 16 years follow-up	61 (mean)	Cause of death, oral health	Dentures = higher risk of CVA mortality CD/RDP highest	HR = 1.0 HR = 1.99
Polzer et al 2012[62]	152 k	Systematic review, meta-analysis	18 to 89	Cause of death, #teeth	Dentures = increased risk of all-cause and circulatory mortality	
Schwahn et al 2013[63]	1803	Cross-sectional, 9.9-year follow-up	63.6 (mean)	Cause of death, #teeth	9+ unreplaced teeth directly related to all-cause mortality	OR = 1.43 OR = 1.88 for CVD
Takata et al 2014[47]	207	Cross-sectional, 10-year follow up	85	Cause of death	Cognitive impairment = increased risk of mortality	OR = 2.6
Liljestrand et al 2015[65]	8446	Cross-sectional 13-year follow-up	25 to 74	Dental status, diabetes, CVD, CHD, mortality rates	Edentulous at greater risk for CVD, CHD, Diabetes mellitus, mortality	HR = 1.4 HR = 1.65 HR = 1.56 HR = 1.68

with one denture) then the partially dentate population, and that if a patient had up to eight remaining natural teeth, these teeth served as a protective mechanism against malnutrition. Saarela et al[19] reported that the denture-wearing patient cohort was better equipped to have an adequate diet, and that complete edentulism without dentures resulted in malnutrition.

Obesity (Table 2)   Obesity has emerged as one of the fastest growing medical conditions in the United States. It affects more than a third of the adult U.S. population. Obesity can lead to a multitude of comorbid conditions, including cardiovascular disease, type 2 diabetes, certain types of cancer, and premature death. The estimated annual cost associated with obesity is a significant part of the expenditures for health care in the United States. The incidence of diabetes appears to be age- and ethnicity-related. The U.S. Centers for Disease Control (CDC) estimates of obesity are shown in Figure 3 for 2011; note how that increased by 2013 (Fig 4). Sadly, it is even worse for non-Hispanic blacks. Also note that in *NO* state is the incidence of obesity less than 20% (U.S. CDC).

In our previous report, only Sheiham et al[20] reported that the edentulous population was at an increased risk for obesity. De Marchi et al[21] found that a 3.28-time higher risk of obesity occurred if fewer than eight natural teeth remained (OR = 3.28). For edentulous patients, Do Nascimento et al[22] reported that the edentulous patient cohort that did not wear dentures were at an increased risk of being obese

(OR = 2.88). Finally, Hamdan et al,[23] in a randomized control trial, compared the nutritional intake of patients with well-fitting complete dentures, and those with implant-retained mandibular overdentures, but found no difference between the cohorts.

Clearly, the evidence appears to support the premise that the edentulous patient appears at risk for poor nutritional intake, malnutrition, and obesity. Our abilities to provide exceptional complete denture prostheses are essential to correct this situation.

Complete Edentulism and Cardiovascular Diseases (Table 3)

Cardiovascular disease is the leading cause of death in the United States, killing more than 370,000 adults annually. The primary risk factors for cardiovascular disease are high blood pressure, high LDL cholesterol levels, and smoking, although other risk factors also play a role in the disease progression (U.S. CDC).

Our previous investigation pointed to the relationship between tooth loss and atherosclerotic plaque formation. Taguchi et al[24] reported that tooth loss increased the risk of hypertension. Desvarieux et al[25] demonstrated that tooth loss was associated with an increase in the formation of carotid artery plaques, and Schwahn et al[26] showed that tooth loss and periodontal disease were associated with increased levels of inflammatory markers in the blood stream. Since that report, two additional studies merit consideration.

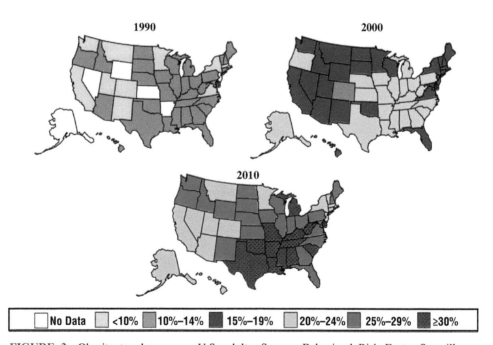

FIGURE 3 Obesity trends* among U.S. adults, Source: Behavioral Risk Factor Surveillance System, US CDC, BRFSS, 1990, 2000, 2010.

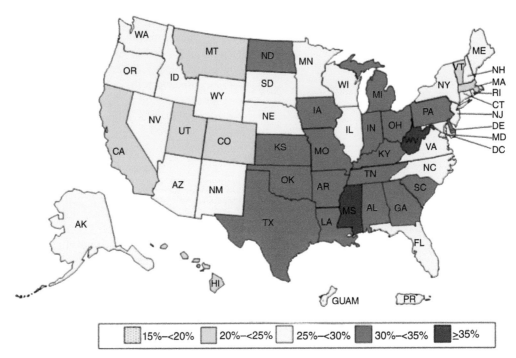

FIGURE 4   Prevalence of self-reported obesity among U.S. adults by state and territory, BRFSS, 2013. U.S. CDC. Note that the scale has changed, with the lower end of the scale set at 15%, and upper end of the scale now set at >35% (previous figure reported <10% and >30%, respectively).

Medina-Solis et al,[27] in a cross-sectional survey of 13,966 participants with a mean age of nearly 51 years, found a rate of complete edentulism of 10.2%. They found that the effect of edentulism on angina pectoris was correlated with age, being more prevalent in the younger age group (OR = 12.93).

Polzer et al[28] conducted a systematic review and meta-analysis to determine whether the number of remaining teeth is associated with circulatory mortality or all-cause mortality, and to determine whether the replacement of missing teeth would provide protection for the patient from mortality. They identified 23 studies that met their inclusion criteria, including five that met moderate to high levels of quality. Their assessment found a relationship between circulatory mortality and the number of remaining teeth, as well as a relationship between all-cause mortality and the number of remaining teeth. Unfortunately, no studies determined whether the replacement of missing teeth protected the patient against mortality. Polzer et al indicated that the effects of denture use on circulatory mortality needed to be studied.

Complete Edentulism and Diabetes (Table 4)

Diabetes is the seventh leading cause of mortality in the United States. In 2012, over 29 million adults were diagnosed with the disease, and it is estimated that one in four people do not know they have the disease. In addition, 86 million are considered prediabetic, and without diet and exercise, up to 30% of these individuals will become type 2 diabetics within 5 years (U.S. CDC). According to the WHO, diabetes is projected to be one of the world's main killers and disablers within the next 25 years. Nearly 171 million globally are estimated to be affected by diabetes. Our previous report suggested that edentulous patients had a higher risk of developing noninsulin dependent diabetes (Cleary and Hutton,[29] and Medina-Solis et al[30]).

More recently, Azogui-Levy and Dray-Spira[31] evaluated this relationship in a French population of 19,231 participants aged 35 and older. They collected data from their patient cohort over three visits in a 2-year period and found that diabetics were older (mean age of 66 years vs. 52 years for nondiabetics), more likely to be obese (35% vs. 12%), and had a higher prevalence of oral health problems (16.4%) than nondiabetics (13.4%). They also determined that diabetics were more likely to experience dental problems (OR = 1.47), and were more than twice as likely to wear removable prostheses (62%) than nondiabetics were (33%; OR = 2.17).

Patel et al[32] analyzed NHANES 2003 to 2004 data of 2508 participants 50 years of age and older. They found the prevalence of edentulism was 28% for the diabetic population, but only 14% for the nondiabetic cohort. Multiple regression analysis indicated that patients with diabetes were more likely to be edentulous than those without diabetes (OR = 2.25).

Complete Edentulism and RA (Table 5)

RA is a systemic inflammatory disease that can manifest itself in numerous joints in the body. The inflammation primarily affects the synovial membrane, leading to cartilage and bone erosions and occasionally, to joint deformity. Common joint manifestations include pain, swelling, and redness. It is believed to be the result of a faulty immune response. RA affects nearly 1.3 million in the United States, with women being affected 2.5 times as frequently as men (U.S. CDC). For a good review of the etiology and pathogenesis of RA, see Culshaw et al.[33] In our previous study, we reported that de Pablo et al[34] found that patients with RA were at a 2.27-time greater risk for being edentulous than those with remaining teeth. This risk was 3.34 times greater when the patient cohorts were adjusted for confounders (sex, age, smoking, and race-ethnicity). In a study of 9702 women using NHANES I data in a cross-sectional analysis, Demmer et al[35] found that completely edentulous patients experienced a statistically significant increase in the risk of incident RA (OR = 1.92) compared to those patients who had lost fewer than five teeth; however, the causality of RA as it relates to complete edentulism has not been demonstrated to date.

Complete Edentulism, Respiratory Diseases, and COPD (Tables 6 and 7)

Chronic obstructive pulmonary disease (COPD) is characterized clinically by the inability to inspire and expire; it is generally associated with inflammation of the lung tissues. The major risk factor is smoking, but poor air quality may be implicated as well. COPD is the third leading cause of death in the United States, and fifth leading cause globally.[36] It is expected to become the fourth leading cause of death globally by 2030.[37] In the United States, COPD affects an estimated 24 million adults, and results in 700,000 hospital admissions and 124,000 deaths annually (U.S. CDC). Individuals with this disease are classified using the Global Initiative for Chronic Obstructive Lung Disease (GOLD) classification system; stages I to IV are identified, based on spirometry assessments.

In our last report, which focused on asthma, we noted that Xie et al[38,39] had reported that asthma was more likely to occur in the edentulous adult, and that the use of inhaled corticosteroids could lead to increased alveolar ridge resorption in the maxillary arch. Six studies were identified that reported on the association between tooth loss and respiratory diseases, including COPD and pneumonia.

Respiratory Infections (Table 6) Several studies have investigated tooth loss and denture use as it relates to the development of upper respiratory tract infections and dysphagia. A plausible mechanism of pneumonia could be associated with aspiration of oral pathogens from the mouth or associated prosthetic appliances.

Sjogren et al[40] conducted a systematic review of the effects of good oral hygiene on respiratory tract infection and pneumonia in hospitals and nursing homes. They estimated that a reduction of 10% of the cases of death from pneumonia in nursing home residents could be associated with improving oral hygiene of the patients.

Iinuma et al[41] investigated a population of community-dwelling elders in Japan. A total of 524 patients age 85+ years were assessed over 36 months. The investigators found that nocturnal denture wear was significantly associated with a higher risk (OR = 2.3) of pneumonia.

Przybylowska et al[42] evaluated the composition of denture plaque biofilm on the oral mucosa in 51 patients, 37 diagnosed with COPD. Of these patients, 62% had complete dentures, 24% had transitional RDPs, and 13.5% had metal-based RDPs. All control group patients had complete dentures. Bacterial sampling was conducted on all patients. The investigators found pathogenic bacteria in 92% of the COPD patients. In addition, 70.3% of the hospitalized patients had denture stomatitis with *C. albicans* infection. Abundant biofilm was detected in 27% of the COPD patients, but only in 7% of the control group. The investigators concluded that poor oral hygiene in the denture-wearing COPD patient can lead to COPD-related events.

Finally, Ortega et al[43] evaluated the oral health status of elderly patients with oropharyngeal dysphagia compared to a control group without swallowing difficulties. The investigators found that 40% of the dysphagia patients were edentulous, 16% of the patients had confirmation of aspiration into the lung tissues, 80% had signs of biofilm penetration into the larynx, and 32% had oropharyngeal residue of the denture biofilm. Ortega et al concluded that elderly patients with oropharyngeal dysphagia had a high risk of developing aspiration pneumonia.

COPD (Table 7) In a prospective 5-year cohort study of 11,387 patients ages 45 to 64, Barros et al[44] studied the inflammatory biomarkers and COPD. They found an increase of IL-6 in the COPD patient cohort, and a significant pathogenic biofilm on dentures; these patients were found to be at higher risk for COPD-related events. Barros et al found that the completely edentulous patient cohort had a 2.37 times higher risk for COPD hospitalization and COPD-related death than the dentate or partially dentate cohorts (OR = 2.37 for GOLD stage 1 and 2).

Offenbacher et al,[45] in a cross-sectional study of 13,465 patients age 45 to 64 (of whom 2084 were completely edentulous) found that 28.3% of the edentulous patient cohort had COPD vs. 19.6% of the dentate patients. The risk (OR) of development of COPD in denture wearers was 1.3 times higher for GOLD stage 2 and 2.5 times higher for GOLD stage 3 COPD.

Complete Edentulism and Cancer (Table 8)

Cancer is the second-leading cause of mortality annually in the United States, resulting in nearly 585,000 deaths in 2011. Currently, the U.S. CDC reports that two of every three individuals diagnosed with cancer lives at least 5 years after their diagnosis. Of great interest to prosthodontists, cancer of the head and neck region (larynx, pharynx, and oral cavity) accounts for 12% of malignancies globally. An estimated 300,000 mortalities are annually associated with head and neck cancer. The leading types of cancer, according to the U.S. CDC, are shown in Figure 5.

Our previous report suggested that complete edentulism was related to various types of cancers, including lung, esophageal, and bladder cancer.[9,46] Three additional studies have been found since our last publication. In the first, by Ansai et al,[47] 656 Japanese community-dwelling participants were studied over 12 years, to determine if tooth loss was associated with orodigestive cancer mortality. A significant association was found between tooth loss and cancer death; however, this became insignificant when adjusted for confounders. Survival rates were lowest in the completely edentulous cohort, especially for female denture wearers, when compared to the dentate cohort having 20 or more remaining teeth $(p = 0.047)$.

Shakeri et al,[48] in a case-controlled study in Iran, studied 309 patients with confirmed diagnoses of gastric adenocarcinoma, and 613 age- and sex-matched controls. They found that participants with eight or more remaining teeth were more likely to have gastric cancer than those with fewer than 8 remaining teeth (OR = 1.6), or those who were edentulous (OR = 1.6); however, the authors reported there was insufficient evidence for a clear pattern of association between the risk of gastric adenocarcinoma and oral health.

Finally, in a similar study, Zeng et al[49] conducted a metaanalysis of 11 articles to determine the association between tooth loss and cancer of the head and neck region. They found a direct association between tooth loss and head and neck cancer. They reported that the loss of 6 to 15 teeth increases the risk (OR = 1.58), the loss of 15 to 19 teeth increases the risk (OR = 1.72), and the completely edentulous condition increases the risk even further (OR = 1.89).

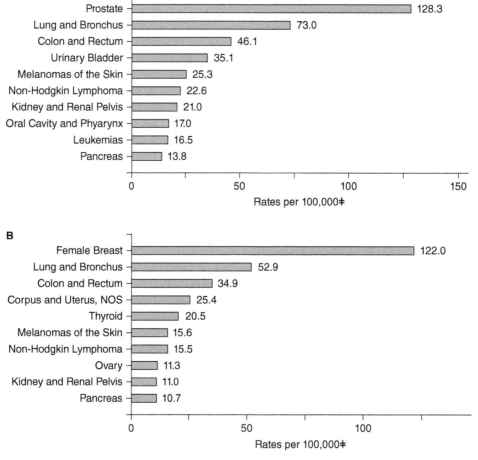

FIGURE 5   (A) Top 10 cancer sites, 2011, U.S. males, all races. (B) Top 10 cancer sites, 2011, U.S. females, all races. U.S. Centers for Disease Control

Complete Edentulism and Cognitive Impairment (Table 9)

Cognitive disorders, also known as dementia, are characterized by memory impairment, as well as marked difficulty in speaking, motor activity, object recognition, and disturbance of executive function (ability to plan, organize, and abstract). Alzheimer's Disease is the most common form of dementia. It is a progressive disease that begins with mild memory loss, and is thought to involve parts of the brain that control thought, memory, and language. The cause remains unclear. In 2013, up to 5 million adults had been diagnosed with Alzheimer's in the United States. The number of individuals with the disease doubles every 5 years after the age of 65. By 2050, the number of affected individuals is projected to rise to 14 million, nearly a three-fold increase above current levels. The best-known risk factor is age, although genetics may play a role. Alzheimer's, and other cognitive disorders, are the sixth leading cause of mortality in the United States. Nearly 84,767 deaths were reported to result from Alzheimer's disease in 2011. In nursing homes in the United States, approximately 48.5% of patients have some level of this disease (U.S. CDC).

In our previous work, we reported on the relationship between tooth loss and cognitive disorders that was first reported by Stein et al.[10] In a prospective longitudinal study of 144 Roman Catholic nuns in Milwaukee, WI, detailed dental records were managed by a single dental practitioner over a 40-year period. In addition, cognitive assessments were performed on the patients over a 12-year period. Finally, cranial tissues were obtained post-mortem, and analyzed by a trained neuropathologist blinded to the nuns' cognitive function scores. The findings were impressive, as 22% of the study participants had one or more copies of the gene for Alzheimer's. In addition, the investigators found a direct correlation between the incidence of dementia and the number of missing teeth. This initial publication has led to additional interest in the relationship between tooth loss and cognitive disorders since 2007.

Okamoto et al[50] evaluated 2335 community-dwelling patients for memory loss as a function of tooth loss in a prospective 5-year clinical trial. They found that the completely edentulous patient experienced a greater decline in cognitive function when compared to the dentate cohort. The risk of decline in cognitive function was 2.39 times greater (OR = 2.39) in the edentulous population. The risk of patients with 1 to 8 remaining teeth becoming edentulous within 5 years was 4.68 times greater than that of patients with more teeth.

Eshkoor et al[51] examined 1210 patients with diagnosed dementia in a national cross-sectional study. They evaluated oral health, gait, and physical and cognitive impairment as a function of tooth loss. They reported that the incidence of falls increased 17% in the edentulous population (OR = 1.58), and that the incidence of falls decreased for those edentulous patients who wore their dentures (OR = 0.66) and for partially dentate patients (OR = 0.59).

Kisely et al[52] conducted a systematic review and meta-analysis of 2784 patients with severe mental illness and a control group of 31,084 patients. Nine studies were selected from 550 citations that met the inclusion criteria. The authors reported that the rate of complete edentulism varied from 3% (India) to 65% (England and Denmark). Patients with severe mental illness had a 3.4-time greater risk of being completely edentulous, and had 6.2 more decayed, missing, and filled surfaces than the control group.

Naorungroj et al[53] used a subset of the Atherosclerosis Risk in Communities study, a community-based study of vascular disease of 558 adult 52- to 75-year olds studied over 8 years. The authors reported that 13.8% of the cohort was edentulous, and that there was a greater, but not clinically significant, decline in cognitive function in the edentulous cohort over the 8-year evaluation period. No causal effect could be determined.

Paganini-Hill et al[54] evaluated the oral health and cognitive abilities of 5468 older community-dwelling adults with a mean age of 81 years over an 18-year period. The authors found that 90% of those patients with inadequate natural masticatory function were edentulous. The edentulous patients who did *not* wear dentures demonstrated a 91% greater risk for dementia (HR = 1.91) than those who were partially dentate. For the partially dentate cohort, poor oral hygiene resulted in a greater risk for dementia (22% to 65%) than those who performed proper brushing daily. The authors concluded that the wearing of removable prostheses appeared to be beneficial in terms of reducing the risk of dementia.

Tsakos et al[55] evaluated cognitive function in 3166 community-dwelling adults 60+ years of age. All assessments were done at baseline and at 5-year intervals (10 years total). Completely edentulous patients were found to recall 0.88 fewer words, and were 0.09 m/sec slower than partially dentate controls. The authors stated that complete edentulism was independently associated with cognitive decline and physical decline in older English adults, and that tooth loss may be a potential early marker of cognitive decline in the elderly.

Zenthofer et al,[56] in a cross-sectional study, assessed oral health related quality of life (OHRQoL) in institutionalized patients. They found that edentulous patients reported lower QoL scores than those with FDPs and RDPs, but higher than those who were edentulous and had no replacement dentures.

Complete Edentulism and Mortality (Table 10)

Current life expectancy in the United States is 78.8 years, and nearly 2.6 million deaths are reported annually, from a multitude of causes (U.S. CDC). In our 2009 paper, there were no reports of the relationship between complete tooth loss, edentulism, and mortality.[9] Although several papers reviewed above[28,40,44,47] have discussed the relationship between tooth loss and mortality, several more deserve consideration.

Brown[57] provided one of the initial studies of the relationship between edentulism and mortality. In a cross-sectional survey of 41,000 adults 18+ years of age. Mortality information was collected after 15 years. He found that 12.3% of the participants were completely edentulous (46% rate at 75+ age cohort), and that complete edentulism that occurred *before* age 65 was associated with all-cause mortality. After adjustment for all confounders, the risk of death was 1.5 times greater for the edentulous patient than for the partially and fully dentate patient cohorts. An association between complete edentulism and cardiovascular mortality was also demonstrated.

Holm-Pedersen et al[58] evaluated 573 nondisabled community-dwelling individuals at baseline, and at 5-year intervals for 20 years. They found that 40% of the entering participants were edentulous, and by 21 years, 88% had died. Edentulous patients had a statistically higher risk for mortality (HR = 1.26) when compared to partially dentate patients. Holm Pedersen et al suggested that tooth loss was independently associated with mortality and that tooth loss may be an early predictor of accelerated aging.

Osterberg et al[59] evaluated whether the number of teeth remaining at age 70 in a Swedish population influenced mortality. In their study of 1803 participants, they found that the 7-year mortality rates were highest in completely edentulous men (42% to 47%). They reported that the number of remaining teeth was an independent, significant 7-year predictor of mortality in both sexes: each remaining tooth reduced 7-year mortality by 4%. The number of remaining teeth was shown to be a significant predictor of mortality in the elderly, regardless of socioeconomic status, health factors, or lifestyle.

Ansai et a[60] studied 656 patients over a 12-year period. They found a significant association between cancer death and tooth loss (HR = 1.03). Survival rates for female patients (only) were lowest in the edentulous patient cohort, and were statistically worse than those with 20 or more teeth.

Janket et al[61] evaluated the role of removable prostheses on cardiovascular survival in a 15-year cross-sectional study. In 256 participants, they found that partially edentulous patients with an RDP had a lower risk for cardiovascular mortality than those who were fully dentate; however, those with complete dentures, or with a complete denture opposing an RDP had a higher risk of mortality. This study suggested that the periodontal health of the remaining teeth, if present, may influence cardiovascular survival; the authors suggested that reducing inflammation of remaining teeth and replacement of missing teeth appears to impact longevity.

Polzer et al[62] conducted a systematic review in which 23 studies were selected. They reported that a relationship existed between the number of remaining teeth and both circulatory and all-cause mortality; however, no study in their investigation demonstrated whether replaced teeth protect the patient against mortality.

In contrast, Schwahn et al[63] studied 1803 patients over a 10-year period to determine if missing, but un-replaced teeth had an effect on mortality. In their patient cohort, 188 had unreplaced missing teeth. They found that having nine or more un-replaced teeth was directly related to all-cause mortality (OR = 1.53) in this patient cohort; those patients with nine or more un-replaced teeth had a two-fold increase for cardiovascular mortality. Interestingly, they demonstrated that an induction period of at least 9 years appears to be required for this relationship to develop. When adjusting for confounders, the OR for all-cause mortality was 1.43, and 1.88 for cardiovascular death. A reduced, but nonreplaced dentition appears to be associated with an increased risk for mortality.

Watt et al[64] studied 12,831 participants for 8 years. After adjusting for confounders, edentulous participants demonstrated a significantly higher risk for all-cause mortality (HR = 1.3 generally, HR = 1.49 for cardiovascular death mortality) compared to participants with natural teeth. Edentulous patients had a 2.97-time greater risk for mortality related to stroke. The authors concluded that being edentulous was shown to be an independent predictor of cardiovascular disease mortality.

Finally, Liljestrand et al,[65] in cross-sectional study of 8446 patients in Finland, evaluated the dental status of their patient cohort at baseline and over the next 13 years. National registers were used to obtain information on various comorbidities and mortality. The authors reported that the edentulous patient was at increased risk for development of cardiovascular disease (HR = 1.40), coronary heart disease (HR = 1.5), diabetes mellitus (HR = 1.56), and death (HR = 1.68). In comparison to patient cohorts with remaining teeth, they were at the greatest risk for death.

CONCLUSIONS

According to the research found and evaluated in this study, it appears that:

(1) Tooth loss, as well as complete edentulism, is associated with a multitude of systemic comorbid conditions.

(2) The edentulous patient is at risk for reduced nutritional intake and for obesity.

(3) Edentulous patients are at an increased risk of COPD-related events.

(4) Poorly maintained removable prostheses may be associated with increases in pneumonia-related hospitalizations.

(5) Tooth loss and complete edentulism may be associated with an increased risk of head and neck cancer.

(6) The risk of decline in cognitive function appears to be greater in the edentulous population.

(7) Edentulism is an independent predictor of cardiovascular disease mortality.

(8) A reduced, but nonreplaced dentition is associated with an increased risk for mortality.

(9) Wearing of optimal removable prostheses may help protect patients against some types of comorbid disease conditions.

(10) We need to educate patients and caregivers as to the potential long-term harmful outcomes of tooth extraction, and of poorly maintained removable prostheses.

REFERENCES

1. Feine JS, Carlsson GE (eds): *Implant Overdentures: The Standard of Care of Edentulous Patients*. Carol Stream, IL, Quintessence, 2003.

2. Nowjack-Ramer RE, Sheiham A: Association of edentulism and diet and nutrition in US adults. *J Dent Res* 2003;82: 122–126.

3. Bouma J, Uitenbroek D, Westert G, et al: Pathways to full mouth extraction. *Community Dent Oral Epidemiol* 1987;15:301–305.

4. Douglas CW, Shih A, Ostry L: Will there be a need for complete dentures in the United States in 2020?. *J Prosthet Dent* 2002;87:5–8.

5. Slade GD, Akinkugbe AA, Sanders AE: Projections of US edentulism prevalence following 5 decades of decline. *J Dent Res* 2014;93:959–965.

6. Wu B, Hybeis C, Liang J, et al: Social stratification and tooth loss among middle-aged and older Americans from 1988–2004. *Community Dent Oral Epidemiol* 2014;42:495–502.

7. Kassebaum NJ, Bernabe E, Dahiya M, et al: Global burden of severe tooth loss: a systematic review and meta-analysis. *J Dent Res* 2014;93:20S–28S.

8. Charlson ME, Pompei P, Ales KL, et al: A new method of classifying prognostic co-morbidity in longitudinal studies: development and validation. *J Chron Dis* 1987;40:373–383.

9. Felton DA: Edentulism and comorbid factors. *J Prosthodont* 2009;18:86–96.

10. Stein PS, Desrosiers M, Donegan SJ, et al: Tooth loss, dementia and neuropathology in the Nun Study. *J Am Dent Assoc* 2007;138:1314–1322.

11. Nowjack-Ramer RE, Sheiham A: Numbers of natural teeth, diet, and nutritional status in US adults. *J Dent Res* 2007;86:1171–1175.

12. Sahyoun NR, Lin C-L, Krall E: Nutritional status of the older adult is associated with dentition status. *J Am Diet Assoc* 2003;103:61–66.

13. Slade GD, Spencer AJ, Roberts-Thomson K: Tooth loss and chewing capacity among older adults in Adelaide. *Aust J Public Health* 1996;20:76–82.

14. Lancker AV, Verhaeghe S, Hecke AV, et al: The association between malnutrition and oral health status in elderly in long-term care facilities: a systematic review. *Int J Nursing Studies* 2012;49:1568–1581.

15. Ioannidou E, Swede H, Fares G, et al: Tooth loss strongly associates with malnutrition in chronic kidney disease. *J Periodontol* 2014;85:899–907.

16. DeMarchi RJ, Hugo FN, Padilha DMP, et al: Edentulism, use of dentures and consumption of fruit and vegetables in south Brazilian community-dwelling elderly. *J Oral Rehabil* 2011;38:533–540.

17. Han SY, Kim CS: Does denture-wearing status in edentulous South Korean elderly persons affect their nutritional intakes? *Gerondontology* 2014 Mar 19. doi: 10. 1111/ger. 12125. [Epub ahead of print].

18. DeMarchi RJ, Hugo FN, Hilgert JB, et al: Association between oral health status and nutritional status in south Brazilian independent-living older people. *Nutrition* 2008;24:546–553.

19. Saarela RK, Soini H, Hiltunen K, et al: Dentition status, malnutrition and mortality among older service housing residents. *J Nurt Health Aging* 2014;18:34–38.

20. Sheiham A, Steele JG, Marcenes W, et al: The relationship between oral health status and Body Mass Index among older people: a national survey of older people in Great Britain. *Br Dent J* 2002;192:703–706.

21. DeMarchi RJ, Hugo FN, Hilgert JB, et al: Number of teeth and its association with central obesity in older Southern Brazilians. *Community Dent Health* 2012;29:85–89.

22. Do Nascimento TLH, Dias SD, Liberalesso NA, et al: Association between underweight and overweight/obesity with oral health among independently living Brazilian elderly. *Nutrition* 2013;29:152–157.

23. Hamdan NM, Gray-Donald K, Awad MA, et al: Do implant overdentures improve dietary intake? A randomized clinical trial. *J Dent Res Clinical Research Supplement* 2013;92:146S–153S.

24. Taguchi A, Sanada M, Suei Y, et al: Tooth loss is associated with an increased risk of hypertension in postmenopausal women. *Hypertension* 2004;43:1297–1300.

25. Desvarieux M, Demmer RT, Rundek T, et al: Relationship between periodontal disease, tooth loss, and carotid artery plaque: The Oral Infections and Vascular Disease Epidemiology Study (INVEST). *Stroke* 2003;34:2120–2125.

26. Schwahn C, Volzke H, Robinson DM, et al: Periodontal disease, but not edentulism, is independently associated with increased plasma fibrinogen levels. *Thromb Haemost* 2004;92:244–252.

27. Medina-Solis CE, Pontigo-Loyola AP, Perez-Campos E, et al: Association between edentulism and angina pectoris in

Mexican adults aged 35 years and older: a multivariate analysis of a population-based survey. *J Periodontol* 2014;85:406–416.

28. Polzer I, Schwahn C, Volzke H, et al: The association of tooth loss with all-cause and circulatory mortanty. If there a benefit of replaced teeth? A systemic review and meta-analysis. *Clin Oral Investig* 2012;16:333–351.

29. Cleary TJ, Hutton JE: An assessment of the association between functional edentulism, obesity, and NIDDM. *Diabetes Care* 1995;18:1007–1009.

30. Medina-Solis CE, Perez-Nunez R, Maupome G, et al: Edentulism among Mexican adults aged 35 years and older and associated factors. *Am J Public Health* 2006;96:1578–1581.

31. Azogui-Levy S, Dray-Sira R: Sociodemographic factors associated with the dental health of persons with diabetes in France. *Spec Care Dentist* 2012;32:142–149.

32. Patel MH, Kumar JV, Moss ME: Diabetes and tooth loss, an analysis of data for the National Health and Nutrition Examination Survey, 2003–2004. *J Am Dent Assoc* 2013;144:478–485.

33. Culshaw S, McInnes IB, Lie FY: What can the periodontal community learn from the pathophysiology of rheumatoid arthritis? *J Clin Peiiodontol* 2011;38:106–113.

34. dePablo P, Dietrich T, McAlindon TE: Association of periodontal disease and tooth loss with rheumatoid arthritis in the US population. *J Rheumatol* 2008;35:70–76.

35. Demmer RT, Jolitor JA, Jacobs DR Jr, et al: Periodontal disease, tooth loss and incident rheumatoid arthritis: Results from the First National Health and Nutrition Examination Survey and its epidemiologic follow-up study. *J Clin Periodontol* 2011;38:998–1006.

36. Corbridge S, Wilken L, Kapella MC, et al: An evidencebased approach to COPD: Part 1. *Am J Nurs* 2012;112:46–57.

37. Wouters EFM: Economic analysis of the confronting COPD survey: an overview of results. *Respir Med* 2003;97:S3–S14.

38. Xie Q, Ainamo A, Tilvis R: Association of residual ridge resorption with systemic factors in home-living elderly subjects. *ActaOdontol Scand* 1997;55:299–305.

39. Xie Q, Ainamo A: Association of edentulous with systemic factors in elderly people living at home. *Community Dent Oral Epidemiol* 1999;27:303–309.

40. Sjogren P, Nilsson E, Forsell M, et al: A systematic review of the preventive effect of oral hygiene on pneumonia and respiratory tract infection in elderly people in hospitals and nursing homes: effect estimates and methodological quality of randomized controlled trials. *J Am Geriatr Soc* 2008;56:2124–2130.

41. Iinuma T, Arai Y, Abe Y, et al: Denture wearing during sleep doubles the risk of pneumonia in the very elderly. *J Dent Res* 2015;94:28S–36S.

42. Przybylowska D, Mierzwinska-Nastalska E, Rubinsztajn R, et al: Influence of denture plaque biofilm on oral mucosal membrane in patients with chronic obstructive pulmonary disease. *Adv Exp Med Biol* 2015;839:25–30.

43. Ortega O, Parra C, Zarcero S, et al: Oral health in older patients with oropharyngeal dysphagia. *Age Ageing* 2014;43:132–137.

44. Barros SP, Suruki R, Loewy ZG, et al: A cohort study of the impact of tooth loss and periodontal disease on respiratory events among COPD subjects: modulatory role of systemic biomarkers of inflammation. *PLoS One* 2013;8: e68592.

45. Offenbacher S, Beck JD, Barros SP, et al: Obstructive airway disease and edentulism in the atherosclerosis risk in communities (ARIC) study. *BMJ Open* 2012;2:e001615.

46. Hiraki A, Matsuo K, Suzuki T, et al: Tooth loss and risk of cancer at 14 comon sites in Japanese. *Cancer Epidemiol Biomarkers Prev* 2008;17:1222–1227.

47. Takata Y, Ansai T, Soh I, et al: Cognitive function and 10 year mortality in an 85 year-old community-dwelling population. *Clinical Interventions in Aging* 2014;9:1691–99.

48. Shakeri R, Malekzadeh R, Etemadi A, et al: Association of tooth loss and oral hygiene with risk of gastric adenocarcinoma. *Cancer Prev Res (Phila)* 2013;6:477–482.

49. Zeng X-T, Luo W, Huang W, et al: Tooth loss and head and neck cancer: a meta-analysis of observational studies. *PLOS One* 2013;8:e79074.

50. Okamoto N, Morikawa M, Tomioka K, et al: Association between tooth loss and the development of mild memory impairment in the elderly: the Fujiwara-kyo study. *J Alzheimer's Dis* 2015;44:777–786.

51. Eshkoor SA, Hamid TA, Nudin SSH, et al: Association between dentures and the rate of falls in dementia. *Med Devices (Auckl)* 2014;4:225–230.

52. Kisely S, Quek L-H, Pais J, et al: Advanced dental disease in people with severe mental illness: systematic review and meta-analysis. *Br J Psychiatry* 2011;199:187–193.

53. Naorungroj S, Shoenbach VJ, Wruck L, et al: Tooth loss, periodontal disease, and cognitive decline in the Atherosclerosis Risk in Communities (ARIC) study. *Community Dent Oral Epidemiol* 2015;43:47–57.

54. Paganini-Hill A, White SC, Atchison KA: Dentition, dental health status, and dementia: the Leisure World cohort study. *J Am Geriatr Soc* 2012;60:1556–1563.

55. Tsakos G, Watt RG, Rouxel PL, et al: Tooth loss associated with physical and cognitive decline in older adults. *J Am Geriatr Soc* 2015;63:91–99.

56. Zenthofer A, Rammelsberg P, Cabrera T, et al: Determinants of oral health-related quality of life of the institutionalized elderly. *Psychogeriatrics* 2014;14:247–254.

57. Brown DW: Complete edentulism prior to age of 65 years is associated with all-cause mortality. *J Pub Health Dent* 2009;69:260–266.

58. Holm-Pedersen P, Schultz-Larsen K, Christiansen N, et al: Tooth loss and subsequent disability and mortality in old age. *J Am Geriatr Soc* 2008;56:429–435.

59. Osterberg T, Carlsson GE, Sundh V, et al: Number of teeth-a predictor of mortality in 70-year old subjects. *Community Dent Oral Epidemiol* 2008;36:258–268.

60. Ansai T, Takata Y, Yoshida A, et al: Association between tooth loss and orodigestive cancer mortality in an 80-year-old community-dwelling Japanese population: a 12-year prospective study. *BMC Public Health* 2013;13:814–819.

61. Janket SJ, Surakka M, Jones JA, et al: Removable dental prostheses and cardiovascular survival: a 15 year follow-up study. *J Dent* 2013;41:740–746.

62. Polzer I, Schwahn C, Volzke H, et al: The association of tooth loss with all-cause and circulatory mortanity. If there a benefit of replaced teeth? A systemic review and meta analysis. *Clin Oral Invest* 2012;16:333–351.

63. Schwahn C, Polzer I, Haring R, et al: Missing, unreplaced teeth and risk of all-cause mortality and cardiovascular mortality. *Int J Cardio* 2013;167:1430–1437.

64. Watt RG, Tsakos G, deOliveira C, et al: Tooth loss and cardiovascular disease mortality risk-results from the Scottish Health Survey. *PLoS One* 2012;7:1–7.

65. Liljestrand JM, Havulinna AS, Paju S, et al: Missing teeth predict incident cardiovascular events, diabetes, and death. *J Dent Res* 2015 May 19. pii: 0022034515586352. [Epub ahead of print].

4

ORAL CANCER: A PROSTHODONTIC DIAGNOSIS

Michael A. Siegel, dds, ms, fds rcs,[1] Michael A. Kahn, dds,[2] and Mitzi J. Palazzolo, dds, ms[3]

[1]Professor and Chair, Department of Diagnostic Sciences, Nova Southeastern University College of Dental Medicine, Fort Lauderdale, FL
[2]Professor and Chair, Department of Oral and Maxillofacial Pathology, Tufts University School of Dental Medicine, Boston, MA
[3]Assistant Professor, Department of Diagnostic Sciences, Nova Southeastern University College of Dental Medicine, Fort Lauderdale, FL

Keywords
Cancer; screen; examination; diagnostic; adjunctive techniques; carcinoma; early diagnosis; recall

Correspondence
Michael A. Siegel, Department of Diagnostic Sciences, Nova Southeastern University College of Dental Medicine, 3200 South University Drive, Fort Lauderdale, FL 33328-2018. E-mail: masiegel@nova.edu

Accepted May 14, 2008

Published in *Journal of Prosthodontics* 2009; Vol. 18, pp. 3–10

doi: 10.1111/j.1532-849X.2008.00373.x

ABSTRACT

The prosthodontic literature is replete with articles addressing the reconstruction, psychological adaption, prosthesis success, quality of life, need for careful follow-up, and many other issues related to the patient who has undergone surgery, radiation, and/or chemotherapy for oral malignant neoplasms. However, in the prosthodontic professional literature, there is a paucity of information related to the early diagnosis and referral of lesions that may represent premalignant or malignant neoplasia. This article will describe the rationale, epidemiology, and appearance of oral premalignant and malignant mucosal lesions as well as the state-of-the-art diagnostic tools currently available to prosthodontists to ensure that their patients are diagnosed at the earliest possible time.

In 2006, approximately 31,000 cases of oropharyngeal cancer were diagnosed in the United States, and about 25% of these patients died from their disease.[1] The preponderance of these tumors represents squamous cell carcinoma of the oral mucous membranes. The combined 5-year survival rate in the United States is approximately 57%, and it has been established that less advanced disease increases the prognosis significantly.[1-4]

The axiom familiar to every dental student—*early detection and diagnosis provide the best prognosis*—remains valid.

According to Campisi, ". . . the development of cancer is almost inevitable as mammalian organisms age."[5] Although the need for prosthodontics was expected to decline with the promotion of preventive measures, it is actually increasing with the aging population.[6] Oral mucosal disease, including malignant neoplasms, is found in higher frequency in an elderly population.[7,8] There is also significant data showing that prosthetic patients suffer significant oral morbidity following cancer therapy that requires close medical and psychological follow-up.[9,10] There are studies suggesting that poor oral hygiene due to infrequent tooth brushing and sores caused by dentures are risk factors for oral precancer and cancer, but this remains controversial and will require larger prospective studies to validate.[11-13] It is recommended that patients at risk for oral cancer be followed carefully for the development of chronic irritation from teeth and appliances (Fig 1).[12]

The prosthodontic literature is replete with articles addressing the reconstruction, psychological adaption, prosthesis success, quality of life, need for careful follow-up, and many other issues related to the patient who has undergone surgery, radiation, and/or chemotherapy for oral malignant neoplasms.[10,14-18]

However, in the professional literature available to the practicing prosthodontist, there is a paucity of information related to the early diagnosis and referral of lesions that may represent premalignant or malignant neoplasia.

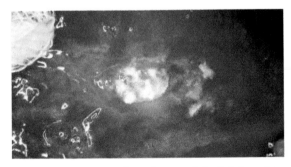

FIGURE 1 Squamous cell carcinoma of the left lateral tongue border in a 67-year-old man. Note the presence of Candida albicans on the surface of the lesion only. This is an ominous prognostic sign, as it may represent an opportunistic infection related to compromised tissue immunity at the site of a neoplasm.

EPIDEMIOLOGY OF ORAL SQUAMOUS CELL CARCINOMA

Oral squamous cell carcinoma, which arises from the mucosal lining of the oral cavity, accounts for over 90% of oral cancers.[3]

Worldwide, more than 500,000 new cases are diagnosed annually.[19,20] Oral cancer accounts for less than 3% of all cancers in the United States, but it is the sixth most common cancer in males and twelfth most common in females.[1] It is estimated that 34,360 new cancer cases of the oral cavity and pharynx will be diagnosed in 2007.[21] The incidence rates are more than twice as high in men as in women; however, the disparity in the male:female ratio has become less pronounced over the past half century. This may be because the exposure to alcohol and tobacco in women has also increased.[22] The incidence of cancer of the oral cavity is greatest in men who are older than 50; however, the average annual incidence and mortality rates vary considerably between different races, genders, and age groups. During the past decade, it has been noted and verified that the incidence rate in persons under the age of 40 is increasing. Over time, the incidence of intraoral cancer has been increasing dramatically for black men in the United States. An estimated 7,550 deaths from oral cancer are expected in 2007.[21] The 5 year relative survival rates vary by race and sex. Black men seem to carry a higher burden, with a survival rate of 35.5% compared to whites (62.8%).[21]

RISK FACTORS ASSOCIATED WITH THE DEVELOPMENT OF ORAL SQUAMOUS CELL CARCINOMA

The cause of oral squamous cell carcinoma is multifactorial.[23] No single causative agent or factor has been clearly defined or accepted. It is likely that multiple factors play a role in malignant transformation.

Tobacco and Alcohol

The strong association between squamous cell carcinoma of the oral cavity with tobacco use is well established.

Epidemiological studies show that the risk of developing oral cancer is 5 to 9 times greater for smokers than for nonsmokers, and this risk may increase to as much as 17 times greater for extremely heavy smokers of 80 or more cigarettes per day.[22] The risk for a second primary carcinoma of the upper aerodigestive tract is 2 to 6 times greater for treated patients with oral cancer who continue to smoke than for those who quit after diagnosis.[22]

Alcohol use has been identified as a major risk factor for cancers of the upper aero-digestive tract. In studies controlled for smoking, moderate-to-heavy drinkers have been shown to

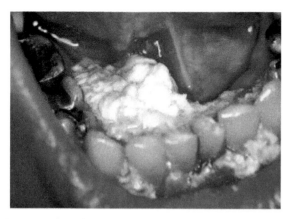

FIGURE 2   Cauliflower-like lesion that clinically represents human papillomavirus-induced verrucous carcinoma in a 59-year-old woman.

have a 3 to 9 times greater risk of developing oral cancer.[22] In addition, alcohol consumption appears to be a significant potentiator or promoter for other causative factors, especially tobacco, and its effects are significant when it is understood that most heavy drinkers are also heavy smokers. The simultaneous use of tobacco products and alcohol abuse results in a multiplicative effect of those two social habits rather than an additive one.

Oncogenic Viruses

Viral agents capable of integration into the host's genetic material may inhibit the ability of the host to regulate the normal growth and proliferation of the infected cell. Recent evidence suggests that human papillomavirus (HPV) is associated with some oral and oropharyngeal cancers. HPV-16 and HPV-18 have been identified in up to 50% of the oral squamous cell carcinomas arising in Waldeyer's tonsillar ring and in 15 to 25% of those in the tongue and other parts of the oral cavity (Fig 2).[24,25]

PREMALIGNANT LESIONS OF THE ORAL CAVITY

Invasive oral squamous cell carcinoma is often preceded by the presence of clinically identifiable premalignant changes of the oral mucosa. These lesions often present as white, red, or mixed patches, known as leukoplakia, erythroplakia, or erythroleukoplakia, respectively.[22] Many cases of oral squamous cell carcinoma are preceded by recognizable premalignant epithelial changes, the most important of which is thought to be the presence of epithelial dysplasia.[26,27] Histopathologic evaluation of the epithelium adjacent to oral squamous cell carcinomas often reveals dysplastic changes, and these changes are frequently multicentric. Severe

dysplasia indicates a very high risk of the subsequent development of cancer.[28]

The proportion of squamous cell carcinomas that develop through clinically recognizable precancerous stages is not known. Histopathologically, these precancerous lesions vary from mild to severe. Prediction of which precancerous lesions will develop into oral carcinoma is difficult. Overall, the proportion of dysplastic epithelial lesions that evolve into cancer is about 16%, and the time period over which this occurs varies from months to beyond 20 years.[27] The average malignant transformation rate has been reported to be 24 to 30 months. Higher grades of dysplasia are generally associated with a higher risk of development of carcinoma. Only 4 to 11% of mild to moderate dysplasia progresses to squamous cell carcinoma, whereas 35% of lesions diagnosed as severe dysplasia progress to squamous cell carcinoma. The presence of dysplasia does not always predict the development of squamous cell carcinoma, which may also develop in the absence of dysplasia.[27]

Leukoplakia

Leukoplakia, as defined by the World Health Organization, is a clinical term that describes "a white patch or plaque that cannot be characterized clinically or pathologically as any other disease" (Fig 3). Therefore, leukoplakia is a clinical term and has no specific histopathologic connotation. The majority of these lesions are detected in individuals aged 60 years or older, although patients of any age may be affected. In men over the age of 70, the prevalence of leukoplakia is 8%. The prevalence in women past the age of 70 is approximately 2%.[22] The male:female predilection is decreasing, with women being affected almost as frequently as men. About half the lesions involve the mandibular mucosa, mandibular sulcus, and buccal mucosa.[29]

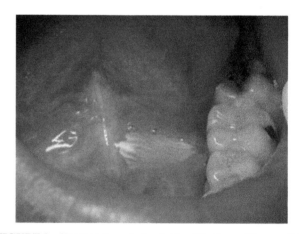

FIGURE 3   Homogeneous leukoplakia of the floor of the mouth in a 36 year-old male patient with a significant cigarette smoking history. Excisional biopsy provided a histopathologic diagnosis of hyperkeratosis and mild dysplasia.

The majority of leukoplakic lesions are physiologic reactions of the mucosa against chronic trauma or irritation. Ill-fitting dentures and parafunctional oral habits such as cheek or tongue chewing are common causes. Factors associated with these white mucosal lesions include, but are not limited to, mechanical and chemical irritants, chronic hyperplastic candidiasis, syphilis, and electro-galvanic reactions.[30] Leukoplakic lesions are frequently noted in patients with a history of tobacco or alcohol use. Leukoplakias may be varied in their appearance. The lesions may appear homogenous or heterogenous with a smooth, fissured, or corrugated surface and colored white, gray, or translucent. Leukoplakias are also variable with regard to size and distribution. These lesions may be barely discernable clinically or cover entire mucosal surfaces. The sites where leukoplakic lesions are commonly encountered are the floor of the mouth, lateral and ventral borders of the tongue, labial and buccal mucosae, gingivae, soft palate, and retromolar areas.

The vast majority (i.e., 80%) of leukoplakias are benign.[29]

The remaining lesions are either premalignant (dysplastic or carcinoma-in-situ) or malignant. The precancerous nature of leukoplakia has been established based on several factors. In various studies, 15.6 to 39.2% of leukoplakia biopsy samples have demonstrated epithelial dysplasia or invasive carcinoma, and more than one third of oral carcinomas have areas of leukoplakia in close proximity.[31] The location of oral leukoplakia has a significant correlation with the frequency of finding dysplastic or malignant changes upon biopsy. The floor of the mouth shows the highest chance of dysplasia or carcinoma (42.9%) presence, while the lateral and ventral tongue is second highest (25%).[22]

Dysplastic lesions are multicentric and are most commonly encountered in the floor of the mouth or on the tongue.[29,32]

Other risk sites for premalignant or malignant leukoplakias include the labial mucosa and vermilion lip, lateral and ventral borders of the tongue, floor of the mouth, soft palate, uvula complex, and retromolar areas. Leukoplakic lesions are prognostically ominous in a patient with a previous history of carcinoma of the tongue. Multiple carcinomas of the oral cavity and oropharynx (116 times greater than expected) have been encountered in patients with a history of tongue carcinoma.[33] The clinician faces the problem of determining which of these lesions are premalignant or malignant and must determine the nature of the white lesion without unreasonably alarming the patient.

Erythroleukoplakia

Leukoplakia with localized speckled red areas or erythroplakia with localized speckled white areas also confer a high risk of oral cancer (Fig 4). Many terms, such as speckled erythroplakia or speckled leukoplakia, have been used to describe these mixed red and white lesions. There is a four-

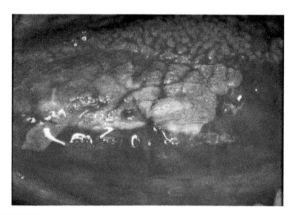

FIGURE 4   Erythroleukoplakia of the left lateral tongue border in a 42 year-old male patient. Biopsy of the lesion disclosed moderate epithelial dysplasia.

fold increased risk that these lesions will undergo malignant transformation when compared to homogeneous leukoplakias.[7] Erythroleukoplakia may occur in any intraoral site. It has a male predilection. Not surprisingly, these lesions are usually found in patients exhibiting poor oral hygiene who use tobacco and alcohol. *Candida albicans*, a commonly encountered intraoral fungal organism, is often found in these lesions and may have a role in the dysplastic changes;[26] however, no studies have documented a direct relationship between candidal involvement and malignant transformation.[31,34] Mixed red and white lesions that have not resolved in 7 to 14 days following removal of any local causative factors should be selected for biopsy due to their increased risk for developing into carcinoma.

Erythroplakia

Erythroplakia is a clinical term used to define a velvety red patch that cannot be characterized as any other condition (Fig 5). These lesions are often asymptomatic and are first recognized during a routine dental examination. Erythroplakias can occur anywhere in the oral cavity but are most commonly encountered in the floor of the mouth, alveolar ridge, and oropharynx. The redness is due to the thinning (erosion) of the overlying epithelium. Incidence is highest in men and women over the age of 60, and both genders are equally affected.

Biopsy of erythroplakic lesions is mandatory, because it has been shown histologically that approximately 90% of these lesions represent severe dysplasia, carcinoma in situ, or carcinoma.[35] The patient must be followed closely, as multiple sites of the oral cavity may be affected, a phenomenon referred to as "field cancerization." In patients with multiple lesions, referral should be made to ensure that representative biopsy specimens are procured from each site.

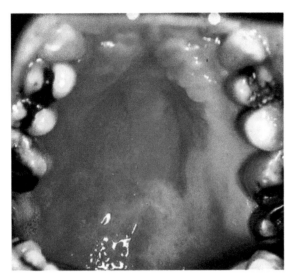

FIGURE 5 Erythroplakia of the right palate in a 76-year-old man; biopsy proven as well-differentiated squamous cell carcinoma.

EXTRAORAL AND INTRAORAL EXAMINATION

The prosthodontist must perform a careful, organized, and reproducible visual and palpation examination of the intraoral soft tissues as well as submandibular and cervical chain lymph node palpation on all new patients as well as patients presenting for recall examination.[36,37] Edentulous patients must be specifically counseled about returning for prescribed, regular recall examinations. They may erroneously think that, as they do not have teeth, they do not need to be regularly followed by a prosthodontist.[38] Following the examination, patients should be advised that they have been examined for oral cancer. Only 28% of patients reported ever having had an oral cancer examination. Of those, 20% had had the examination in the preceding year.[39,40] Patients who use tobacco products must be encouraged to quit. The prosthodontist may be instrumental in helping a patient quit smoking either by direct counseling or by referral to a smoking cessation program.[41] Geriatric alcoholism is rising, so the prosthodontist may also be influential in advising patients of the necessity of limiting their alcohol intake, especially if there are intraoral signs of alcohol abuse.[42,43] The highest risk of developing oral cancer is in adults over the age of 40 who use both tobacco and alcohol.[34]

The initial step in the treatment of leukoplakia or erythroplakia is to eliminate any source of chronic irritation or trauma, such as a sharp tooth or denture border. Induration, rolled borders, locations such as the lateral surface of the tongue or floor of mouth, a red component to the lesion, or a nonhomogeneous granular surface may increase the suspicion of the prosthodontist performing the examination. However, it must be kept in mind that even the most innocuous-looking homogeneous leukoplakia may be histopathologically malignant, so clinical appearance alone should not be the only criterion for the decision to refer for a biopsy. Controversy exists as to whether a therapeutic trial of medication such as a topical steroid or retinoid is appropriate prior to the performance of a biopsy, which remains the "gold standard" for the diagnosis of these lesions.[44] If the leukoplakic lesion has not resolved within a reasonable time period following the removal of local etiologic factors, the prosthodontist should refer these patients to a specialist colleague for biopsy and should follow up with that colleague to ensure that the patient has been seen and managed appropriately. In the event the lesion is found to be dysplastic or malignant, for the first 2 to 3 years, the patient should be followed up four times yearly. The prosthodontist and surgeon should coordinate a recall schedule so that the patient is alternatively seen by the two treating specialists. For example, the oral and maxillofacial surgeon can evaluate the patient in January and July, while the prosthodontist alternatively evaluates the patient in April and October. In this way, there is frequent evaluation of the patient following the diagnosis of a premalignant or malignant lesion as well as continuity of care between the two treating specialists. Any suggestion of lesion recurrence, ulceration, leukoplakia, or erythroplakia should be rebiopsied at the earliest possible time.

ORAL CANCER SCREENING DEVICES AND ADJUNCTIVE DIAGNOSTIC TECHNIQUES

Recently, several companies have marketed devices [following obtainment of FDA Class I (501c) device approval] intended to aid the dentist in the early detection and diagnosis of premalignant oral lesions. Among those intended to be used as oral cancer screening devices are Vizilite Plus® (Zila Pharmaceuticals, Inc., Phoenix, AZ), MicroLux-DL® (AdDent, Inc., Danbury, CT), Orascoptic® DK (Orascoptic by the Kerr Company, Middleton, WI), and VELscope® (L. E. D. Dental, Inc., White Rock, BC, Canada). Procedures intended for adjunctive diagnosis of oral premalignancies include The BrushTest®(formerly called the brush biopsy; OralCDx, Suffern, NY) and liquid-based cytology technology, ThinPrep® and SurePath® (TriPath, Burlington, NC, and Cytyc Corp., Boxborough, MA, respectively). It should be noted that the techniques described below have limitations, including falsepositive and false-negative results, depending on the character and site of the lesion in question. Most prosthodontists do not have ready access to these tools, but should know that they are available for the care of their patients as well as to be able to interpret the results of these adjunctive techniques. A specialist such as an oral and maxillofacial surgeon is well trained in these technologies and can use them in appropriate situations when deemed necessary; however, the scalpel biopsy is still the gold standard for definitive histopathologic diagnosis, so if the prosthodontist is especially concerned with the clinical presentation of a lesion, a routine excisional or incisional biopsy should be specifically requested.

Tissue Reflectance with Chemiluminescence and Vital Dye Marking

Following the conventional incandescent light soft tissue head and neck examination described above, the Vizilite Plus system (single use, disposable kit) uses a 30- to 60-second prerinse, nontoxic 1% acetic acid swish and spit mouth rinse (raspberry flavored) followed by the bending of a plastic lightstick that when shaken results in an endothermic blue-white lightproducing reaction (with peak wavelength outputs near 430, 540, and 580 nm). During the ensuing 10 minutes, with the operatory ambient lights significantly dimmed, the illuminated lightstick is shined throughout the oral cavity following its placement into a two-piece plastic retractor. The mild acetic acid rinse is reported to prepare the oral mucosa by dehydration for the detection of epithelial cells with the increased nuclear/cytoplasmic ratio, including those that may be dysplastic, following the use of the diffuse blue-white light.[45,46]

If the suspicious oral lesion (i.e., leukoplakia, erythroplakia, erythroleukoplakia) noted during the routine operatory white light examination becomes visibly enhanced in coloration (e.g., leukoplakic) or darkened (erythroplakic), then it is considered a positive finding. Reports in the literature indicate that premalignant lesions (verified by subsequent surgical biopsy) that were not seen by dental experts in a high-risk patient population have been discovered following use of the Vizilite Plus system.[47–51]

The second step of this system includes a visual marking of the identified lesion by use of a metachromatic vital dye, toluidine blue (toloniun chloride), which has a reported affinity for DNA and, thus, binds to epithelial cells with the increased nuclear cytoplasmic ratio. Zila Pharmaceuticals, Inc., has produced a pharmaceutical grade of this vital dye and includes it in this system with the trade name TBlue[630] (Zila tolonium chloride). Therefore, the clinician has the option of a three-step marking of the suspicious lesion with TBlue[630] for documentation and as an aid in biopsy/cytology sampling or by referral to a dental colleague. It should be emphasized that TBlue[630] is only FDA -approved for use in the Vizilite Plus system *after* the use of the chemiluminescent lightstick step.

Tissue Reflectance with Luminescence

There are two FDA-approved Class I light-emitting devices similar to the first step of the Vizilite Plus system—Micro-Lux-DL® and Orascoptic DK®. These oral cancer screening aids are manufactured by the same company (AdDent, Inc., Danbury, CT) but marketed by two different companies, hence their different trade names. Both devices are reusable,

batteryoperated light emitting diode dental transilluminators that have been adopted to emit a diffuse blue-white light (assumed to be the same wavelength as the Vizilite) by removing the transilluminator light tip and replacing it with a sterilizable, translucent glass tip. As with the Vizilite Plus system, patients prepare their oral mucosa by rinsing and spitting with the same 1% acetic acid rinse, but, unlike Vizilite, the battery-containing handle creates the diffuse blue light in a manner similar to the common flashlight. These adjunctive devices, as with the Vizilite Plus system, are to only be used following the conventional incandescent light intraoral examination with a positive finding defined as visual enhancement of a suspicious lesion.

Narrow-Emission Tissue Fluorescence

The VELscope is an oral premalignant screening device that emits a concentrated blue light (peak wavelength outputs of 405 and 436 nm) that creates a natural fluorescence. In North America, it is powered by a 120-V AC electric current and emits a blue light by use of a replaceable metal halide bulb, a series of dichromatic mirrors, and a flexible fiber optic cable. In addition, the blue light emitter handpiece has an optical inline ocular eyepiece through which the clinician observes the oral mucosa tissue. A series of optical filters are located between the clinician's eye and the emitted light. The emitted blue light emission excites natural substances, fluorophores, within the oral epithelium and underlying lamina propria (connective tissue). When exited, fluorophores autofluoresce and emit an apple green color that can be appreciated by the clinician due to the filters contained within the eyepiece. As with other oral cancer light screening devices, the VELscope is only to be used following a conventional incandescent light intraoral examination. The clinician repeats the intraoral examination, after dimming the ambient operatory light, with the activated VELscope; normal oral mucosa will appear green. If an area of black (i.e., loss of fluorescence) is seen, it can correlate to a suspicious premalignant lesion previously appreciated during the incandescent light examination or, in some reported cases, an area of lost fluorescence is seen despite being unable to appreciate a suspicious lesion with the naked eye.[52,53] The VELscope is reported to exhibit loss of fluorescence in the presence of dysplasia due to the destruction of the naturally occurring fluorophores in the affected epithelium and/or connective tissue. Oral lesions have also been documented in which the loss of fluorescence extends beyond the clinically visible lesion, and subsequent biopsy of the extended dark areas revealed the presence of microscopic dysplasia or squamous cell carcinoma.[54]

Adjunctive Diagnostic Procedures

During the late 1950s and 1960s many dental investigators attempted to adopt the Pap smear, the early 1950s' highly successful adjunctive diagnostic technique for uterine cervical cancer, for use within the oral cavity. This was an exfoliative cytology procedure in which surface epithelial cells were scraped in a minimally invasive manner and immediately transferred ("smeared") to a glass microscope slide that was subsequently sprayed with an alcohol-based fixative to preserve the collected cells. The cells were then coverslipped following the use of Papanicolaou stain and examined with the light microscope. A pathology report was issued indicating that if any of the cells exhibited atypical morphological characteristics that could indicate the clinical presence of epithelial dysplasia or squamous cell carcinoma. Unfortunately, the Pap smear proved to be unreliable when used within the oral cavity, since there were numerous reports of unacceptably high incidence of false-positive and false-negative results.[55] Thus, this noninvasive potential adjunctive oral diagnostic technique was not actively pursued for nearly 30 years. In 1999, the brush biopsy technique (recently renamed the BrushTest) was introduced to dentistry. It was reported to be an efficacious, sensitive, and specific diagnostic adjunct in which a transepithelial collection (from surface to basal cell layer) of disaggregated oral mucosa epithelial cells was removed by a helical-shaped, stiff nylon bristle brush and immediately transferred ("smeared") to a clear glass microscope slide.[56] The collected cells were fixed with an alcohol solution and, following drying, were placed in a plastic protective case and sent to a central laboratory for computer-assisted analysis followed by examination of computer-selected areas by a trained cytopathologist. The cells were to be collected in a painless or mildly uncomfortable manner verifying obtainment of all epithelial levels by the clinical sight of pinpoint bleeding and redness of the upper vascular plexus with the superficial underlying connective tissue. Subsequent to the seminal report of this technique, there has been a series of case reports and investigations that either tout or dispute the technique's accuracy.[57–62] There have also been reports that all techniques that attempt to transfer collected cells from a brush device to the planar surface of a microscope slide can fail to transfer up to 80% of the cells distributed on the brush's bristles.[63,64] There has also been controversy about the cost/benefit ratio of the brush biopsy, since a positive or atypical finding of possible epithelial dysplasia would mandate a second procedure, the gold standard surgically invasive biopsy.

During the 1990s a revolutionary new Pap smear technique garnered FDA approval following several large phase-3 clinical trials.[64–67] The adjunctive diagnostic technique, known as liquid-based cytology, is reported to increase the accuracy of Pap smears.[67] The major technical improvement is that the brush-collected cells are directly transferred into a container with methanol- or ethanol-based liquid preservative/fixative; the brush's bristle head is also placed in the liquid container. Upon arrival of the solution at the pathology laboratory, a patented machine then filters, disperses,

collects, and transfers the epithelial cells of the solution to a glass slide. The cells are placed in a monolayer greatly reducing overlapping epithelial cells; in addition, obscuring elements such as inflammation, debris, mucous, and blood are also removed. Lastly, the cells are stained (Papanicolaou) and coverslipped prior to microscopic examination by a boarded medical pathologist.

More recently, the liquid-based technology has been adopted for use in nongynelogical clinical settings including within the oral cavity.[64] As with cervical mucosa, this technique utilized to obtain a transepithelial sampling of oral mucosa has the same potential to result in an improved evaluation of the disaggregated cells obtained from a clinically suspicious premalignant lesion whether detected during the incandescent light examination or during one of the above-mentioned adjunctive oral cancer screening techniques.

CONCLUSION

Prosthodontists are in a unique position to significantly impact their patients' overall health, not only via their expertise in the art and science of prosthodontics but also by virtue of their access to patients at risk for oral cancer and the influence they may exert. The performance of careful soft tissue intraoral examination, lymph node palpation, identification of suspect lesions, use of adjunctive diagnostic techniques, and early referral for biopsy will ensure that patients are afforded state-of-the-art prosthodontic health care along with a decreased risk of morbidity and mortality.

REFERENCES

1. American Cancer Society: *Cancer Facts and Figures 2006.* American Cancer Society, Atlanta, 2006. Available at http://www.cancer.org (accessed on June 5, 2008)

2. Shiboski CH, Shiboski SC, Silverman S Jr: Trends in oral cancer rates in the United States, 1973–1996. *Community Dent Oral Epidemiol* 2000;28:249–256.

3. Silverman S Jr: Demographics and occurrence of oral and pharyngeal cancers: the outcomes, the trends, the challenge. *J Am Dent Assoc* 2001;132 (suppl):7S–11S.

4. National Cancer Institute: Surveillance, Epidemiology, and End Results Program Public-Use-Data, 1973–1998. Rockville, MD, National Cancer Institute, Division of Cancer Control and Population Sciences, Surveillance Research Program, Cancer Statistics Branch, 2001

5. Campisi J: Cancer, aging and cellular senescence. *In Vivo* 2000;14:183–188.

6. Chaytor DV: Prosthodontics 1966–2042: changes in prosthodontic education, past and future. *J Can Dent Assoc* 2005;71:329.

7. Correa L, Frigerio ML, Sousa SC, et al: Oral lesions in elderly population: a biopsy survey using 2250 histopathological records. *Gerodontology* 2006;23:48–54.

8. Jainkittivong A, Aneksuk V, Langlais RP: Oral mucosal conditions in elderly dental patients. *Oral Dis* 2002;8:218–223.

9. Gellrich NC, Schramm A, Bockmann R, et al: Follow-up in patients with oral cancer. *J Oral Maxillofac Surg* 2002;60:380–388.

10. Rogers SN, McNally D, Mahmoud M, et al: Psychologic response of the edentulous patient after primary surgery for oral cancer. *J Prosthet Dent* 1999;82:317–321.

11. Velly AM, Franco EL, Schlecht N, et al: Relationship between dental factors and risk of upper aerodigestive tract cancer. *Oral Oncol* 1998;34:284–291.

12. Lockhart PB, Norris CM Jr, Pulliam C: Dental factors in the genesis of squamous cell carcinoma of the oral cavity. *Oral Oncol* 1998;34:133–139.

13. Morse DE, Katz RV, Pendrys DG, et al: Mouthwash use and dentures in relation to oral epithelial dysplasia. *Oral Oncol* 1997;33:338–343.

14. Schoen PJ, Reinsema H, Bouma J, et al: Quality of life related to oral function in edentulous head and neck cancer patients posttreatment. *Int J Prosthodont* 2007;20:469–477.

15. Roumanas ED, Garrett N, Blackwell KE, et al: Masticatory and swallowing threshold performances with conventional and implant-supported prostheses after mandibular fibula free-flap reconstruction. *J Prosthet Dent* 2006;96:289–297.

16. Garrett N, Roumanas ED, Blackwell KE, et al: Efficacy of conventional and implant-supported mandibular resection prostheses: study overview and treatment outcomes. *J Prosthet Dent* 2006;96:13–24.

17. Weischer T, Mohr C: Implant-supported mandibular telescopic prostheses in oral cancer patients: an up to 9-year retrospective study. *Int J Prosthodont* 2001;14:329–334.

18. Weischer T, Schettler D, Mohr C: Implant-supported telescopic restoration in maxillofacial prosthetics. *Int J Posthodont* 1997;10:287–292.

19. Sanderson RJ, Ironside JA: Squamous cell carcinomas of the head and neck. *BMJ* 2002;325:822–827.

20. Vokes EE, Weichselbaum RR, Lippman SM, et al: Head and neck cancer. *N Engl J Med* 1993;328:184–194.

21. Ries LAG, Melbert D, Krapcho M, et al (eds): SEER Cancer Statistics Review, 1975–2004. Bethesda, MD, National Cancer Institute, http://seer.cancer.gov/csr/1975_2004/, based on November 2006 SEER data submission, posted to the SEER web site, 2007 (accessed June 5, 2008)

22. Neville BW, Day TA: Oral cancer and precancerous lesions. *CA Cancer J Clin* 2002;52:195–215.

23. Binnie WH, Rankin KV, Mackenzie IC: Etiology of oral squamous cell carcinoma. *J Oral Pathol* 1983;12:11–29.

24. Kreimer AR, Clifford GM, Boyle P, et al: Human papillomavirus types in head and neck squamous cell carcinomas worldwide: a systematic review. *Cancer Epidemiol Biomarkers Prev* 2005;14:467–475.

25. Paz I, Cook N, Odom-Maryom T, et al: Human papillomavirus (HPV) in head and neck cancer. An association of HPV 16 with squamous cell carcinoma of Waldeyer's tonsillar ring. *Cancer* 1997;79:595–604.

26. Scully C, Cawson RC: Potentially malignant lesions. *K Epidemiol Biostat* 1996;1:3–12.

27. Lumerman H, Freedman P, Kerpel S: Oral epithelial dysplasia and the development of invasive squamous cell carcinoma. *Oral Surg Oral Med Oral Pathol Oral Radiol Endod* 1995;79:321–329.

28. Bouquot JE, Ephros H: Erythroplakia: the dangerous red mucosa. *Pract Periodontics Aesthet Dent* 1995;7:59–67.

29. Waldron CA, Shaffer WG: Leukoplakia revisited: a clinical immunopathologic study of 3256 oral leukoplakias. *Cancer* 1975;36:1386–1392.

30. Langlais RP, Miller CS: *Color Atlas of Common Oral Diseases* (ed 1). Philadelphia, PA, Lea and Febiger, 1992, pp. 54–55.

31. Silverman S, Jr, Gorsky M, Lozada F: Oral leukoplakia and malignant transformation. A follow-up study of 257 patients. *Cancer* 1984;53:563–568.

32. Lumerman H, Friedman P, Kerpel S: Oral epithelial dysplasia and the development of invasive squamous carcinoma. *Oral Surg Oral Med Oral Pathol Oral Radiol Endod* 1995;79:321–329.

33. Shibuya H, Amagasa T, Seto K, et al: Leukoplakia-associated multiple carcinomas in patients with tongue carcinoma. *Cancer* 1986;57:843–846.

34. Silverman S Jr: *Oral Cancer* (ed 5). Hamilton, BC, Decker, 2003, pp. 40–42.

35. Shafer WG, Hine MK, Levy BM: *A Textbook of Oral Pathology* (ed 4). Philadelphia, PA, Saunders, 1983, pp. 108.

36. Glazer HS: Spotting trouble: without an oral cancer screening, no dental exam is complete. *AGD Impact* 2003;31:18–19.

37. Sciubba JJ: Oral cancer ands its detection: history-taking and the diagnostic phase of management. *J Am Dent Assoc* 2001;132 (Suppl): 12S–5S.

38. John MT, Szentpetery A, Steele JG: Association between factors related to the time of wearing complete dentures and oral health-related quality of life in patients who maintained a recall. *Int J Prosthodont* 2007;20:31–36.

39. Horowitz AM, Canto MT, Child WL: Maryland adults' perspectives on oral cancer prevention and early detection. *J Am Dent Assoc* 2002;133:1058–1063.

40. Horowitz AM, Moon HS, Goodman HS, et al: Maryland adults' knowledge of oral cancer and having oral cancer examinations. *J Public Health Dent* 1998;58:281–287.

41. Cruz GD, Ostroff JS, Kumar JV, et al: Preventing and detecting oral cancer: oral health care providers' readiness to provide health behavior counseling and oral cancer examinations. *J Am Dent Assoc* 2005;136:594–601.

42. Friedlander AH, Marder SR, Pisegna JR, et al: Alcohol abuse and dependence. *J Am Dent Assoc* 2003;134:731–740.

43. Friedlander AH, Norman DC: Geriatric alcoholism. *J Am Dent Assoc* 2006;137:330–337.

44. Brown RS, Bottomley WK, Abromovich K, et al: Immediate biopsy versus a therapeutic trial in the diagnosis of vesiculo-bullous/vesiculoerosive oral lesions. *Oral Surg Oral Med Oral Pathol* 1992;73:694–697.

45. Huber MA, Bsoul SA, Terezhalmy GT: Acetic acid wash and chemiluminescent illumination as an adjunct to conventional oral soft tissue examination for the detection of dysplasia: a pilot study. *Quintessence Int* 2004;35:378–384.

46. Lingen MW, Kalmar JR, Karrison T, et al: Critical evaluation of diagnostic aids or the detection of oral cancer. *Oral Oncol* 2008;44:10–12.

47. Ram S, Siar CH: Chemiluminescence as a diagnostic aid in the detection of oral cancer and potentially malignant epithelial lesions. *Int J Oral Maxillofac Surg* 2005;34:521–527.

48. Epstein JB, Gorsky M, Lonky S, et al: The efficacy of oral lumenoscopy (Vizilite) in visualizing oral mucosal lesions. *Spec Care Dent* 2006;26:171–174.

49. Kerr AR, Sirois DA, Epstein JB: Clinical evaluation of chemi-luminescent lighting: an adjunct for oral mucosal examinations. *J Clin Dent* 2006;17:59–63.

50. Oh ES, Laskin DM: Efficacy of the ViziLite system in the identification of oral lesions. *J Oral Maxillofac Surg* 2007;65:424–426.

51. Epstein JB, Silverman S Jr, Epstein JD, et al: Analysis of oral lesion biopsies identified and evaluated by visual examination, chemiluminescence and toluidine blue. *Oral Oncol* 2008;44:538–544.

52. Lane PM, Gilhuly T, Whitehead P, et al: Simple device for the direct visualization of oral cavity tissue fluorescence. *J Biomed Opt* 2006;11:024006

53. Poh CF, Williams PM, Zhang L, et al: Direct fluorescence visualization of clinically occult high-risk oral premalignant disease using a simple hand-held device. *Head Neck* 2007;29:71–76.

54. Poh CF, Zhang L, Anderson SW, et al: Fluorescence visual-ization detection of field alterations in tumor margins of oral cancer patients. *Clin Cancer Res* 2006;12:6716–6722.

55. Kahn MA: Oral cancer screening aids. *Inside Dentistry* 2007;3:24–27.

56. Sciubba JJ, US Collaborative OralCDx Study Group: Improv-ing detection of precancerous and cancerous oral lesions. Computer-assisted analysis of the oral brush biopsy. *J Am Dent Assoc* 1999;2130:1445–1457.

57. Svirksy JS, Burns JC, Carpenter WM, et al: Comparison of computer-assisted brush biopsy results with follow up scalpel biopsy and histology. *Gen Dent* 2002;40:829–834.

58. Poate TW, Buchanan JA, Hodgson TA, et al: An audit of the efficacy of the oral brush biopsy technique in a specialist Oral medicine unit. *Oral Oncol* 2004;40:829–834.

59. Potter TJ, Summerlin DJ, Campbell JH: Oral malignancies associated with negative transepithelial brush biopsy. *J Oral Maxillofac Surg* 2003;61:674–677.

60. Rick GM: Oral brush biopsy: the problem of false positives. *Oral Surg Oral Med Oral Pathol Oral Radiol Endod* 2003;96:252.

61. Christian DC: Computer-assisted analysis of oral brush biop-sies at an oral cancer screening program. *J Am Dent Assoc* 2002;133:357–362.

62. Scheifele C, Schmidt-Westhausen AM, Dietrich T, et al: The sensitivity and specificity of the OralCDx technique: evaluation of 103 cases. *Oral Oncol* 2004;40:824–828.

63. Bernstein ML, Miller RL: Oral exfoliative cytology. *J Am Dent Assoc* 1978;96:625–629.

64. Kujan O, Desai M, Sargent A, et al: Potential applications of oral brush cytology with liquid-based technology: results from a cohort of normal oral mucosa. *Oral Oncol* 2006;42:810–818.

65. Hayama FH, Motta AC, Silva Ade P, et al: Liquid-based preparations versus conventional cytology: specimen adequacy and diagnostic agreement on oral lesions. *Med Oral Pathol Oral Cir Bucal* 2005;10:115–122.

66. Hoelund B: Implementation of liquid-based cytology in the screening programme against cervical cancer in the county of Funen, Denmark, and status for the first year. *Cytopathology* 2003;14:269–274.

67. Schledermann D, Ejersbo D, Hoelund B: Improvement of diagnostic accuracy and screening conditions with liquid-based cytology. *Diagn Cytopathol* 2006;34:780–785.

5

THE CURRENT AND FUTURE TREATMENT OF EDENTULISM

LYNDON F. COOPER, DDS, PHD, FACP
Department of Prosthodontics, University of North Carolina School of Dentistry, Chapel Hill, NC

Keywords
Denture quality; morbidity; edentulism prevention; residual ridge resorption; oral mucosal health; maladaptive patients; implants.

Correspondence
Lyndon F. Cooper, Department of Prosthodontics, UNC School of Dentistry, CB 7450, Chapel Hill, NC 27599. E-mail: lyndon_cooper@dentistry.unc.edu

Presented as part of the FDI 2008 World Dental Congress: "Facing the Future of Edentulism: 21st Century Management of Edentulism—A World of Challenges in a Universe of Helpful Technologies." September 26, 2008, Stockholm, Sweden.

Accepted December 3, 2008

Published in *Journal of Prosthodontics* 2009; Vol. 18, Issue 2, pp. 116–22

doi: 10.1111/j.1532-849X.2009.00441.x

ABSTRACT

The purpose of this review and summary is to focus the clinician's attention on existing potential limitations regarding the management of edentulism. The current published data and opinions concerning the need for treating edentulism, the quality of dentures, related morbidity, and alternative or related therapeutics (e.g., dental implants) suggest there are opportunities for improvement in the treatment of the edentulous population. This may be achieved by adopting a broader therapeutic strategy focused not solely on technical aspects of an oral prosthesis. Instead, a wider array of clinical features of the edentulous patient should be addressed. A contemporary strategy may include concerns for prevention of tooth loss, evaluation of residual alveolar ridge resorption, and related issues of denture function, continual evaluation of oral mucosal health, compassionate management of maladaptive patients, a rationale for timely replacement of dentures, and continued development of dental implant therapies. The importance of therapeutic technical quality can be underscored, but should not overwhelm the broader concerns for assuring the overall health and well-being of the edentulous population.

Journal of Prosthodontics on Complete and Removable Dentures, First Edition. Edited by Jonathan P. Wiens, Jennifer Wiens Priebe, and Donald A. Curtis.
© 2018 American College of Prosthodontists. Published 2018 by John Wiley & Sons, Inc.

The future success of edentulous patient care is dependent on the development of shared goals for both the edentulous patient and the clinical team. This requires careful elucidation of a goal and strategies to reduce or eliminate edentulism, of new and improved standards for management of edentulism, and of innovation in the delivery of denture care. Success will be achieved when therapeutic success is similarly viewed by the clinician and the patient. The selective use of technology to improve denture fabrication should be guided by factors that improve the process and outcome of denture fabrication and use as viewed by the denture wearer.

The causes of edentulism are many. While largely the result of genetic or microbial diseases that have strong individual and behavioral influences, total tooth loss can be the result of iatrogenic, traumatic, or therapeutic causes. Unfortunately, in addition to patient neglect and poor oral hygiene, the failure of prostheses is a real issue facing individuals and populations with comprehensively restored dentitions.

The truth about edentulism is that it has not disappeared nor is it disappearing. Eklund and Bert[1] indicated that in the United States, future edentulism may be predicted based on the degree of partial edentulism, but not other variables. Such statistical predictions suggest that for approximately 150 million adults, over 10 million new cases of edentulism will be presented in the next decade. Other investigators suggest there are reductions in edentulism in various parts of the world (i.e., continental Europe[2]). Mojon et al[3] indicated that reductions in edentulism are to be expected in Scandinavian countries; however, these and similar reports from developed nations and small populations of interest (compared to larger centers of developing nations such as China and India), may not fully represent the worldwide status of edentulism. Edentulism remains an individual concern, a professional responsibility, and a prominent public health issue. Many reports claim that while the prevalence of tooth loss is diminishing with each generation, the longevity of populations worldwide and the potential accommodation to sugar-rich diets and Western lifestyles contribute to sustaining the actual number of edentulous individuals throughout the world.

Public health strategies to prevent edentulism include maintenance of optimal levels of fluoride in community water supplies, oral health promotion for all age groups, and expansion of dental insurance coverage, particularly for older persons. Other preventive measures include the appropriate use of fluoridecontaining or antibacterial agents such as dentifrices, topical gels, mouth rinses, and varnishes. In addition, improved access to clinical dental services and expanded community tobaccocontrol activities can help prevent total tooth loss. These suggestions are largely based on knowledge of existing populations and studies performed on mobile, active adults. As a new generation of institutionalized elderly grows, it will be important to understand how and if it is possible to prevent edentulation of individuals with failing tooth- (or implant-) supported prostheses.

Fortunately, the variability in total tooth loss reported throughout the world and the sociodemographic variation in tooth loss suggests edentulism is not an inevitable outcome of aging. Moreover, the impact of oral health promotion (hygiene, smoking cessation, etc.) and public actions such as water fluoridation suggest that edentulism is preventable. Douglass et al[4] summarized their findings of the prevalence of edentulism in the United States by stating that a sizable minority of the population will continue to need complete denture services, and if dental education supporting these services is eliminated, millions of patients will seek alternative providers.

FACING THE REALITY OF EDENTULISM

Edentulism exists, it will remain prevalent (>20% in some socioeconomic sectors of the population), and its management is beneficial to the affected population and society. It has been elegantly stated that "the predicament of being both elderly and edentulous undermines life quality for both patient and dentist. The former suffer because of morphological and functional compromises, the latter because of a dearth of safe and predictably successful clinical techniques."[5] The global management of edentulism as a socially relevant public health issue requires that clinicians examine edentulism as a chronic oral condition with relationships to chronic oral diseases and significant links to chronic systemic conditions. Mignogna and Fedele[6] reported that chronic oral diseases, despite not being life threatening, result in pain and suffering and reduce the overall quality of life. They are costly, and these costs are often out-of-pocket expenses. Importantly, chronic oral diseases that result terminally in edentulism are associated with the prevalent chronic diseases of developed nations (cardiovascular disease, cancer, chronic respiratory disease, and diabetes) due to common risk factors (dietary factors, tobacco, and alcohol misuse). *The prevention of edentulism is a primary aspect of any broad-based contemporary strategy in the global management ofedentulism.*

Edentulation may represent an intervention (or interventions) in a lifelong process of managing chronic oral diseases. While effective in removing the focus of dentoalveolar infections, it creates other chronic conditions that require additional clinical care and pose other clinical risks. Edentulism results in a reduction in oral and social functions (both measured and perceived). It is managed, perhaps incompletely, by the provision of complete dentures.

Complete denture therapy is further associated with an entire set of related complications and associated clinical manifestations of denture use. Examples include denture stomatitis, traumatic ulcers, irritation-induced hyperplasia, altered taste perception, burning mouth syndrome, and gagging. Residual ridge resorption leads to unfavorable dimensional changes to the lower third of the face when dentures do not compensate properly. In addition to treatment-related morbidity, treatment outcomes may not meet the physiological, psychological, or social needs of the individual.[7]

Residual Ridge Resorption

It is well known that removal of teeth leads to alveolar bone resorption.[8,9] This response varies in extent among individuals,[10] but appears to be a general occurrence that is inevitable for the majority of individuals experiencing complete tooth loss. The continued reduction in alveolar bone volume leads to unstable clinical conditions that require awareness of the process and accommodation to it.

Tooth extraction in the mandible will result in continual reduction in alveolar bone volume. It is more dramatic in the mandible than the maxilla. The continued resorption of the mandibular alveolar bone is associated with greater difficulty with mandibular denture construction, use, and satisfaction. This absence of teeth is also associated with reduced social and physiologic function.[11–13]

Oral implant placement may prevent the continued resorption of bone and has been associated with increased mandibular bone height distal to the implant location.[14] Wright et al[15] described an increase in posterior mandible bone height in response to functioning with implant-supported fixed dentures, but not overdentures. Subsequent contradictory findings indicated that implant-supported overdenture use was associated with mandibular bone resorption.[16] Although positive bone responses are widely recognized following implant placement in the parasymphyseal mandible, the extent of this benefit remains controversial and merits additional investigation. Posterior mandibular alveolar ridge resorption should be anticipated. The management of the edentulous patient by well-trained clinicians is necessary and involves the continued monitoring of residual alveolar ridge resorption and related issues of denture function. Clinical management of residual alveolar bone mass must be addressed. *Beyond the promise of endosseous implants, the prevention or management of residual alveolar ridge resorption should be the second part of a contemporary strategy in the treatment of edentulism.*

Oral Mucosal Lesions

The prevalence of oral mucosal lesions among edentulous subjects is not fully defined. It is sufficient to acknowledge its presence in the population and to understand the causes and associated risk factors and to appreciate the need for intervention, management, or treatment. At the most simple level, denture wearers may exhibit a significantly higher prevalence of oral mucosal conditions than individuals without dentures.

The literature implies that the comparator group is the dentate, and this suggests there has not been a focused effort to understand the differences between edentulous individuals wearing dentures and those who have no prostheses. It is suggested that denture use, not edentulism, is associated with the prevalence of oral mucosal lesions.

The results presented in the third National Health and Nutrition Examination Survey (NHANES III) involving over 17,000 individuals 17 years and older demonstrated that denture-related lesions accounted for 8.4% of all oral mucosal lesions.[17] Commonly reported denture-related problems include traumatic ulcers, denture stomatitis, and angular cheilitis.[18] In addition, denture-induced inflammatory fibrous hyperplasia may occur in approximately one-third of denture wearers.[19] Inflammatory fibrous hyperplasia was associated with duration of prosthesis use[20] and appears to occur more frequently in women.[19] Inflammatory fibrous hyperplasia is frequently associated with pain.

Most recently, evaluations of elderly patients revealed a high incidence of denture stomatitis.[20,21] The incidence may be higher when denture use is associated with comorbid disease states such as HIV and irradiation.[22] Diabetes is implicated as a cofactor in the severity of periodontitis, but when 30 diabetic and nondiabetic denture wearers were evaluated, no significant differences were observed in denture retention or oral mucosal lesions.[23] The relationship of oral inflammation of edentulous individuals with chronic systemic diseases should be further investigated.

The etiology of denture stomatitis is controversial. Zissis et al[24] reported that denture stomatitis was significantly related to the years of denture-wearing experience and the current denture's useage. Continuous denture wearing was highly related to denture stomatitis prevalence. When 200 Croatian patients were examined, denture wearing habits, hygiene, and denture cleanliness had significant influence on the degree of denture stomatitis in denture wearers. A clear correlation between denture plaque accumulation and denture stomatitis was defined;[25] however, Barbeau et al[26] and Emami et al[27] suggest that denture cleanliness and presence of *Candida* species are not significant risk factors for denture stomatitis. Moreover, when Emami et al[27] evaluated possible causes of denture stomatitis among 173 edentulous elders, it was observed that the risk of denture stomatitis was 4.5 times greater in individuals wearing conventional dentures than in those who wore an implant-retained overdenture ($p < 0.00001$). The authors suggest that denturerelated trauma leading to inflammation is reduced by use of endosseous oral implants. Additional data indicated that there were no differences in denture cleanliness or frequency of denture cleaning. Beyond the type of prosthesis, only nocturnal use of the prosthesis was associated with the frequency of denture stomatitis. Nocturnal or continuous use of the denture may mitigate the protective effect of saliva, oxygenation of the mucosa, and the positive biological features of the keratinized mucosa. It is of further importance to note that there may be little relationship between patients' perceptions of denture stability or stomatitis and the ability to wear a denture. *The continual surveillance of oral mucosal health, including the concern for both inflammatory and malignant lesions, may be included as a third feature of contemporary management of the edentulous patient.*

There is only limited information concerning the oral mucosal biofilm of denture wearers. An understanding of the microbiota of the edentulous adult with complete dentures has only recently received detailed attention.[20] From a group of 61 edentulous subjects using maxillary and mandibular complete dentures, samples of the oral mucosa were analyzed by DNA probe analysis of 41 species. The total bacterial counts were highest for the tongue and attached gingiva. Equal bacterial counts were found in saliva samples and on the denture hard palate. An important finding was that the periodontal pathogens *A. actinomycetemcomitans* and *P. gingivalis* were found in samples of the edentulous subjects. The authors suggested that complete denture patients may be at some risk for systemic diseases possibly associated with these periodontal pathogens.

The relationship of denture adherent biofilm to oral health is poorly understood. Yet, the cleanliness of dentures is suspect. When Dikbas et al[29] examined 234 denture patients, they observed few clean dentures (11.9%). Moreover, older dentures were dirtier than newer dentures and had an accompanying higher incidence of denture stomatitis. Most denture wearers did not clean their dentures well and indicated that their dentists did not inform them how to clean their dentures. Similar findings were reported for 321 Jordanian patients; there was a high percentage of unclean dentures and a significant relationship between stomatitis and denture hygiene.[30]

The microbiology of denture plaque has received little attention in comparison with dental plaque. It differs in location and composition. Oral bacteria have been implicated in bacterial endocarditis, pneumonia, chronic obstructive pulmonary disease, and gastrointestinal infection, and dentures offer a reservoir for microorganisms associated with these infections.[31] *Candida albicans* figures prominently in the etiology of oral mucosal inflammation and is frequently part of any differential diagnosis. The acquisition of *Candida*-containing species in denture retentive plaque is associated with stomatitis.[32]

It may be possible to directly control oral microbial infection by management of the denture surface. A simple management strategy is the cleaning of dentures. Recent literature suggests a renewed and growing interest in developing denture cleaning aids. The simple act of mechanical debridement of denture adherent plaque is a recurrent theme in these reports. When the ability of ambulatory denture wearers to clean biofilm from dentures was evaluated, Salles et al[33] demonstrated that mechanical cleaning of a denture with a designated denture cleaning agent was effective in removing biofilm. One portion of the denture-wearing population includes the institutionalized elderly who may not have the capacity to achieve mechanical cleaning of the dentures and who unfortunately do not receive sufficient assistance.[34] Denture hygiene improvements are indicated and may benefit from additional development of denture cleaning agents and devices.

Further improvement in control of denture biofilm and related oral mucosal inflammation may be possible. Milillo et al[35] illustrated this possibility using a varnish containing 5% amorolfine (antifungal agent used for onychomycosis). In this pilot study, treatment of the denture with the amorolfine varnish suppressed nystatin-resistant denture stomatitis. Other agents that may be useful in controlling denture stomatitis by treating the denture base include typical anti-mycotic agents (nystatin, fluconazole, etc.), several denture cleaners, and an innovative application of salivary proteins. Edgerton et al[36] showed that polymethylmethacrylate resin could be modified and loaded to affect the controlled release of histatin 5 in an effort to control *Candida albicans* adhesion.

The eventual control of chronically accumulated denture biofilm is an important goal. When complete denture renewal was investigated as a means of controlling (eliminating) existing denture biofilm, few parameters related to denture function changed; however, the main effects of denture renewal were observed for patient satisfaction and improved condition of the oral mucosa.[37]

It has become apparent that the denture is an important factor affecting oral biofilm. As denture use continues without proper denture hygiene, changes in oral biofilm and oral mucosal health may be evident. Pursuing optimal oral health requires that the denture be evaluated and treated as necessary. Contemporary denture therapy must include periodic denture evaluation and management of denture-adherent biofilm. The replacement of existing dentures every 5 years is suggested to effectively meet the many clinical challenges of the edentulous denture wearer. *Contemporary denture therapy should, as a fourth strategy, include the rational replacement of existing dentures based on defined criteria and the future development of dentures as therapeutic devices that aid in control of (not the exacerbation of) oral mucosal lesions.*

Maladaptation to Dentures

Successful accommodation of patients to dentures is a frequently acknowledged challenge to many clinicians. The mindset that clinical management of the patient can be guided by technical features of the denture or its construction is suggested by clinical behavior of clinicians; however, recent data strongly suggest that patient-based measures of denture success may differ from those of clinicians. Both the clinician and the patient are quick to identify individual features of the denture as the cause of dissatisfaction.

When new dentures are provided, the patient's reported satisfaction did not correlate with the method of denture fabrication.[38] Brunello and Mandikos[39] examined 100 patients with ongoing denture dissatisfaction. They too observed an association with denture design faults and the condition of the patient's mucosa. Most of the patients experienced poor denture retention. Interestingly, approximately one-third of the subjects showed mucosal irritation. Among the most prevalent problems recorded were: (a) underextension of the denture bases and (b) incorrect jaw relationships. Less frequently, incorrect occlusal vertical dimension and inadequate posterior palatal seal were noted. They concluded that complete denture patients present with complaints only when there is a real design fault or a tissue problem. When patient complaints were considered in the context of dentist-observed denture faults, Dervis[40] indicated that there were significant relationships between denture construction faults, the condition of the bearing mucosa, and patient complaints. These observations were reiterated in a review of literature concerning patients who experienced ongoing difficulties with new complete dentures.[41]

The notion that key features of the denture itself underscore dissatisfaction strongly implies that clinical success is dependent on technique of fabrication, design, and quality of the denture. A spectrum of functional impairments that range from reduced masticatory function, to impaired phonetic ability, to claims of lowered social function including sexuality are all associated with mandibular edentulism and associated denture instability.[42,43] While several investigators have shown that patient-based and clinician attitudes about denture quality and use are not well correlated, the aforementioned studies that address denture quality directly suggest that worldwide improvement in therapy requires enhanced clinical ability. Both educational and technological advances should be explored by organized dentistry if these observations are taken at face value.

Dissatisfaction with mandibular dentures has a multifactorial basis. When considering the self-reported satisfaction regarding complete denture use, patients have described instability and discomfort as key reasons for dissatisfaction. Comparison of outcomes for mandibular versus maxillary denture use has revealed that stability and comfort are the features that distinguish maxillary denture acceptance from more generalized mandibular denture dissatisfaction.[44] Suggested is the possibility that stability of the prosthesis may be a key feature of denture acceptance.

The importance of denture base stability may underscore the present interest in pursuing treatment of edentulism using oral implants. When oral implants are beyond the capacity of the clinician, health care system, or patient's desire, few techniques are left to aid the patient. The use of neutral zone impressions, altered occlusal forms, and the use of denture adhesives have been advocated.

Recent interest in the use of denture adhesives is obvious in the literature. For example, de Baat et al[45] used a measure of incisal force before dislodgement of maxillary denture dislodgement to objectively score the effect of denture adhesive on maxillary denture retention. They observed a benefit of the denture adhesive, particularly for existing (vs. new) dentures. This confirms observations made by clinicians earlier.[46] When patients were polled regarding their assessment of denture adhesives, all subjects responded that retention of their dentures was better when using an adhesive paste.[47] In a similar study comparing five denture adhesives, the majority of subjects also declared benefit from the use of adhesive pastes.[48]

In a further key paper by Fenlon and Sherriff,[49] a refined patient satisfaction structural model revealed strong relationships between the quality of mandibular residual alveolar ridges, new denture quality, and patient satisfaction with the new dentures. The accuracy of jaw relations was indicated as a key variable in the model. In turn, this affected mandibular denture security and mandibular anatomy. This work strongly suggests that the process of fabricating a denture— that is, the quality of the individual procedural steps— influences denture satisfaction by influencing mandibular denture stability. Other approaches to increasing mandibular denture stability include detailed emphasis on the neutral zone technique[50] that aims to establish muscular control over the denture.

Other technical aspects of denture construction are often viewed passionately as factors affecting success. Most investigations fail to show any preference by the patient for dentures fabricated using different impression techniques, various tooth arrangements or occlusal designs, or articulator preferences.[51] Yet the delivery of a denture is often not fully explored. Irrespective of how a denture may be constructed, its delivery may help to harmonize the prosthesis with the recipient. Shigli et al[52] compared the fabrication and delivery of dentures with and without laboratory and clinical remount procedures and revealed that remount procedures and occlusal corrections reduced the number of postinsertion visits and resulted in enhanced patient comfort. Again, there may be some reason to carefully evaluate the curricular content of denture techniques, education, and practice. While current thought is intensely focused on endosseous oral implants to provide denture stability, it must be recognized that not every patient desires nor can afford to obtain such treatment.

Alternatively, a long-standing assumption is that a subset of patients may not adapt to denture use, irrespective of the technique or quality of the denture. Historical reference to patient dissatisfaction and its management is well known.[53] There may be more than anecdotal value to this understanding. Bolender et al[54] investigated effects of patient personality on satisfaction with complete dentures in 402 patients and found a significant association between high neuroticism scores and patient dissatisfaction. Fenlon et al, however, found significant negative associations between Neuroticism (but not Extrovertism or Psychotism) and all aspects of satisfaction with new dentures. In an interesting report, depression and denture satisfaction were associated in the general population of older adults examined in a cross-sectional study.[55] Depression represents a comorbid condition that may influence our ability to treat individual patients. It is critical that management of edentulism be expansive and not restricted to the technical aspects of denture construction. Contemporary denture therapeutic success must comprehensively embrace technical, patient, and socioeconomic features of the treatment scenario. Furthermore, there is need to examine new materials, techniques, and clinical business models for delivery of excellent complete dentures. *Both the detailed quality of denture technique and patient management represent essential educational and professional mandates that comprise a fifth aspect of contemporary denture therapy.*

Given the therapeutic limitations addressed above, are dentures the solution to edentulism? Fortunately and unfortunately, the answers to this question include both yes and no. The ability to replace missing teeth for various anticipated and expected reasons using a seemingly simple device such as a removable denture has been available to the edentate person for centuries. In fact, much of the technology we depend on to create dentures for individual patients has not changed at all. Unfortunately, the rehabilitation of the edentate person using dentures can be incomplete. The historically recent advent of endosseous oral implants and the refinement of methods for implant-supported dentures offer limited improvements for a limited set of individuals.

ENDOSSEOUS ORAL IMPLANTS FOR TREATMENT OF EDENTULISM

Brånemark and coworkers provided a fixed solution for mandibular edentulism. The advantages of this prosthodontic therapy using oral implants include both stability and comfort of the fixed prostheses. Importantly, it offers a perception that the prosthesis is fixed to the mandible. Biological advantages suggested for this approach include the induction of posterior mandibular bone apposition[15] and increased masticatory function;[56] however, relative disadvantages include potential maladaptation to the complex intraoral appliance, inability to perform necessary oral hygiene, and cost.

Implant-supported or -retained removable prostheses offer alternative advantages for rehabilitation of the edentulous mandible. The selection of the overdenture versus a fixed implant prosthesis may be favored on initial cost advantages.[57] Other advantages such as access for hygiene, avoidance of food impaction, and support of facial profile by the denture flange are commonly cited as factors that favor a removable prosthesis supported by mandibular implants.[58]

It remains an unfortunate fact that too few edentulous individuals worldwide are able to benefit from this therapy.

Burns[59] indicated that there is consensus among investigators that: (i) retention and stability problems negatively influence treatment outcomes for conventional mandibular dentures; (ii) oral implant success in the anterior mandible is generally excellent; (iii) implant-retained or -supported mandibular overdentures offer many benefits compared with conventional denture treatment; (iv) implants in the anterior mandible can slow the process of physiological bone resorption; (v) periimplant mucosal and osseous responses to mandibular implant overdenture treatment are favorable; (vi) treatment complications are a concern, especially during the first year of treatment service, and there is need for routine recall and follow-up evaluation and treatment; and (vii) data indicate significant increases in patient satisfaction with mandibular implant overdenture treatment when compared with conventional denture treatment.

Positive long-term outcomes for implant-supported overdentures were reported by in a 10- to 19-year review of 42 consecutively treated mandibular overdenture patients.[60] In addition to observing that the prosthetic and implant cumulative survival rates were greater than 90%, the authors further noted a requirement for relining, on average, every 4 years. In fact, the majority of investigations that considered the implant and prosthetic outcomes of mandibular implant overdenture therapy indicated similar high implant survival rates, low biological complication rates as well as the important requirement for prosthetic intervention. Mandibular edentulism treatment using implantretained overdentures with ball abutment-retained overdentures is cost-effective and highly accepted.[61]

The treatment of the edentulous patient using implants to retain mandibular overdentures has been suggested to be a standard of care.[62] Fitzpatrick[63] argues that prosthodontists should consider a broader range of therapeutic choices and that the "standard of care" for the treatment of edentulous mandibles is to offer choice. Informed decision making at the individual level requires that choices are based on a wide range of factual data, patient perceptions, and economic factors. Addressing edentulism as a condition affecting diverse populations worldwide requires further distillation of information driving policies that affect professional education, prevention, and therapy. Oral implants are firmly established among the other aforementioned strategies to comprehensively address the treatment of edentulism.

Despite the highly successful outcomes for the implant-supported overdenture, it seems that a majority of edentulous individuals have not pursued implant-based rehabilitation of mandibular function and self-esteem. Among the reasons cited for this discrepancy between highly successful therapy and its acceptance are the cost of treatment and the process of treatment. Newer immediate provisionalization/loading protocols for implant-retained mandibular overdentures may address the perceptions of lengthy treatment. Although every patient will not consent to receive oral implants, Walton and MacEntee[64] suggest that pain, perceptions of poor chewing function and speech, and dissatisfaction with appearance motivated patients to choose oral implants. Endosseous oral implants have been used to improve the function, physiology, and perceived outcomes of treatment of mandibular edentulism. Promotion of oral implant therapy is recognized as a first choice treatment strategy; however, the worldwide acceptance of oral implant treatment for mandibular edentulism faces both educational and economic challenges. *A sixth feature of contemporary strategies in the management of edentulism is the continued development of oral implant technology and worldwide enhancement of educational standards concerning oral implant-supported prosthesis therapy.*

SUMMARY

Contemporary management of the edentulous population should include improvements in the general oral health of edentate patients. Clearly, prevention of edentulism is foremost as a public health strategy; however, the management of tens of millions of edentulous people requires renewed focus. In particular, organized dentistry must reinforce (1) *prevention*, (2) *the continued monitoring of residual alveolar ridge resorption and related issues of denture function*, (3) *the continual surveillance of oral mucosal health including the concern for both inflammatory and malignant lesions and development of dentures as therapeutic devices*, (4) *a rationale for timely replacement of existing dentures based on defined criteria*, (5) *clinical responses to maladaptive denture patients be expansive and not solely restricted to the technical aspects of denture construction*, and (6) *the management of edentulism by the continued development of oral implant technology and worldwide enhancement of educational standards concerning oral implant overdenture therapy and denture quality.*

TIPS FOR THE PRACTICING DENTIST

1. Emphasize prevention for the dentate patient.
2. Continually monitor residual alveolar ridge resorption and related issues of denture function.
3. Continually monitor oral mucosal health, with a particular emphasis on both inflammatory and malignant lesions.
4. Develop a rationale for timely replacement of existing dentures based on defined criteria.

5. Respond to maladaptive denture patients not solely through the technical aspects of denture construction but also through patient personality and socioeconomic features.
6. Remain up-to-date on the latest oral implant technology, and educate patients on the benefits of this treatment.

REFERENCES

1. Eklund SA, Burt BA: Risk factors for total tooth loss in the United States; longitudinal analysis of national data. *J Public Health Dent* 1994;54:5–14.
2. Müller F, Naharro M, Carlsson GE: What are the prevalence and incidence of tooth loss in the adult and elderly population in Europe? *Clin Oral Implants Res* 2007;18:2–14. Review. Erratum in: Clin Oral Implants Res 2008;19:326–328.
3. Mojon P, Thomason JM, Walls AW: The impact of falling rates of edentulism. *Int J Prosthodont* 2004;17:434–440.
4. Douglass CW, Shih A, Ostry L: Will there be a need for complete dentures in the United States in 2020? *J Prosthet Dent* 2002;87:5–8.
5. Zarb GA, Schmitt A: Implant therapy alternatives for geriatric edentulous patients. *Gerodontology* 1993;10:28–32.
6. Mignogna MD, Fedele S: The neglected global burden of chronic oral diseases. *J Dent Res* 2006;85:390–391.
7. MacEntee MI, Nolan A, Thomason JM: Oral mucosal and osseous disorders in frail elders. *Gerodontology* 2004;21:78–84.
8. Atwood DA: Reduction of residual ridges: a major oral disease entity. *J Prosthet Dent* 1971;26:266–279.
9. Tallgren A: The continuing reduction of the residual alveolar ridges in complete denture wearers: a mixed-longitudinal study covering 25 years. *J Prosthet Dent* 1972;27:120–132.
10. Carlsson GE: Clinical morbidity and sequelae of treatment with complete dentures. *J Prosthet Dent* 1998;79:17–23.
11. Musacchio E, Perissinotto E, Binotto P, et al: Tooth loss in the elderly and its association with nutritional status, socioeconomic and lifestyle factors. *Acta Odontol Scand* 2007;65:78–86.
12. Stein PS, Desrosiers M, Donegan SJ, et al: Tooth loss, dementia and neuropathology in the Nun study. *J Am Dent Assoc* 2007;138:1314–1322.
13. Fiske J, Davis DM, Frances C, et al: The emotional effects of tooth loss in edentulous people. *Br Dent J* 1998;184:90–93.
14. Davis WH, Lam PS, Marshall MW, et al: Using restorations borne totally by anterior implants to preserve the edentulous mandible. *J Am Dent Assoc* 1999;130:1183–1189.
15. Wright PS, Glantz PO, Randow K, et al: The effects of fixed and removable implant-stabilised prostheses on posterior mandibular residual ridge resorption. *Clin Oral Implants Res* 2002;13:169–174.

16. Blum IR, McCord JF: A clinical investigation of the morphological changes in the posterior mandible when implant-retained overdentures are used. *Clin Oral Implants Res* 2004;15:700–708.

17. Shulman JD, Beach MM, Rivera-Hidalgo F: The prevalence of oral mucosal lesions in U.S. adults: data from the Third National Health and Nutrition Examination Survey, 1988–1994. *J Am Dent Assoc* 2004;135:1279–1286.

18. Jainkittivong A, Aneksuk V, Langlais RP: Oral mucosal conditions in elderly dental patients. *Oral Dis* 2002;8: 218–223.

19. Macedo Firoozmand L, Dias Almeida J, Guimarães Cabral LA: Study of denture-induced fibrous hyperplasia cases diagnosed from 1979 to 2001. *Quintessence Int* 2005;36:825–829.

20. Freitas JB, Gomez RS, De Abreu MH, et al: Relationship between the use of full dentures and mucosal alterations among elderly Brazilians. *J Oral Rehabil* 2008;35:370–374.

21. Mujica V, Rivera H, Carrero M: Prevalence of oral soft tissue lesions in an elderly Venezuelan population. *Med Oral Patol Oral Cir Bucal* 2008;13:E270–E274.

22. Davies AN, Brailsford SR, Beighton D: Oral candidosis in patients with advanced cancer. *Oral Oncol* 2006;42:698–702.

23. Cristina de Lima D, Nakata GC, Balducci I, et al: Oral manifestations of diabetes mellitus in complete denture wearers. *J Prosthet Dent* 2008;99:60–65.

24. Zissis A, Yannikakis S, Harrison A: Comparison of denture stomatitis prevalence in 2 population groups. *Int J Prosthodont* 2006;19:621–625.

25. Celić R, Knezović Zlatarić D, Baucić I: Evaluation of denture stomatitis in Croatian adult population. *Coll Antropol* 2001;25:317–326.

26. Barbeau J, Séguin J, Goulet JP, et al. : Reassessing the presence of Candida albicans in denture-related stomatitis. *Oral Surg Oral Med Oral Pathol Oral Radiol Endod* 2003;95:51–59.

27. Emami E, de Grandmont P, Rompré PH, et al: Favoring trauma as an etiological factor in denture stomatitis. *J Dent Res* 2008;87:440–444.

28. Sachdeo A, Haffajee AD, Socransky SS: Biofilms in the edentulous oral cavity. *J Prosthodont* 2008;17:348–356.

29. Dikbas I, Koksal T, Calikkocaoglu S: Investigation of the cleanliness of dentures in a university hospital. *Int J Prosthodont* 2006;19:294–298.

30. Khasawneh S, al-Wahadni A: Control of denture plaque and mucosal inflammation in denture wearers. *J Ir Dent Assoc* 2002;48:132–138.

31. Coulthwaite L, Verran J: Potential pathogenic aspects of denture plaque. *Br J Biomed Sci* 2007;64:180–189.

32. Radford DR, Challacombe SJ, Walter JD: Denture plaque and adherence of Candida albicans to denture-base materials in vivo and in vitro. *Crit Rev Oral Biol Med* 1999;10: 99–116.

33. Salles AE, Macedo LD, Fernandes RA, et al: Comparative analysis of biofilm levels in complete upper and lower dentures after brushing associated with specific denture paste and neutral soap. *Gerodontology* 2007;24:217–223.

34. De Visschere LM, Grooten L, Theuniers G, et al: Oral hygiene of elderly people in long-term care institutions—a cross-sectional study. *Gerodontology* 2006;23:195–120.

35. Milillo L, Lo Muzio L, Carlino P, et al: Candida-related denture stomatitis: a pilot study of the efficacy of an amorolfine antifungal varnish. *Int J Prosthodont* 2005;18:55–59.

36. Edgerton M, Raj PA, Levine MJ: Surface-modified poly (methyl methacrylate) enhances adsorption and retains anti-candidal activities of salivary histatin 5. *J Biomed Mater Res* 1995;29:1277–1286.

37. Peltola MK, Raustia AM, Salonen MA: Effect of complete denture renewal on oral health—a survey of 42 patients. *J Oral Rehabil* 1997;24:419–425.

38. Ellis JS, Pelekis ND, Thomason JM: Conventional rehabilitation of edentulous patients: the impact on oral health-related quality of life and patient satisfaction. *J Prosthodont* 2007;16:37–42.

39. Brunello DL, Mandikos MN: Construction faults, age, gender, and relative medical health: factors associated with complaints in complete denture patients. *J Prosthet Dent* 1998;79:545–554.

40. Dervis E: Clinical assessment of common patient complaints with complete dentures. *Eur J Prosthodont Restor Dent* 2002;10:113–117.

41. Laurina L, Soboleva U: Construction faults associated with complete denture wearers' complaints. *Stomatologija* 2006;8:61–64. Review

42. Awad MA, Lund JP, Dufresne E, et al: Comparing the efficacy of mandibular implant-retained overdentures and conventional dentures among middle-aged edentulous patients: satisfaction and functional assessment. *Int J Prosthodont* 2003;16:117–122.

43. Heydecke G, Klemetti E, Awad MA, et al: Relationship between prosthodontic evaluation and patient ratings of mandibular conventional and implant prostheses. *Int J Prosthodont* 2003;16:307–312.

44. Fenlon MR, Sherriff M, Walter JD: Agreement between clinical measures of quality and patients' rating of fit of existing and new complete dentures. *J Dent* 2002;30:135–139.

45. de Baat C, van't Hof M, van Zeghbroeck L, et al: An international multicenter study on the effectiveness of a denture adhesive in maxillary dentures using disposable gnathometers. *Clin Oral Investig* 2007;11:237–243.

46. Grasso JE, Rendell J, Gay T: Effect of denture adhesive on the retention and stability of maxillary dentures. *J Prosthet Dent* 1994;72:399–405.

47. Kulak Y, Ozcan M, Arikan A: Subjective assessment by patients of the efficiency of two denture adhesive pastes. *J Prosthodont* 2005;14:248–252.

48. Kelsey CC, Lang BR, Wang RF: Examining patients' responses about the effectiveness of five denture adhesive pastes. *J Am Dent Assoc* 1997;128:1532–1538.

49. Fenlon MR, Sherriff M: An investigation of factors influencing patients' satisfaction with new complete dentures using structural equation modelling. *J Dent* 2008;36:427–434.

50. Gahan MJ, Walmsley AD: *The neutral zone impression revisited. Br Dent J* 2005;198:269–272.

51. Carlsson GE: Facts and fallacies: an evidence base for complete dentures. *Dent Update* 2006;33:134-136, 138-140, 142. Review

52. Shigli K, Angadi GS, Hegde P: The effect of remount procedures on patient comfort for complete denture treatment. *J Prosthet Dent* 2008;99:66–72.

53. Koper A: Difficult denture birds. *J Prosthet Dent* 1967;17:532–539.

54. Bolender CL, Swoope CC, Smith DE: The Cornell Medical Index as a prognostic aid for complete denture patients. *J Prosthet Dent* 1969;22:20–29.

55. Fenlon MR, Sherriff M, Newton JT: The influence of personality on patients' satisfaction with existing and new complete dentures. *J Dent* 2007;35:744–748.

56. Fueki K, Kimoto K, Ogawa T, et al: Effect of implant-supported or retained dentures on masticatory performance: a systematic review. *J Prosthet Dent* 2007;98:470–477. Review

57. Zitzmann NU, Marinello CP, Sendi P: A cost-effectiveness analysis of implant overdentures. *J Dent Res* 2006;85:717–721.

58. Zitzmann NU, Marinello CP: A review of clinical and technical considerations for fixed and removable implant prostheses in the edentulous mandible. *Int J Prosthodont* 2002;15:65–72. Review

59. Burns DR: Mandibular overdenture treatment: consensus and controversy. *J Prosthodont* 2000;9:37–46.

60. Attard NJ, Zarb GA: Long-term treatment outcomes in edentulous patients with implant overdentures: the Toronto study. *Int J Prosthodont* 2004;17:425–433.

61. Sadowsky SJ: Mandibular implant-retained overdentures: a literature review. *J Prosthet Dent* 2001;86:468–473.

62. Feine JS, Carlsson GE, Awad MA, et al: The McGill Consensus Statement on Overdentures. *Int J Prosthodont* 2002;15:413–414. Review

63. Fitzpatrick B: Standard of care for the edentulous mandible: a systematic review. *J Prosthet Dent* 2006;95:71–78. Review

64. Walton JN, MacEntee MI: Choosing or refusing oral implants: a prospective study of edentulous volunteers for a clinical trial. *Int J Prosthodont* 2005;18:483–488.

6

IMPACT OF DIFFERENT PROSTHODONTIC TREATMENT MODALITIES ON NUTRITIONAL PARAMETERS OF ELDERLY PATIENTS

KOPAL GOEL, MDS,[1] SAUMYENDRA V. SINGH, MDS,[2] POORAN CHAND, MDS,[1] JITENDRA RAO, MDS,[1] SHUCHI TRIPATHI, MDS,[1] LAKSHYA KUMAR, MDS,[1] ABBAS ALI MAHDI, PHD,[2] AND KALPANA SINGH, MD[2]

[1]Department of Prosthodontics, Faculty of Dental Sciences, King George's Medical University UP, Lucknow, India
[2]Department of Biochemistry, King George's Medical University UP, Lucknow, India

Keywords

Edentulism; elderly; diet; nutritional status; prosthodontic rehabilitation

Correspondence

Saumyendra V. Singh, 2/273 Viram Khand, Gomtinagar, Lucknow, UP, India. 226010. E-mail: saumyendravsingh@rediffmail.com

The authors deny any conflicts of interest.

Accepted September 9, 2014

Published in *Journal of Prosthodontics* 2016; Vol. 25, Issue 1, pp. 21–7

doi: 10.1111/jopr.12283

ABSTRACT

Purpose: To assess dietary and nutritional changes among the elderly following prosthodontic rehabilitation. Another objective was to study the relationship, if any, between diet and nutrition, with extent of edentulism and different types of prosthodontic treatment.

Materials and Methods: One hundred and thirty-five patients who satisfied the inclusion and exclusion criteria and agreed to be a part of the study after informed consent were recruited to this longitudinal study. Following selection, they were investigated on four aspects: dental examination, dietary assessment, anthropometric assessment, and serum biochemical assessment. All measurements were collected twice, first at baseline and then 6 months following prosthodontic rehabilitation. Treatment modalities included were complete denture (CD), removable partial denture (RPD), and fixed partial denture (FPD). The RPD group was of two types: distal extension prosthesis (RPDD) and tooth-supported prosthesis (RPDT). Change (post-pre) in outcome measures was compared by one-way ANOVA, and significance of mean difference between the groups was done by Tukey's honestly significance difference post hoc test.

Results: The improvement in diet was found to be: CD > RPDD > RPDT > FPD. Significant improvement in weight

($p < 0.001$), BMI ($p < 0.001$), protein ($p < 0.001$), carbohydrate ($p = 0.021$), calorie ($p < 0.001$), iron ($p = 0.002$), and vitamin B ($p < 0.001$) in group CD as compared to partially edentulous patients (group RPDD + RPDT + FPD) was noted. The protein and calorie intake increased significantly

in group RPD as compared to group FPD in partially edentulous patients.
Conclusion: Prosthetic rehabilitation becomes increasingly important as the level of edentulism increases to improve dietary, anthropometric, and biochemical parameters.

Nutrition is defined by the Council of Foods and Nutrition of the American Medical Association as "the science of food, the nutrients and other substances therein, their actions, interactions, and balance in relation to health and disease and the processes by which the organism ingests, digests, absorbs, transports, utilizes, and excretes food substances."[1]

Edentulism can significantly impact oral and general health and quality of life, including nutrition and enjoyment of food.[2] Even with dentures, the loss of all teeth reduces chewing efficiency and affects food taste, preferences, and consumption patterns.

The relationship between oral health conditions, dietary intake, nutritional and general health status in older adults is complex, with many interrelating factors.[3] Many elderly patients have an increased risk for malnutrition compared with other adults. It is estimated that between 2% to 16% of community-dwelling elderly are nutritionally deficient in protein and calories.[4] Malnutrition, in turn, is associated with a decrease in functional skills, increased susceptibility to infection, increased hospitalization and higher mortality. Therefore, maintaining good nutritional status is important in geriatric patients. The elderly often have multiple comorbidities that contribute to overall nutritional compromise. Given these complex contributing factors, a careful nutritional assessment is necessary for successful diagnosis of malnutrition and development of an appropriate treatment plan.[5] According to a study, one in five older people reported that their oral condition prevented them from eating foods they would choose, 15% took longer time to complete their meal, and enjoyment of food was limited by their oral condition. Five percent avoided eating certain foods because of chewing problems.[6] Dietary guidance, based on assessment of the edentulous patient's nutritional history and diet, should therefore be an integral part of prosthodontic treatment.[7] Therefore, a longitudinal study was done to assess dietary and nutritional changes in aging patients following prosthodontic rehabilitation.

MATERIALS AND METHODS

One hundred and thirty-five patients who satisfied the inclusion and exclusion criteria were selected for this longitudinal study after statistical calculation of sample size, over a period

of 4 months. The study was approved by the institutional ethics committee of King George's Medical University UP, Lucknow, India. After taking informed consent, the purpose of the study and procedures involved were explained to the patients. All measurements were collected twice, first at baseline and then 6 months following prosthodontic rehabilitation. To examine whether level of edentulism and its rehabilitation were independently associated with nutritional status, selection was based on the following inclusion criteria: (1) Age 60 years and above (this was done to minimize variations in study results due to extreme differences in age. A 40-year old, for example, may have different nutritional parameters and response compared to a 70-year old);[8] (2) physically healthy participants free of difficulties from daily living activities and lower extremity functional limitations (defined as difficulty in walking 0.4 km or climbing 10 steps without resting);[2] (3) no history of nutritional, systemic, or metabolic disease or medication for these; (4) psychologically healthy participants with normal mental functioning evaluated by the Short Portable Mental Status Questionnaire.[9] The exclusion criteria were: (1) education below high school; (2) financial status below poverty line defined as less than Indian currency in Rupees (Rs) 28.65 daily consumption in cities and Rs 22.42 in rural areas;[10] (3) patients with addictions such as smoking, chewing tobacco, alcohol consumption, as manifested by three (or more) of the WHO criteria, occurring at any time in the same 12-month period;[11–13] and (4) patients needing different prosthodontic treatment modalities in upper and lower arches, as it would not be possible to decide which modality actually affected the nutritional status. Following selection, the patient was investigated on four aspects: dental examination, dietary assessment, anthropometric assessment, and serum biochemical assessment.

The dental examination recorded the distribution of present teeth (distal extension or not), number of missing teeth (excluding third molars), and prosthesis recommended. Participants were categorized into groups according to dental status (group CE: completely edentulous, group PE: partially edentulous), number of missing teeth in PE group: (group 1: fewer than 8, group 2: 8 to 18, group 3: more than 18), and type of prosthesis recommended (group CD: complete denture, group RPD: removable partial denture, group FPD: fixed partial denture). Group RPD was further subdivided into group RPDD: distal extension prosthesis (Kennedy class I, II) and group RPDT: tooth-supported prosthesis (Kennedy class III, IV). Implant-supported prosthesis patients were excluded as they were few in number.

For measuring nutritional assessment, detailed information about quantity of foods and nutrients consumed was collected. Participants were asked to keep a last-three-meals diary record of all food and drink consumed, both in and out of home in terms of standard bowl, cup, glass, teaspoon, and tablespoon sizes according to Indian Council of Medical Research guidelines.[14] Written and oral instructions for completion of records by the participants were provided: 1 cup = 200 ml, 1 bowl = 200 g, 1 glass = 200 ml, 1 teaspoon = 5 ml, 1 tablespoon = 15 ml. For certain dishes with multiple food items, the main ingredients were identified. Data were tabulated on energy (fats, carbohydrates, proteins, and kilocalorie [kcal] consumption) and nutrient (iron, calcium, vitamin A, vitamin B, and vitamin C) values.[15–19]

Anthropometric assessment was done by calculating body mass index (BMI) using baseline weight and standing height measurements. Weight was measured in kilograms and standing height in meters.[8,20–22]

Biochemical assessment was done by collecting 5 ml fasting blood (participants were asked not to eat or drink anything except water for 10–12 hours) from participants at the baseline visit through venipuncture using standard protocol. Blood was collected into tubes containing plain polystyrene crystals. Within 4 hours of blood draw, tubes were sent to the laboratory for serum analysis. Serum albumin and total serum cholesterol were used as biochemical markers for undernutrition. Albumin levels were tested using the BCG Dye Binding Method and cholesterol with the cholesterol oxidase method.[20,23]

The patients were rehabilitated prosthetically, and these tests were repeated 6 months after baseline tests. Whether there was any variation in these parameters after rehabilitation was assessed. Statistics were analyzed by summarizing the data. Changes (post/pre) in outcome measures were compared by one-way ANOVA, and the significance of mean difference between groups was done by Tukey's honestly significance difference post hoc test after ascertaining normality by Shapiro-Wilk test and homogeneity of variance by Levene's test. Groups were also compared by independent Student's i-test. A two-sided ($\alpha = 2$) $p < 0.05$ was considered statistically significant. All analyses were performed on STATISTICA for Windows v6.0 (StatSoft Inc., Tulsa, OK).

RESULTS

Out of 135 subjects recruited, 16 were not considered as they did not come for follow-up or provided ambiguous dietary records. The dental status of patients is summarized in

TABLE 1 Dental status

Characteristics	No. (n = 119) (%)
Dentition status	
Completely edentulous (CE)	52 (43.7%)
Partially edentulous (PE)	67 (56.3%)
Prosthesis recommended	
Complete denture (CD)	52 (43.7%)
Distal extension prosthesis (RPDD)	20 (16.8%)
Tooth-supported prosthesis (RPDT)	19 (16.0%)
Fixed partial denture (FPD)	28 (23.5%)
Missing teeth:	
Group 1	44 (37.0%)
Group 2	16 (13.4%)
Group 3	7 (5.9%)
RPDD + RPDT	39 (32.8%)
FPD	28 (23.5%)
CD + RPDD + RPDT	91 (76.5%)
FPD	28 (23.5%)

Table 1. Outcome measures are shown in Table 2. The mean change at 6 months postbaseline for most variables was highest in group CD followed by groups RPDD, RPDT, and FPD. On comparing pre- versus postmean change in variables for all four prosthesis groups (Table 3), ANOVA revealed significant ($p < 0.05$) change in weight, BMI, protein, carbohydrate, calorie, iron, and vitamin B among the groups; however, the mean change in serum albumin, serum cholesterol, fat, calcium, vitamin A, and vitamin C did not differ statistically. Furthermore, Tukey's test revealed significantly different and greater pre- versus postchange in weight and BMI variables of group CD as compared to RPDD, RPDT, and FPD groups.

The mean change in protein, iron, and vitamin B variables was also significantly higher in group CD as compared to both RPDT and FPD groups. The mean pre- versus postchange in the protein variable was significantly higher in RPDD and RPDT groups compared to group FPD. The mean change in carbohydrate and calorie variables was also significantly higher in group CD as compared to group FPD (pre vs. post).

On comparing change in variable values for the three missing teeth groups (Tables 4 and 5), significant change in protein and vitamin B was found. Table 6 shows significant pre- versus postmean variable change in weight, BMI, protein, carbohydrate, calorie, calcium, iron, vitamin B, and vitamin C in group CD as compared to group PE. Protein and calorie variables changed significantly in group RPD as compared to group FPD (Table 7). Table 8 shows significant mean pre- versus postchange in weight, BMI, protein, carbohydrate, calorie, iron, and vitamin B variables in the removable prosthesis group (CD + RPDD + RPDT) as compared to group FPD.

TABLE 2 Mean change in variables in different prosthetic groups, 6 months from baseline

Variables	CD (n = 52)	RPDD (n = 20)	RPDT (n = 19)	FPD (n = 28)
Anthropometric variables				
Weight (kg)	1.64 ± 1.45	0.50 ± 1.83	0.47 ± 0.75	0.36 ± 1.11
BMI (kg/m^2)	0.66 ± 0.58	0.20 ± 0.66	0.23 ± 0.35	0.13 ± 0.43
Biochemical variables				
S. albumin (g/dl)	0.68 ± 0.28	0.05 ± 0.22	−0.01 ± 0.33	0.06 ± 0.33
S. cholesterol (mg/dl)	1.80 ± 8.86	3.36 ± 8.33	2.56 ± 6.40	0.45 ± 10.28
Nutrients				
Protein (g)	24.58 ± 7.30	19.50 ± 7.51	18.23 ± 8.72	10.03 ± 7.57
Fat (g)	2.75 ± 11.47	2.05 ± 8.65	2.70 ± 12.30	1.78 ± 11.54
Carbohydrate (g)	5.02 ± 2.11	4.10 ± 2.06	3.93 ± 1.71	3.75 ± 1.64
Calorie (kcal)	40.57 ± 7.46	38.04 ± 7.76	35.59 ± 7.62	32.12 ± 8.51
Calcium (mg)	4.89 ± 1.77	4.26 ± 1.46	4.21 ± 1.58	4.07 ± 1.65
Iron (mg)	6.62 ± 6.12	5.83 ± 6.32	1.30 ± 8.09	2.49 ± 4.05
Vitamin A (µg)	512.88 ± 1346.74	235.07 ± 1431.86	−2.97 ± 1338.76	36.01 ± 757.19
Vitamin B (mg)	0.67 ± 0.53	0.54 ± 0.50	0.26 ± 0.41	0.19 ± 0.44
Vitamin C (mg)	26.59 ± 60.05	8.40 ± 63.17	−2.47 ± 64.48	5.98 ± 37.74

TABLE 3 Significance (p-value) of mean change in variables in different prosthetic groups, 6 months from baseline

Comparison	CD vs. RPDD	CD vs. RPDT	CD vs. FPD	RPDD vs. RPDT	RPDD vs. FPD	RPDT vs. FPD	F (3.155DF)	*p*-value
Anthropometric variables								
Weight (kg)	0.010	0.010	<0.001	1.000	0.984	0.992	7.73	<0.001
BMI (kg/m^2)	0.007	0.015	<0.001	0.999	0.973	0.934	8.09	<0.001
Biochemical variables								
S. albumin (g/dl)	0.837	0.809	0.795	1.000	1.000	1.000	0.49	0.690
S. cholesterol (mg/dl)	0.908	0.989	0.913	0.992	0.673	0.851	0.47	0.702
Nutrients								
Protein (g)	0.061	0.013	<0.001	0.954	<0.001	0.003	22.18	<0.001
Fat(g)	0.995	1.000	0.983	0.998	1.000	0.993	0.06	0.982
Carbohydrate (g)	0.275	0.161	0.030	0.993	0.925	0.989	3.37	0.021
Calorie (kcal)	0.606	0.085	<0.001	0.759	0.052	0.443	7.55	<0.001
Calcium (mg)	0.470	0.421	0.156	1.000	0.981	0.992	1.92	0.130
Iron (mg)	0.961	0.008	0.024	0.101	0.249	0.914	5.11	0.002
Vitamin A (µg)	0.832	0.416	0.366	0.933	0.948	1.000	1.29	0.281
Vitamin B (mg)	0.728	0.011	<0.001	0.287	0.083	0.971	7.21	<0.001
Vitamin C (mg)	0.620	0.233	0.415	0.933	0.999	0.959	1.63	0.187

DISCUSSION

Proper nutrition is essential to the health and comfort of oral tissues to enhance the possibility of successful prosthodontic treatment of the elderly. Proper nutritional assessment and suitable dietary advice is often more appropriate in coping with malnutrition than merely instituting prosthodontic therapy.[24]

According to Marshall et al[25] the presence of natural teeth and well-fitting dentures were associated with higher and more varied nutrient intake and greater dietary quality. Muller et al[27] found that complete denture patients had significantly lower ratings regarding difficulty in chewing.

There was a significant improvement in weight and BMI in group CD as compared to the RPDD, RPDT, and FPD groups in this study. Improved mastication, comminution, and absorption from the gastrointestinal tract may be responsible for weight gain in this group; however, in a study conducted by Kanehisa et al[20] conducted 6 months after prosthodontic treatment, body weight changes were significantly different between wearers and nonwearers, regardless

TABLE 4 Mean change in variables in groups categorized according to number of missing teeth 6 months from baseline

Variables	Group 1 (n = 44)	Group 2 (n = 16)	Group 3 (n = 7)
Anthropometric variables			
Weight (kg)	0.28 ± 1.10	0.63 ± 1.64	0.93 ± 1.43
BMI (kg/m^2)	0.13 ± 0.43	0.19 ± 0.63	0.46 ± 0.37
Biochemical variables			
S. albumin (g/dl)	0.04 ± 0.33	0.01 ± 0.25	0.09 ± 0.14
S. cholesterol (mg/dl)	1.63 ± 9.05	1.30 ± 9.34	5.09 ± 4.29
Nutrients			
Protein (g)	12.96 ± 8.91	18.22 ± 7.28	22.17 ± 7.84
Fat (g)	1.73 ± 12.04	1.96 ± 7.17	4.98 ± 10.66
Carbohydrate (g)	3.72 ± 1.59	4.56 ± 2.29	3.56 ± 1.34
Calorie (kcal)	35.02 ± 8.76	35.79 ± 6.15	31.84 ± 10.17
Calcium (mg)	4.08 ± 1.63	4.64 ± 1.50	3.60 ± 0.93
Iron (mg)	2.22 ± 6.12	6.03 ± 6.68	2.44 ± 4.88
Vitamin A (μg)	36.95 ± 1026.54	296.91 ± 913.42	-103.30 ± 2178.05
Vitamin B (mg)	0.22 ± 0.43	0.57 ± 0.47	0.33 ± 0.53
Vitamin C (mg)	2.44 ± 50.81	10.37 ± 41.26	2.16 ± 94.06

Group 1: fewer than 8 missing teeth, group 2: 8 to 18 missing teeth, group 3: more than 18 missing teeth.

TABLE 5 Significance (p-value) of mean changes in variables in groups categorized according to number of missing teeth 6 months from baseline

Comparisons	Group 1 vs. 2	Group 1 vs. 3	Group 2 vs. 3	F (2.64DF)	p-value
Anthropometric variables					
Weight (kg)	0.633	0.434	0.859	1.01	0.370
BMI (kg/m^2)	0.892	0.224	0.454	1.41	0.253
Biochemical variables					
S. albumin (g/dl)	0.956	0.895	0.828	0.17	0.842
S. cholesterol (mg/dl)	0.991	0.601	0.611	0.52	0.599
Nutrients					
Protein (g)	0.092	0.026	0.562	4.93	0.010
Fat (g)	0.997	0.747	0.816	0.27	0.765
Carbohydrate (g)	0.237	0.974	0.428	1.49	0.233
Calorie (kcal)	0.947	0.622	0.554	0.56	0.573
Calcium (mg)	0.431	0.728	0.304	1.29	0.281
Iron (mg)	0.094	0.996	0.408	2.30	0.108
Vitamin A (μg)	0.725	0.953	0.728	0.40	0.675
Vitamin B (mg)	0.024	0.811	0.467	3.65	0.032
Vitamin C (mg)	0.872	1.000	0.941	0.13	0.878

of denture type. Shah et al[8] studied the correlation between oral health parameters and sociodemographic variables, diet, and BMI and found that BMI was not correlated with level of edentulousness. The present findings are in contrast to Sahyoun et al[21] who concluded that edentulous elderly subjects had elevated BMI because they tended to eat foods high in caloric density with a consequent increase in weight. Tsai and Chang[22] found that removable denture wearers had lower self-perceived nutritional status and BMI compared to fixed denture wearers.

Serum albumin values improved after prosthetic rehabilitation, especially in cases of the complete denture prosthesis group, but this was found to be statistically insignificant. Kanehisa et al[20] found that 6 months after prosthodontic treatment, serum albumin level significantly increased among individuals using partial dentures in either or both jaws; however, Wöstmann et al[23] stated that despite significant improvement in masticatory ability after optimization of dentures, no improvement was observed in albumin, zinc, and mininutritional assessment values.

TABLE 6   Mean changes in variables in completely and partially edentulous patients 6 months from baseline

Variables	Complete (CD; n = 52)	Partial (RPDD + RPDT + FPD; n = 67)	t-value (DF = 117)	p-value
Anthropometric variables				
Weight (kg)	1.64 ± 1.45	0.43 ± 1.28	4.84	<0.001
BMI (kg/m^2)	0.66 ± 0.58	0.18 ± 0.48	4.92	<0.001
Biochemical variables				
S. albumin (g/dl)	0.68 ± 4.28	0.04 ± 0.30	1.22	0.225
S. cholesterol (mg/dl)	1.80 ± 8.86	1.91 ± 8.72	0.07	0.946
Nutrients				
Protein (g)	24.58 ± 7.30	15.18 ± 8.95	6.15	<0.001
Fat (g)	2.75 ± 11.47	2.12 ± 10.84	0.30	0.762
Carbohydrate (g)	5.02 ± 2.11	3.90 ± 1.77	3.14	0.002
Calorie (kcal)	40.57 ± 7.46	34.87 ± 8.32	3.88	<0.001
Calcium (mg)	4.89 ± 1.77	4.16 ± 1.55	2.38	0.019
Iron (mg)	6.62 ± 6.12	3.15 ± 6.28	3.02	0.003
Vitamin A (μg)	512.88 ± 1346.74	84.38 ± 1150.49	1.87	0.064
Vitamin B (mg)	0.67 ± 0.53	0.31 ± 0.47	3.87	<0.001
Vitamin C (mg)	26.59 ± 60.05	4.31 ± 53.71	2.13	0.035

TABLE 7   Mean change in variables in removable partial versus fixed partial prosthesis groups 6 months from baseline

Variables	Removable partial (RPDD + RPDT; n = 39)	Fixed partial (FPD; n = 28)	t-value (DF = 65)	p-value
Anthropometric variables				
Weight (kg)	0.49 ± 1.39	0.36 ± 1.11	0.41	0.684
BMI (kg/m^2)	0.21 ± 0.52	0.13 ± 0.43	0.67	0.506
Biochemical variables				
S. albumin (g/dl)	0.02 ± 0.28	0.06 ± 0.33	0.55	0.587
S. cholesterol (mg/dl)	2.97 ± 7.36	0.45 ± 10.28	1.17	0.246
Nutrients				
Protein (g)	18.88 ± 8.04	10.03 ± 7.57	4.55	<0.001
Fat (g)	2.37 ± 10.45	1.78 ± 11.54	0.22	0.829
Carbohydrate (g)	4.02 ± 1.87	3.75 ± 1.64	0.61	0.542
Calorie (kcal)	36.85 ± 7.70	32.12 ± 8.51	2.37	0.021
Calcium (mg)	4.23 ± 1.50	4.07 ± 1.65	0.42	0.674
Iron (mg)	3.62 ± 7.50	2.49 ± 4.05	0.73	0.471
Vitamin A (μg)	119.11 ± 1374.27	36.01 ± 757.19	0.29	0.773
Vitamin B (mg)	0.40 ± 0.47	0.19 ± 0.44	1.81	0.075
Vitamin C (mg)	3.11 ± 63.21	5.98 ± 37.74	0.21	0.831

Improvement in nutrient intake was greater in group CD than groups RPDD, RPDT, and FPD. Krall et al[6] stated that nutrient intakes of men who had teeth replaced with RPDs were comparable to those of men with intact dentition and consistently better than those of men with missing unreplaced teeth or full dentures.

We found significant improvement in protein intake in the CD group compared to the RPDT and FPD groups. This may be because non-rehabilitated edentulous individuals prefer soft diet, high in carbohydrates and low in protein.

The mean change in carbohydrates and calorie intake was significantly higher in group CD compared to group FPD. A study by Seman et al[15] showed that "elderly subjects with good dentures (noncompromised functional dentition) seemed to have a better chance of having adequate calorie intake as compared to those without dentures or with defective dentures (compromised functional dentition)." In addition, Lamster[16] and Walton et al[17] supported the fact that defective and ill-fitting dentures adversely affect chewing efficiency. Hence, adequacy of dental prostheses in an

TABLE 8   Mean change in variables in removable prosthesis versus fixed prosthesis groups 6 months from baseline

Variables	Removable (CD + RPDD + RPDT) (n = 91)	Fixed partial (FPD) (n = 28)	t-value (DF = 117)	p-value
Anthropometric variables				
Weight (kg)	1.15 ± 1.53	0.36 ± 1.11	2.53	0.013
BMI (kg/m^2)	0.47 ± 0.60	0.13 ± 0.43	2.76	0.007
Biochemical variables				
S. albumin (g/dl)	0.40 ± 3.25	0.06 ± 0.33	0.54	0.588
S. cholesterol (mg/dl)	2.30 ± 8.23	0.45 ± 10.28	0.98	0.328
Nutrients				
Protein (g)	22.14 ± 8.10	10.03 ± 7.57	7.02	<0.001
Fat (g)	2.58 ± 10.98	1.78 ± 11.54	0.33	0.738
Carbohydrate (g)	4.59 ± 2.06	3.75 ± 1.64	1.98	0.050
Calorie (kcal)	38.98 ± 7.74	32.12 ± 8.51	4.00	<0.001
Calcium (mg)	4.61 ± 1.68	4.07 ± 1.65	1.49	0.138
Iron (mg)	5.33 ± 6.87	2.49 ± 4.05	2.08	0.040
Vitamin A (μg)	344.12 ± 1365.13	36.01 ± 757.19	1.14	0.257
Vitamin B (mg)	0.55 ± 0.52	0.19 ± 0.44	3.31	0.001
Vitamin C (mg)	16.52 ± 62.18	5.98 ± 37.74	0.85	0.398

edentulous person is important for an optimal nutritional status.[18] This study differed from Papas et al[19] who reported that people with compete dentures consumed fewer calories and lower levels of several specific nutrients than did those who had partial dentures or natural dentition.

Mean intake of calcium was significantly improved in all groups. Sheiham et al[26] associated higher calcium intake with the presence of natural teeth and increased number of natural teeth. In this study, vitamins A and C uptake did not increase significantly among different prosthetic groups. Greksa et al[28] concluded that full denture wearers consumed significantly lower levels of vitamins A and C than did dentate people.

This study concluded that consumption of fruits, vegetables, and salads increased after rehabilitation with all prostheses provided. Tsai and Chang[22] said that nondenture and removable denture wearers had poorer masticatory ability and greater nutritional risk. Such subjects consumed fruits and vegetable less often compared to fixed denture wearers.

Reduction in number of teeth was associated with poor diet quality among older adults in this study. Hildebrandt et al[29] observed that number of functional units (any opposing pair of natural or fixed prosthetic teeth) was related to food avoidance and difficulties in chewing. Sahyoun et al,[21] Shinkai et al,[30] and Sheiham et al[26] examined the role of missing posterior functional units in relation to dietary intake of specific nutrients and overall diet quality. The fewer teeth an individual had, the more likely he or she had a compromised nutritional status.

Results revealed significant increase in weight, BMI, protein, carbohydrate, calorie, iron, and vitamin B in the removable prosthesis group compared to the fixed prosthesis

group. This differed from a study by Tsai and Chang[22] who found that nondenture and removable denture wearers had poorer masticatory ability and greater nutritional risk compared to fixed denture wearers.

The main limitation of this study was the method used to evaluate the intake of energy and nutrients from standard portions. This may not be exact enough to detect small changes. Moreover, all dietary data were self-reported. An improvement in dietary habits might also be ascribed to an increased interest in diet as a result of participating in the study. Further study is required for evaluating changes in the given parameters with a longer follow-up period and more participants.

CONCLUSIONS

Within the limitations of this study, the following conclusions could be drawn:

1. The improvement in diet was highest in rehabilitated completely edentulous participants followed by participants with distal extension RPDs and toothsupported RPD and least in participants with FPDs.
2. Significant improvement in body weight, BMI, protein, carbohydrate, calorie, calcium, iron, and vitamins B and C in completely edentulous participants was seen compared to partially edentulous participants.
3. A significant increase in body weight, BMI, protein, carbohydrate, calorie, iron, and vitamin B in patients rehabilitated by removable prostheses was seen compared to fixed prostheses.

4. Among partially edentulous patients, protein and calorie intake increased significantly in individuals rehabilitated by RPDs compared to FPDs.

This study emphasized that prosthetic rehabilitation becomes increasingly important as the level of edentulism increases to improve dietary, anthropometric, and biochemical parameters.

REFERENCES

1. Barone JV: Nutrition-phase one of the edentulous patient. *J Prosthet Dent* 1978;40:122–126.

2. Lee JS, Weyant RJ, Corby P, et al: Edentulism and nutritional status in abiracial sample of well-functioning, communitydwelling elderly: the Health, Aging, and Body Composition Study. *Am J Clin Nutr* 2004;79:295–302.

3. Pla GSW: Oral health and nutrition. *Prim Care* 1994;21:121–133.

4. Whitehead C, Finucane P: Malnutrition in elderly people. *Aust NZ J Med* 1997;27:68–74.

5. Wells JV, Dumbrell AC: Nutrition and aging: assessment and treatment of compromised nutritional status in frail elderly patients. *Clin Interv Aging* 2006;1:67–79.

6. Krall E, Hayes C, Garcia R: How dentition status and masticatory function affect nutrient intake. *J Am Dent Assoc* 1998;129:1261–1269.

7. Palmer CA. Gerodontic nutrition and dietary counseling for prosthodontic patients. *Den Clin North Am* 2003;47:355–371.

8. Shah N, Parkash H, Sunderam KR: Edentulousness, denture wear and denture needs of Indian elderly-a community-based study. *J Oral Rehabil* 2004;31:467–476.

9. Pfeiffer E: A short portable mental status questionnaire for the assessment of organic brain deficit in elderly patients. *J Am Geriatr Soc* 1975;23:433–441.

10. Planning Commission Further Lowers Poverty Line to Rs. 28/Day. India Today, March 19, 2012. New Delhi, India. Available online at http://indiatoday.intoday.in/story/india-poverty-line-now-lowered-to-rs-28-per-day/1/178483.html. Accessed June 13, 2014.

11. Goldstein MG: Pharmacotherapy for smoking cessation. In Abrams DB, Niaura R, Brown RA, et al (eds): *The Tobacco Dependence Treatment Handbook: A Guide to Best Practice.* New York, Guilford Press, 2003, pp. 230–248.

12. *Diagnostic and Statistical Manual of Mental Disorders*, ed 4 Washington, DC, American Psychiatric Association, 2000.

13. DSM-IV Criteria for Alcohol Abuse and Alcohol Dependence. Available online at http://www.alcoholcostcalculator.org/business/about/dsm.html Reference for the whole section. Accessed June 13, 2014.

14. Gopalan C, Rama Sastri BV, Balasubramanian SC: *Nutritive Value of Indian Foods. Revised and updated by Narasinga Rao BS, Deosthale YG, and Pant KC.* Hyderabad, National Institute of Nutrition, 1996.

15. Seman K, Manaf HA, Ismail AR: Association between functional dentition with inadequate calorie intake and underweight in elderly people living in "Pondok" in Kelantan. *Arch Orofac Sci* 2007;2:10–19.

16. Lamster IB: Oral health care services for older adults: a looming crisis. *J Am Public Health* 2004;94:699–702.

17. Walton JC, Miller J, Tordecilla L: Elder oral assessment and care. *Medsurg Nursing* 2001;10:37–44.

18. Brodeur JM, Laurine D, Vallee R, et al: Nutrient intake and gastrointestinal disorders related to masticatory performance in the edentulous elderly. *J Prosthet Dent* 1993;70:468–473.

19. Papas AS, Palmer CA, Rounds MC, et al: Longitudinal relationships between nutrition and oral health. *Ann NY Acad Sci* 1989;561:124–142.

20. Kanehisa Y, Yoshida M, Taji T, et al: Body weight and serum albumin change after prosthodontic treatment among institutionalized elderly in a long-term care geriatric hospital. *Community Dent Oral Epidemiol* 2009;37:534–538.

21. Sahyoun NR, Lin CL, Krall E: Nutritional status of the older adult is associated with dentition status. *J Am Diet Assoc* 2003;103:61–66.

22. Tsai AC, Chang TL: Association of dental prosthetic condition with food consumption and the risk of malnutrition and follow-up 4-year mortality risk in elderly Taiwanese. *J Nutr Health Aging* 2011;15:265–270.

23. Wöstmann B, Michel K, Brinkert B, et al: Influence of denture improvement on the nutritional status and quality of life of geriatric patients. *J Dent* 2008;36:816–821.

24. N'Gom P, Woda A: Influence of impaired mastication on nutrition. *J Prosthet Dent* 2002;87:667–673.

25. Marshall TA, Warren JJ, Hand JS, et al: Oral health, nutrient intake and dietary quality in the very old. *J Am Dent Assoc* 2002;133:1369–1379.

26. Sheiham A, Steele JG, Marcenes W, et al: The relationship among dental status, nutrient intake, and nutritional status in older people. *J Dent Res* 2001;80:408–413.

27. Muller K, Morais J, Feine J: Nutritional and anthropometric analysis of edentulous patients wearing implant overdentures or conventional dentures. *Braz Dent J* 2008;19:145–150.

28. Greksa LP, Parraga IM, Clark CA: The dietary adequacy of edentulous older adults. *J Prosthet Dent* 1995;73:142–145.

29. Hildebrandt GH, Dominguez BL, Schork MA, et al: Functional units, chewing, swallowing, and food avoidance among the elderly. *J Prosthet Dent* 1997;77:588–595.

30. Shinkai RSA, Hatch JP, Sakai S, et al: Oral function and diet quality in a community-based sample. *J Dent Res* 2001;80:1625–1630.

7

CONVENTIONAL REHABILITATION OF EDENTULOUS PATIENTS: THE IMPACT ON ORAL HEALTH-RELATED QUALITY OF LIFE AND PATIENT SATISFACTION

JANICE S. ELLIS, PHD, BDS, FDS RCS, PGCE,[1] NANITA D. PELEKIS, DDP, MSC,[2] AND J. MARK THOMASON, PHD, BDS, FDS RCS[3]

[1]Senior Lecturer, School of Dental Sciences, University of Newcastle upon Tyne, UK
[2]Postgraduate Student, School of Dental Sciences, University of Newcastle upon Tyne, UK
[3]Professor, School of Dental Sciences, University of Newcastle upon Tyne, UK

Keywords
Edentulism; conventional dentures; duplicate dentures; OHIP-20; satisfaction

Correspondence
Janice S. Ellis, PhD, BDS, FDS RCS, PGCE, School of Dental Sciences, Framlington Place, Newcastle upon Tyne, NE2 4BW, United Kingdom. E-mail: j.s.ellis@ncl.ac.uk

Accepted August 25, 2005

Published in *Journal of Prosthodontics* 2007; Vol. 16, Issue 1, pp. 37–42

doi: 10.1111/j.1532-849X.2006.00152.x

ABSTRACT

Purpose: This study examined patient satisfaction and oral health-related impacts on the quality of life of patients restored with complete conventional or duplicate dentures.

Materials and Methods: Forty patients (aged 55 to 85 years) were assigned to receive new complete maxillary and mandibular dentures using either a conventional or duplication technique according to clinical need. Patients rated their satisfaction with their dentures on 100-mm visual analogue scales before treatment and 1 month after delivery of their new dentures. Their oral health-related quality of life was determined by completion of an Oral Health-Related Impacts on Quality of Life questionnaire (OHIP-20) at the same time points.

Results: Both groups of patients had similar satisfaction and OHIP ratings at the beginning of the study and 1 month after delivery of their new dentures. The two groups were comparable with regard to age and gender. Statistically significant improvement in the OHIP domains of functional limitation and physical and psychological disability was seen in both groups. The conventional group also showed significant improvement with regard to handicap, whereas the duplicate denture group showed significant improvement in the patients' rating of pain and psychological discomfort. Patient satisfaction improved significantly in both groups across all variables except ease of cleaning and ability to speak. The duplication technique resulted in patients being less satisfied with the esthetics of their new dentures.

Conclusion: In this study, the provision of new dentures either with a conventional technique or with a duplication technique resulted in an overall improvement in oral health-related quality of life and satisfaction. These improvements were statistically significant for some domains, which varied depending on the technique used for construction of the new dentures. Neither technique was seen to be superior, which may be a reflection of the patients' treatment expectations at the outset. Patients' reported satisfaction with their dentures and the impact that dentures have on their quality of life may not be useful measures for determining the most appropriate technique for providing new dentures.

Studies have shown that there is a poor correlation between patient satisfaction and clinical variables[1] and that clinicians' assessment of the quality of denture-supporting tissues are poor predictors of patients' satisfaction.[2] Prosthodontists and patients also show poor agreement when it comes to the evaluation of individual prostheses.[3] Traditionally, clinicians have assessed prostheses using predetermined criteria for success which usually do not take into account the needs and attitudes of individual patients, for example, resistance to displacement away from the tissues and balanced occlusion.[4,5] The primary goal in therapies for chronic conditions such as edentulism is improvement in that condition rather than cure, and therefore it is patient-based outcomes that are most important.[4]

Parameters such as the patient's personality, the relationship between patient and dentist, and the attitude toward new dentures appear to be significant for determining satisfaction when providing new dentures.[6] Success with complete dentures depends largely on the patient's capacity to surmount the many limitations of dentures by the process of habituation.[7,8] The notion that duplicating favorable features of the patient's previous dentures and in particular, the polished surface shape, would facilitate this adaptation process has resulted in the development of duplication techniques.[9,10] The evidence to support this belief is limited, and much is based on clinical observation.[11]

When considering elective treatment, the use of patient-centered outcomes is of particular importance.[12] Patients' satisfaction with their dentures is likely to be affected by their ability to perform certain tasks with them.[13] In these instances the use of patient satisfaction as a primary outcome is appropriate.[14] Feine et al have written, "patient satisfaction with therapy is likely to be the distinguishing outcome of many treatments for chronic diseases for which living with treatment is a more realistic objective than cure."[15] The problems patients encounter with dentures impact on their quality of life, and as these issues are at the forefront of public health policy, their consideration is pertinent.

Patient satisfaction and oral health-related quality-of-life instruments have been developed for use in clinical settings and studies. A validated patient satisfaction instrument has been developed by asking both patients and prosthodontists to list and rank factors they felt determined the success of complete dentures.[16,17] Several studies investigating implant-supported prostheses have used both this and quality-of-life measures to describe the effects of rehabilitation of edentulous patients using implants.[18–20]

Quality-of-life measures assess the impact of disease on peoples' quality of life.[21–23] The OHIP subjective indicator, developed and validated by Slade and Spencer, has been used in many clinical trials.[24–26] The OHIP-20 comprises 20 statements grouped in seven subscales and involves questions concerning the functional limitation, the physical and psychological discomfort, the physical and psychological disability, the social effect of denture wearing on the individual's everyday life, and finally, the degree of handicap. The answers are given by the patients in a Likert response format.[26]

Studies in edentulous subjects strongly support the concept that patient-based measures are more sensitive than functional measures for detecting differences between treatments.[16,17,27]

The aim of the current study was to assess the impact of new complete dentures made by conventional and duplication techniques on patient satisfaction and oral health-related quality of life, the null hypothesis being that neither treatment method will be superior.

MATERIALS AND METHODS

The study, which had received appropriate ethical approval, was undertaken within the Prosthodontic Unit of the School of Dental Sciences in Newcastle University. Patients were seen in a restorative diagnostic clinic where they were examined and placed on a predoctoral student waiting list. Patients were assigned to students for the replacement of existing dentures using either a conventional or a duplication technique.

Using data from a previous study, it was estimated that 20 patients per group would provide 80% power to detect an effect size of 0.86, assuming a type I error rate of 0.05.

TABLE 1 **Inclusion Criteria**

- Age between 55 and 85 years
- Edentulous for more than 5 years
- Currently wearing upper and lower complete dentures
- No known history of temporomandibular joint disorders or clenching
- Able to understand and respond to the instruments

Patients were invited to take part if, during their first appointment, they fulfilled the inclusion criteria given in Table 1.

Patients were provided with full written information, and written consent was obtained. Sociodemographic data, including age and gender, were collected. A standardized denture assessment was undertaken under the following headings: occlusal surfaces, polished surfaces, retention, and stability. Patients were asked to rate their level of general satisfaction with their dentures, and then as separate entities, comfort and stability, ability to chew, clean, and speak with their prostheses. This was marked on a 100-mm visual analogue scale (anchored by the words "completely dissatisfied" at one end of the scale to "completely satisfied" at the other end). They also completed an OHIP-20 instrument.

Administration of these instruments was undertaken by the author (NDP), who was not involved with treatment. Data were collected using custom-made data collection sheets. They were completed by the subjects and verified by the author.

Conventional and duplication dentures were provided using standard hospital protocols.

Patients were reviewed, and minor adjustments were made to their dentures as required. When no further adjustment was required or indicated, patients were asked to return for a further review 1 month later. At this visit they were asked to repeat the two instruments.

Data were transcribed onto a spreadsheet and analyzed with available statistical packages (SPSS, SPSS Inc., Chicago, IL). The mean and the SD were calculated as summary statistics for all variables. Between-group variations of the principal outcome measures of patient satisfaction and OHIP scores were tested with independent two sample t-test. The within-group variables were compared using the paired t-test.

RESULTS

Forty-nine patients were recruited to the study, of which 29 received conventional dentures. Nine patients from the conventional denture group were lost from the study; 5 failed to return; 2 were unable to return for health reasons; and 2 refused to complete the second questionnaire. All the 20 patients who received duplicate dentures completed the study.

There was no significant difference between groups for age $(p = 0.665$; conventional group mean age 74.2 ± 7.29 years, duplicate denture group 73.1 ± 8.61 years) or gender distribution $(p = 0.514)$.

The pre- and posttreatment patient satisfaction scores and OHIP-20 ratings of the two groups are shown in Tables 2 and 3. There was no significant difference between the groups at the start of treatment $(p > 0.05)$.

Both groups showed an improvement across all aspects of the patient satisfaction instrument. With the exception of ease of cleaning and the speaking ability scores, the improvements were all significant. OHIP-20 ratings showed a similar trend with improvements across all domains except social disability in the duplicate group. In the conventional group improvements were significant for functional limitation, physical disability, psychological disability, and handicap. In the duplicate group, functional limitation, pain, psychological discomfort, and physical and psychological disability demonstrated significant improvement. Nevertheless, posttreatment, the two groups had similar ratings for satisfaction and OHIP-20 $(p > 0.05)$.

The pre- and posttreatment changes for satisfaction and OHIP-20 scores are shown in Table 4. The only area in which one treatment offered a significant advantage over the other was with regard to handicap, where the conventional group

TABLE 2 **Pre- and Posttreatment Patient Satisfaction Scores for Both Groups with p Values for Within-Group Difference**

Variables	Conventional Group–Mean (SD)			Duplicate Group–Mean (SD)		
	Pretreatment	Posttreatment	p Value	Pretreatment	Posttreatment	p Value
Ease of cleaning	83 (27)	89 (11)	0.34	88 (22)	90 (7)	0.58
General satisfaction	33 (41)	63 (28)	**0.014**	39 (40)	77 (26)	**0.001**
Speaking ability	64 (36)	75 (27)	0.19	73 (36)	86 (14)	0.165
Comfort	20 (31)	62 (30)	**0.000**	42 (41)	68 (32)	**0.010**
Esthetics	53 (43)	77 (21)	**0.041**	57 (38)	38 (19)	**0.007**
Stability	32 (52)	68 (25)	**0.000**	29 (35)	60 (33)	**0.007**
Chewing ability	32 (36)	64 (32)	**0.004**	34 (35)	62 (33)	**0.005**

$p \leq 0.05$ shown in bold.

TABLE 3   Pre- and Posttreatment OHIP-20 Scores for Both Groups with *p* Values for Within-Group Difference

Variables	Conventional Group–Mean (SD)			Duplicate Group–Mean (SD)		
	Pretreatment	Posttreatment	p Value	Pretreatment	Posttreatment	p Value
Functional limitation	13.10 (3.74)	9.85 (4.20)	**0.03**	12.25 (4.22)	8.45 (3.76)	**0.01**
Pain	15.25 (5.09)	12.90 (5.26)	0.14	14.70 (6.52)	10.90 (4.69)	**0.03**
Psychological discomfort	6.55 (3.59)	5.30 (2.72)	0.13	6.22 (4.00)	4.70 (2.32)	**0.10**
Physical disability	14.55 (5.75)	10.00 (4.71)	**0.005**	12.55 (6.29)	8.90 (4.17)	**0.01**
Psychological disability	6.85 (3.32)	4.25 (2.74)	**0.001**	6.05 (3.65)	4.05 (1.93)	**0.01**
Social disability	6.15 (4.23)	4.95 (2.01)	0.27	4.50 (2.35)	5.00 (2.03)	0.38
Handicap	5.45 (3.40)	3.30 (1.42)	**0.01**	3.95 (2.24)	3.65 (1.95)	0.69

$p \leq 0.05$ shown in bold.

TABLE 4   Between-Group Comparison of Pre- and Posttreatment Changes in Patient Satisfaction and OHIP-20

Variable	Posttreatment Change in Patient Satisfaction–Mean (SD)			Variable	Posttreatment Change in OHIP-20–Mean (SD)		
	Conventional	Duplicate	p Value		Conventional	Duplicate	p Value
Ease of cleaning	6 (29)	3 (20)	0.63	Functional limitation	−3.25 (6.20)	−3.80 (5.91)	0.81
General satisfaction	30 (49)	38 (46)	0.60	Pain	−2.35 (6.88)	−3.80 (7.15)	0.52
Speaking ability	12 (38)	13 (39)	0.92	Psychological discomfort	−1.25 (3.57)	−1.50 (3.93)	0.41
Comfort	42 (40)	26 (42)	0.25	Physical disability	−4.50 (6.38)	−3.60 (5.90)	0.30
Esthetics	24 (48)	−24 (35)	0.10	Psychological disability	−2.60 (2.96)	−2.00 (3.18)	0.09
Stability	45 (36)	31 (46)	0.28	Social disability	−1.20 (4.73)	0.50 (2.46)	0.08
Chewing ability	32 (44)	27 (31)	0.71	Handicap	−2.15 (3.42)	−0.30 (3.31)	**0.05**

$p < 0.05$ shown in bold.

demonstrated a significantly greater improvement over the duplicate group.

DISCUSSION

In this study, all denture treatments were undertaken by predoctoral dental students. The outcome of treatment was analyzed after only 1 month of function. Other studies using the same patient satisfaction instrument have reviewed patients treated by experienced clinicians 2 and 6 months posttreatment. Similar pre- and posttreatment patient satisfaction scores for patients receiving conventional replacement dentures were reported.[16] The similarity of these results suggests that the use of a shortened review period to determine pre- and posttreatment changes in patient satisfaction is appropriate. The only exception to this is the improvement in speaking ability.

The compliance of patients recruited to the duplicate group was 100%, whereas nearly one-third of patients in the conventional denture group were lost (9 of the original 29 patients). This represents an area of weakness in the study. Five of the "lost patients" failed to return for 1-month review. It is possible to interpret this in one of two ways; either these

patients were entirely satisfied with their replacement dentures, or alternatively, they were totally dissatisfied and did not wish to waste more time. An additional two patients were unable to return due to ill health, and the last two refused to complete the second set of questionnaires. It is interesting that the nine who failed to complete the study were from the conventional denture group. The reasons for the differences between the two groups are unclear and purely speculative, but may be related to patients' previous interactions with the dental profession.

In this nonrandomized study, there was no significant difference in satisfaction or OHIP-20 between the two treatment groups at the beginning of treatment. There was, however, a trend that the conventional group had higher OHIP-20 and lower patient satisfaction scores pretreatment as compared with the duplicate denture group. An assumption was made that the patients allocated to the duplicate group had dentures that demonstrated a higher degree of technical "correctness" as assessed by the referring clinician. A consultant in restorative dentistry allocated the patients within this study to treatment groups, and criteria for allocation were not recorded. A subjective analysis of the degree of clinical correctness of the current denture and the clinician's perceived level of patient satisfaction is, however, likely to have influenced their decision. Nevertheless, the previous findings of Heydecke,[2,3] suggest that a clinician's assessment of dentures is a poor predictor of patients' satisfaction. The pretreatment differences demonstrated in this study were not significant when assessed by patient-based measures.

Both groups showed significant increase in all aspects of the patient satisfaction instrument, apart from ease of cleaning and speaking ability, and for the duplicate group, esthetics. The first finding was to be expected as this domain was included in order to provide quality control for the instrument and confirmed that patients could use a visual analogue scale. When the techniques for duplicating dentures were first described, one of the advantages of the technique was claimed to be its ability to reproduce the polished surface shape of the previous dentures and therefore facilitate the adaptive process.[9,10] It was therefore not surprising that no significant changes in the ability to speak were seen, when the polished surface shape had been duplicated in the duplicate dentures. However, speech is a complex skill requiring prolonged adaptation to changes in polished surface shape, thus the lack of significant improvement may very well be due to a shorter review period. Similar failure to see significant improvements in speech has been reported in other studies at early review,[27] whereas studies using a 6-month review period demonstrated significant differences pre- and posttreatment with conventional dentures.[28,29]

A significant decrease in the patients' satisfaction with their duplicate denture esthetics is less easy to understand. Maintenance of the polished surface shape and incisal plane position may have resulted in a degree of disappointment if there was an expectation of change that did not materialize. Alternatively, limitations of the duplication technique may have resulted in inadvertent increase in vertical dimension and, in particular, a lowering of the incisal plane in the maxillary arch.[30]

Both groups also showed an improvement trend across all domains of the OHIP-20 instrument except for social disability in the duplicate group. The magnitude of improvements tended to be greater for the duplicate group in relation to functional limitation, pain, and psychological discomfort. It is suggested that patients attending for replacement of previously satisfactory dentures largely do so because the dentures have become uncomfortable/painful due to ongoing alveolar resorption, poor tissue adaptation, and a tendency toward overextension. Correction of only the fitting surface with duplicate dentures should result in reestablishment of correct extensions and good tissue adaptation. This should reduce pain and functional limitations that occur as a result of pain. Patients wearing dentures that have no beneficial qualities are more likely to experience impacts on their quality of life relating to actual disability. Correction of all aspects is more likely to produce a greater level of improvement in conventional dentures than is seen with duplication techniques.

The differences between treatments were only significant in relation to handicap where the conventional approach appeared to offer advantages over the duplication technique.

There is a belief held by many prosthodontists that patients will adapt better to duplicated dentures, and yet, comparison of the conventional and duplication technique with regard to the number of reviews required shows no difference related to technique.[31] It is also debatable as to what extent the duplication technique is limited in its ability to truly duplicate the previous denture.[30]

Patients' interpretation of the difficulties they experience with their dentures is inherently personal and therefore highly subjective. For comparison, they only have to recall their own dentate or partially dentate state, or their perception of how others manage their complete dentures.

Analysis of patients' satisfaction with dentures and/or the impact dentures have on their oral health-related quality of life is perhaps related more to the extent of their acceptance of denture limitations than it is to the technical correctness of their dentures. What one patient accepts as a normal level of discomfort or handicap, may to another be unbearable. Ultimately, both groups reported improvements in their perception of their oral condition as recorded by the posttreatment satisfaction and OHIP scores. While both techniques offer improvements for deficient aspects of the patients' current dentures, they were both unable to alter the patients' level of acceptance of the generic shortcomings of complete dentures.

CONCLUSIONS

One month after delivery, the edentulous patients in this study who received maxillary and mandibular complete dentures using either conventional or duplication techniques showed similar improvements in terms of overall patient satisfaction and oral health-related quality of life. These improvements were statistically significant for some domains and varied depending on the technique used for construction of the new dentures.

Patients' reported satisfaction with their dentures and the impact dentures had on their quality of life might not be useful measures for determining the most appropriate technique for providing new dentures.

REFERENCES

1. van Waas MA: The influence of clinical variables on patient satisfaction with complete dentures. *J Prosthet Dent* 1990;63:307–310.
2. Heydecke G, Locker D, Awad MA, et al: Oral and general health-related quality of life with conventional and implant dentures. *Community Dent Oral Epidemiol* 2003;31:161–168.

3. Heydecke G, Klemetti E, Awad MA, et al: Relationship between prosthodontic evaluation and patient ratings of mandibular conventional and implant prostheses. *Int J Prosthodont* 2003;16:307–312.

4. Silverman WA: Doing more good than harm. *Ann N Y Acad Sci* 1993;703:5–11.

5. Stephens RJ, Hopwood P, Girling DJ, et al: Randomized trials with quality of life endpoints: are doctors' ratings of patients' physical symptoms interchangeable with patients' self-ratings? *Qual Life Res* 1997;6:225–236.

6. Sheiham A, Steele JG, Marcenes W, et al: The impact of oral health on stated ability to eat certain foods; findings from the national diet and nutrition surveyofolder people in Great Britain. *Gerodontology* 1999;16:11–20.

7. Carlsson GE: Clinical morbidityand sequelae of treatment with complete dentures. *J Prosthet Dent* 1998;79:17–23.

8. Langer A, Michman J, Seifert I: Factors influencing satisfaction with complete dentures in geriatric patients. *J Prosthet Dent* 1961;11:1019–1031.

9. Chick AO: The copying of full dentures. *Dent Practit* 1962;13:96–98.

10. Liddelow KP: The prosthetic treatment of the elderly. *Br Dent J* 1964;117:307–315.

11. Anderson JD: The need for criteria on reporting treatment outcomes. *J Prosthet Dent* 1998;79:49–55.

12. Carlsson GE, Otterland A, Wennstrom A, et al: Patient factors in appreciation of complete dentures. *J Prosthet Dent* 1967;17:322–328.

13. Feine JS, Awad MA, Lund JP: The impact of patient preference on the design and interpretation of clinical trials. *Community Dent Oral Epidemiol* 1998;26:70–74.

14. Weaver M, Patrick DL, Markson LE, et al: Issues in the measurement of satisfaction with treatment. *Am J Manag Care* 1997;3:579–594.

15. Feine JS, Carlsson GE, Awad MA, et al: The McGill consensus statement on overdentures. Mandibular two-implant overdentures as first choice standard ofcare for edentulous patients. *Gerodontology* 2002;19:3–4.

16. Feine JS, de Grandmont P, Boudrias P, et al: Withinsubject comparisons of implant-supported mandibular prostheses: choice of prosthesis. *J Dent Res* 1994;73:1105–1111.

17. Feine JS, Maskawi K, de Grandmont P, et al: Withinsubject comparisons of implant-supported mandibular prostheses: evaluation of masticatory function. *J Dent Res* 1994;73:1646–1656.

18. Thomason JM, Lund JP, Chehade A, et al: Patient satisfaction with mandibular implant overdentures and conventional dentures 6 months after delivery. *Int J Prosthodont* 2003;16:467–473.

19. Allen F, Locker D: A modified short version of the oral health impact profile for assessing health-related quality oflife in edentulous adults. *Int J Prosthodont* 2002;15:446–450.

20. Atchison KA, Dolan TA: Development of the geriatric oral health assessment index. *J Dent Educ* 1990;54:680–687.

21. Deber RB: Physicians in health care management: 7. The patient-physician partnership: changing roles and the desire for information. *CMAJ* 1994;151:171–176.

22. Allen PF, McMillan AS: The impact of tooth loss in a denture wearing population: an assessment using the oral health impact profile. *Community Dent Health* 1999;16:176–180.

23. Allen PF, McMillan AS, Locker D: An assessment ofsensitivity to change of the oral health impact profile in a clinical trial. *Community Dent Oral Epidemiol* 2001;29:175–182.

24. Slade GD, Spencer AJ: Development and evaluation of the oral health impact profile. *Community Dent Health* 1994;11:3–11.

25. Allen PF, Locker D: Do item weights matter? An assessment using the oral health impact profile. *Community Dent Health* 1997;14:133–138.

26. de Grandmont P, Feine JS, Tache R, et al: Within-subject comparisons of implant-supported mandibular prostheses: psychometric evaluation. *J Dent Res* 1994;73:1096–1104.

27. Awad MA, Lund JP, Shapiro SH, et al: Oral health status and treatment satisfaction with mandibular implant overdentures and conventional dentures: a randomised clinical trial in a senior population. *Int J Prosthodont* 2003;16:390–396.

28. Muller F, Hasse-Sander I, Hupfauf L: Studies on adaptation to complete dentures. Part I. Oral and manual motor ability. *J Oral Rehabil* 1995;22:501–507.

29. Muller F, Heath MR, Ott R: Maximum bite force after the replacement of complete dentures. *Gerodontology* 2001;18:58–62.

30. Clark RK, Radford DR, Fenlon MR: The future ofteaching ofcomplete denture construction to undergraduates in the UK: is a replacement denture technique the answer? *Br Dent J* 2004;196:571–575.

31. Davis DM, Watson RM: A retrospective study comparing duplication and conventionally made complete dentures for a group of elderly people. *Br Dent J* 1993;175:57–60.

8

DENTURES ARE A RESERVOIR FOR RESPIRATORY PATHOGENS

Lindsay E. O'Donnell, bsc,[1] Karen Smith, bsc, phd,[2] Craig Williams, mb, md,[2] Chris J. Nile, bsc, phd,[1] David F. Lappin, bsc, phd,[1] David Bradshaw, bsc, phd,[3] Margaret Lambert, bsc, msc,[3] Douglas P. Robertson, phd, bds (hons), mfds, fhea,[1] Jeremy Bagg, phd, fds, frcpath, ffph,[1] Victoria Hannah, bsc, bds, phd,[1] and Gordon Ramage, bsc, phd, frcpath[1]

[1]*Infection and Immunity Research Group, Glasgow Dental School, School of Medicine, College of Medical, Veterinary and Life Sciences, University of Glasgow, UK*
[2]*Institute of Healthcare Associated Infection, School of Health, Nursing and Midwifery, University of the West of Scotland, Paisley, UK*
[3]*GlaxoSmithKline, Weybridge, Surrey, UK*

Keywords
Denture plaque; Staphylococcus aureus; Pseudomonas aeruginosa; respiratory; biofilm

Correspondence
Gordon Ramage, Infection and Immunity Research Group, Glasgow Dental School, School of Medicine, College of Medical, Veterinary and Life Sciences, University of Glasgow, 378 Sauchiehall Street, Glasgow, G2 3JZ, UK. E-mail: gordon.ramage@glasgow.ac.uk

Conflict of Interest Statement: We thank the BBSRC and GlaxoSmithKline for supporting the PhD studentship of Lindsey O'Donnell. We also thank the Royal College of Physicians and Surgeons of Glasgow for awarding Victoria Hannah the TC White Prize to support this work. Authors David Bradshaw and Margaret Lambert are employees of GlaxoSmithKline.

Accepted May 5, 2015

Published in *Journal of Prosthodontics* 2016; Vol. 25, pp. 99–104

doi: 10.1111/jopr.12342

ABSTRACT

Purpose: Recent studies have established a relationship between dental plaque and pulmonary infection, particularly in elderly individuals. Given that approximately one in five adults in the UK currently wears a denture, there remains a gap in our understanding of the direct implications of denture plaque on systemic health. The aim of this study was to undertake a comprehensive evaluation of putative respiratory pathogens residing upon dentures using a targeted quantitative molecular approach.

Materials and Methods: One hundred and thirty patients' dentures were sonicated to remove denture plaque biofilm from the surface. DNA was extracted from the samples and was assessed for the presence of respiratory pathogens by qunatitative polymerase chain reaction (qPCR). Ct values were then used to approximate the number of corresponding colony forming equivalents (CFEs) based on standard curves.

Results: Of the dentures, 64.6% were colonized by known respiratory pathogens. Six species were identified: *Streptococcus aureus, Streptococcus pneumoniae, Pseudomonas aeruginosa, Haemophilus influenzae B, Streptococcus pyogenes*, and *Moraxella catarrhalis*. *P. aeruginosa* was the most abundant species followed by *S. pneumoniae* and *S. aureus* in terms of average CFE and overall proportion of denture plaque. Of the participants, 37% suffered from denture stomatitis; however, there were no significant differences in the prevalence of respiratory pathogens on dentures between healthy and inflamed mouths.

Conclusions: Our findings indicate that dentures can act as a reservoir for potential respiratory pathogens in the oral cavity, thus increasing the theoretical risk of developing aspiration pneumonia. Implementation of routine denture hygiene practices could help to reduce the risk of respiratory infection among the elderly population.

Globally, 810 million people are aged 60 years or over, a figure that is expected to reach two billion by 2050 (22% of the entire global population).[1] With this ever-increasing elderly population, there will inevitably be greater challenges for both systemic and oral health care delivery. Clear associations between oral and systemic disease have been reported, for example with rheumatoid arthritis, cardiovascular disease, and respiratory infection.[2,3] Many of these aging individuals will experience a general decline in oral health. Current estimates suggest that around 20% of the US and UK population wear some form of removable denture.[4,5] Dentures have been shown to support the growth of biofilms known as denture plaque, which are complex polymicrobial consortia of bacteria, and yeasts. Given a denture's close proximity to the respiratory tract, denture wearers are potentially at an increased risk of aspirating opportunistic pathogens from the denture into their lungs.

Aspiration pneumonia (AP) is a potentially life-threatening respiratory infection associated with entry into the bronchial tree of contaminated foreign material such as gastric or oropharyngeal contents, including food debris, dental and/or denture plaque, and saliva. Pneumonia is the leading cause of death attributable to infection in patients aged 65 years and older, costing the NHS in excess of £440 million annually.[6]

Moreover, it has been found that aspiration of oropharyngeal contents is a common occurrence in healthy individuals, of whom approximately 45% aspirate material into the lungs during sleep.[7] Risk factors for AP, such as dysphagia and chronic obstructive pulmonary disease, are more common in the elderly, thus putting this subpopulation at an increased risk of infection.[8] Poor oral hygiene has been linked to respiratory infection with common pathogens being identified in dental plaque.[9] The microbial composition of dental plaque has been well characterized, and these oral bacteria have been linked with systemic infections.[10] However, a gap remains in our understanding of the direct implications of denture plaque. The aim of this study was to undertake a comprehensive evaluation of putative respiratory pathogens residing upon dentures using a targeted quantitative molecular approach.

MATERIALS AND METHODS

Patient Sampling

Samples for the study were obtained from 130 denture wearers attending the Glasgow Dental Hospital and School, UK, for treatment. Written informed consent was obtained from all participants. Ethical approval for recruitment of study participants was granted by the West of Scotland Research Ethics Service (12/WS/0121). A dentist was responsible for the collection of clinical samples. The presence or absence of denture stomatitis (DS) was assessed by the clinician, and those patients with DS were grouped according to Newton's classification.[11] Demographic data, including age, gender, and oral hygiene habits were recorded. Patients were excluded from the study if they had been receiving antimicrobial/antifungal treatment or using prescription mouthwashes within 6 weeks prior to sampling.

Collection of Denture Plaque

Dentures were removed from the patient's mouth and placed in sterile bags (Fisher Scientific, Loughborough, UK) filled with 50 ml PBS (Sigma-Aldrich, Dorset, UK) then placed in a sonic bath (Ultrawave, Cardiff, UK) for 5 minutes to remove biofilm from the surface. The denture sonicate was transferred to a 50 ml tube and transported to a category II laboratory where it was centrifuged for 10 minutes at 3700 g. The plaque pellet was then resuspended in 2 ml of RNAlater® (QIAgen, Manchester, UK) and stored at −80 °C.

Microbial Culture and DNA Extraction

For identification of respiratory pathogens in this study we took a targeted approach. Bacterial type strains of nine pathogens known to cause respiratory infection were selected and grown in appropriate media and atmospheric conditions for 24 hours as outlined in Table 1. Bacteria were subsequently washed in PBS and standardized to 1×10^8 CFU/ml, prior to serially diluting in preparation for calibrated standard curve analysis. These samples and denture plaque sonicates were centrifuged for 10 minutes at 10,000 g, resuspended in proteinase K extraction buffer, and incubated at 55 °C for 20 minutes. DNA was extracted using the QIAmp mini DNA Extraction Kit (Qiagen) according to manufacturer's instructions, with a minor modification to include a mechanical disruption step with sterile acid-washed glass beads of 0.5 mm diameter (Thistle Scientific, Glasgow, UK). This was achieved by vortexing for 3×30 seconds on a Mini-BeadBeater (Sigma-Aldrich, Gillingham, UK), although intermittently being placed on ice. DNA quality and quantity was then quantified by NanoDrop® (Thermo Scientific, Loughborough, UK).

Quantitative PCR

Primers were either taken from published literature or designed using the web-based GenScript real-time PCR primer design software (https://www.genscript.com/ssl-bin/app/primer). Primer sequences were checked for specificity to each target organism using the NIH-BLAST database. PCR amplification efficiencies of all primer sets were optimized prior to gene expression analysis, with efficiencies ranging from 90% to 110%. Details of the oligonucleotide primers (Eurogentec, Southampton, UK) used in this study are listed in Table 2. Two hundred ng of DNA was used in a mastermix containing SYBR® GreenER™ (Life Technologies, Paisley, UK), UV-treated RNase-free water, and forward/reverse primers (10 μM), following manufacturers' instructions. qPCR was carried out using the step one plus real-time PCR unit (Applied Biosciences, Paisley, UK), under the following conditions;

50 °C for 2 minutes, 95 °C for 2 minutes, followed by 40 cycles of 95 °C for 3 seconds and 59 °C for 30 seconds. Data analysis was carried out using StepOne software V2.3 (Life Technologies). Baseline threshold values of the samples were adjusted to correspond with the equivalent standard curve; Ct values were then used to approximate the number of corresponding colony forming equivalents (CFEs) based on standard curves created from serial two-fold dilutions of each bacterial species.

Statistical Analysis

Graph production, data distribution, and statistical analysis were performed using GraphPad Prism (v.4; La Jolla, CA, USA) or IBM SPSS statistics (v.21; Chicago, IL). Since continuous data including real-time qPCR determination of bacterial cell numbers on dentures did not conform to a normal distribution, the Mann-Whitney U-test was used for comparisons between the different denture-wearer subsets. The Spearman bivariate correlation analysis was used to determine relationships between the Newton Grade of inflammation and bacterial numbers.

RESULTS

Patient Demographics

Of the 130 patients that participated in this study, 84 were female. The mean patient age was 70.4 years, with an average denture age of 4.5 years. Clinical diagnoses indicated that 37% of participants were suffering from DS. The majority of patients (68%) wore complete maxillary dentures, whereas 32% had a partial maxillary denture with ≥1 natural teeth remaining.

Detection of Respiratory Pathogens

The dentures of 84 patients (64.6%) carried potential respiratory pathogens. The following six were identified: *S. aureus, S. pneumoniae, P. aeruginosa, H. influenzae B, S. pyogenes,* and *M. catarrhalis* (Table 1). *S. aureus* was the most prevalent, with 67 patients (51.2%) being shown to carry this pathogen. Of these 67 isolates, retesting using primers specific for the *mecA* gene demonstrated that two (3%) were MRSA. *H. influenzae B, Pseudomonas aeruginosa, S. pneumoniae, Streptococcus pyogenes,* and *Moraxella catarrhalis* were also detected within denture plaque of our patients (Table 2). Fifty-eight patients (44.6%) had dentures colonized by a single pathogen, 24 patients (18.5%) were colonized by two pathogens, and two patients (1.5%) were colonized by three. None of the samples were shown to be positive for *Legionella pneumophila, Chlamydia pneumonia,* or *Klebsiella pneumoniae.*

TABLE 1   **Respiratory pathogen primers used for qPCR**

Species	Type strain	Media/conditions	Gene	Primer sequence	Amplicon size
S. aureus	DSMZ 1104	BHI, aerobic	SAR0134	F - ATTTGGTCCCAGTGGTGTGGGTAT R - GCTGTGACAATTGCCGTTTGTCGT	143
MRSA		BHI, aerobic	MecA	F - AACCACCCAATTTGTCTGCC R - TGATGGTATGCAACAAGTCGTAAA	135
H. influenzae B	DSMZ 11969	MHB + 0.4% hemophilus test medium, 5% CO_2	GryB	F - CTTACGCTTCTATCTCGGTGATTAATAA R - TGTTCGCCATAACTTCATCTTAGC	138
P. aeruginosa	PA14	LB, aerobic	RpoD	F - GGGCGAAGAAGGAAATGGTC R - CAGGTGGCGTAGGTGGAGAA	178
S. pneumoniae	DSMZ 14377	BHI, 5% CO_2	CspA	F - ACGCAACTGACGAGTGTGAC R- GATCGCGACACCGAACTAAT	352
M. catarrhalis	DSMZ 11994	BHI, aerobic	OmpCD	F - ACACGCAACTCTTGACGAAG R - CTGAGCCTGTCATTGAGGAA	180
S. pyogenes	DSMZ 20565	BHI, 5% CO_2	SpeB	F - TGC TAAAGTCGCTACGGTTG R - GAATTGATGGCTGATGTTGG	148
C. pneumoniae	ATCC VR-1360D DNA	NA	MomP	F - TTACTTAAAGAAACGTTTGGTAGTTCATTT R - TAAACATTTGGGATCGCTTTGAT	154
K. pneumoniae	DSMZ 12059	TSB, anaerobic	PhoE	F - AGAATTCAGATTCCCAACGG R - ACAAGAACGCGAACAAACTG	167
L. pneumophila	DSMZ 25038	YEB with BCYE supplement, 5% CO_2	Mip	F - CAATGTCAACAGCAATGGCTGCAAC R - CTCATAGCGTCTTGCATGCCTTTAGCC	160
16S			16S	F - ACTCCTACGGGAGGCAGCAGT R - TATTACCGCGGCTGCTGGC	198

TABLE 2   **Prevalence and quantity of respiratory pathogens colonizing dentures**

Species	Positive samples	Prevalence (%)	Average CFE	Average total 16S CFE	Proportion of 16S (%)
S. aureus[*]	67	51.2	1.3×10^5	4.5×10^{10}	2.8×10^{-4}
H. influenzae B	20	15.3	2.4×10^4	1.7×10^{10}	1.4×10^{-4}
P. aeruginosa	15	11.5	4.3×10^6	3.34×10^{10}	1.5×10^{-2}
S. pneumoniae	9	6.9	2.5×10^5	4.4×10^{10}	6.3×10^{-4}
M. catarrhalis	1	0.8	2×10^3	7.97×10^9	2.5×10^{-5}
S. pyogenes	1	0.8	3.7×10^4	3.2×10^{10}	1.2×10^{-4}
C. pneumoniae	ND[**]	ND	ND	ND	ND
K. pneumoniae	ND	ND	ND	ND	ND
L. pneumophila	ND	ND	ND	ND	ND

[*]Two S. aureus samples were found to be MRSA positive.
[**]ND, not detected.

Quantifying Respiratory Pathogens

Standard curves of known quantities of bacteria were prepared for each pathogen; R^2 values ranged from 0.97 to 0.99. Table 2 shows the mean CFE counts of each organism detected on dentures. In terms of overall proportion of denture plaque, P. aeruginosa was found to be the most abundant, with a mean count of 4.3×10^6 CFE when present. This was followed by S. pneumoniae and S. aureus, which were detected at relatively high levels of 2.5×10^5 CFE per denture and 1.3×10^5 CFE per denture, respectively.

Conversely, H. influenzae B, S. pyogenes, and M. catarrhalis where present, were all detected at levels lower than 10^5 CFE per denture. The total number of bacteria residing on dentures shown to harbor respiratory pathogens was calculated using the 16S gene, with mean quantities ranging between 7.97×10^9 and 4.5×10^{10} CFE per denture. As a proportion of the overall plaque, P. aeruginosa was most abundant contributing to $1.5\% \times 10^{-2}\%$ of the total. The remaining pathogens all contributed to less than 0.001% of the complete plaque sample.

TABLE 3 **Prevalence of respiratory pathogens in plaque of patients with healthy palatal mucosa and those with denture stomatitis**

Species	Healthy		Denture stomatitis	
	Patients	Prevalence (%)	Patients	Prevalence (%)
S. aureus	40	49.4	27	55.1
H. influenzae B	16	19.8	4	8.2
P. aeruginosa	10	12.3	5	10.2
S. pneumoniae	3	3.7	6	12.2
M. catarrhalis	ND*	ND	1	2.0
S. pyogenes	ND	ND	1	2.0
C. pneumoniae	ND	ND	ND	ND
K. pneumoniae	ND	ND	ND	ND
L. pneumophila	ND	ND	ND	ND
MRSA	ND	ND	2	4.1
Overall	69	85.2	44	89.8

*ND, not detected.

The relationship between DS, denture hygiene, and presence of respiratory pathogens was investigated. In relation to DS, we determined the prevalence of respiratory pathogens among healthy and diseased patients, based on clinical presentation using Newton's classification (Table 3). The overall prevalence of these was similar between the healthy and diseased groups. Variation between individual species was also investigated; however, no statistical significance was found. In terms of denture hygiene, a greater proportion of dentures left in patients' mouths overnight were found to carry S. pneumoniae, and an increased median number of S. pneumoniae were detected on those dentures ($p = 0.041$ and $p = 0.038$, respectively). In contrast, the proportion of dentures positive for P. aeruginosa and numbers of P. aeruginosa found on dentures left in overnight was lower than dentures that were removed ($p = 0.038$ and $p = 0.04$, respectively).

DISCUSSION

Improvements in health care in the last 100 years have led to a growing population of elderly residents. This aging population, particularly those aged 65 and over, are more susceptible to developing pneumonia, accounting for approximately 90% of deaths in the elderly.[6] Many cases of pneumonia are related to oral bacteria emanating from the oropharynx.[12] Given that 70% of UK adults older than 75 years old wear dentures, it is clear that these individuals are at greater risk of developing life-threatening infections due to putative respiratory pathogens residing upon their denture.[13] This recent study showed that patients who wear their denture overnight double their risk of pneumonia. In this article, using qPCR for the first time on denture plaque from a large cohort of denture

wearers, we report that almost 65% of these individuals harbored significant quantities of pathogens capable of causing respiratory infections. This was regardless of existing oral disease status, and therefore suggests that even denture wearers with healthy palatal mucosa and good oral hygiene may harbor respiratory pathogens on their dentures.

Given the dense and complex microbial population of the oral cavity, the presence of similar genera and species is problematic for accurate quantitative microbial counts on selective agars.[14] Therefore, we adopted an alternative nonculture-based method, which employed a qPCR-based approach to identify a panel of defined respiratory pathogens. This targeted molecular approach enabled us to rapidly assess the presence and quantity of defined respiratory pathogens.[15,16] Although there are numerous putative respiratory pathogens, our study focused on nine key bacterial pathogens widely implicated in respiratory infections. We showed that almost 65% of patients' dentures were positive for one or more of these pathogens. This is in line with a recent report indicating that 64% of the healthy patient group contained respiratory pathogens based on culture-based methodology, though only nine patients were assessed in this study.[17] It is possible that other microorganisms capable of causing pneumonia were not detected due to the limitation of a targeted qPCR approach, as colonization and infection of the respiratory tract is possible by a wide variety of human pathogens. Indeed, microbiome analysis of the entire denture specimen would enable a detailed characterization of potential pathogens, though to date no studies have reported this information. Nonetheless, our qPCR approach gives an initial insight into the risk associated with colonized dentures.

qPCR has proved an important tool, as in this study we have shown a high prevalence of S. aureus (51.2%), which an earlier culture-based study of 50 patients' dentures reported as only 10%.[14] This disparity is likely due to improved detection abilities of qPCR, as in our parallel study using culture techniques S. aureus was detected in only 20% of samples (data not shown). H. influenzae was also detected in 15.3%, whereas Sumi et al[14] were unable to detect this organism at all. P. aeruginosa was also detected in significant levels (11.5%), similar to a study of institutionalized and hospitalized patients. S. pneumoniae was detected on dentures from 6.9% of patients, which is much lower than the prevalence reported by Abe et al[15] (63%); however, this discrepancy is probably due to the nonspecific nature of the primers in Abe's study.[15] We used the cspA gene specifically, instead of the generic primers, to minimize detection of closely related streptococcal species. Collectively, these organisms were detected in relatively low abundance in relation to total bacterial flora ($< 6\% \times 10^{-4}\%$), indicating that these bacteria only occupied limited niches upon the denture surface. Interestingly though, P. aeruginosa comprised 0.015% of the total denture microbiome, which may relate to its resistance to standard mechanical and chemical cleaning methods when grown on denture acrylic.[18]

DS is a disease affecting between 30% and 70% of denture wearers. The etiology of DS is complex, and the microbial composition of denture plaque is not yet fully understood.[19] We were interested to identify whether respiratory pathogen colonization of denture plaque was a more common occurrence in those with DS; however, our results revealed a similar prevalence of respiratory pathogens between healthy and diseased individuals (89.2% and 85.8%, respectively), suggesting that DS had no influence on the likelihood of respiratory pathogen colonization. Thus, despite published studies showing the prevalence of AP to be higher in patients who do not follow adequate dental hygiene measures.[20,21] Our study found no difference in the prevalence of respiratory pathogen carriage in those with and without signs of DS, suggesting that the presence of the denture was sufficient risk in itself.

The high prevalence of *S. aureus* residing on dentures is a concern, particularly in light of the emergence of drug-resistant strains. In this study we found two patients positive for the methicillin resistant S. aureus (MRSA) *mecA* gene (1.5%). Our prevalence rate is low, but similar to a previous study conducted in Scotland in which 5% of denture wearers were found to carry MRSA in their oral cavity.[22] This may be cause for concern, as many over-the-counter oral hygiene antimicrobials are ineffective against MRSA biofilms.[23] *S. pneumoniae* was shown to be significantly more abundant on dentures that were kept in their owner's mouths overnight, a habit practiced by a large proportion (55%) of the patients in this study. This is particularly important given that presently 20% to 30% of *S. pneumoniae* worldwide are multidrug resistant.[24] In addition, 11.5% of patients were carriers of *P. aeruginosa*, a notorious cause of life-threatening pneumonia for intensive care patients with a mortality rate of 44.5%.[25] Oropharyngeal *P. aeruginosa* isolates have also been shown to have a high rate of antibiotic resistance.[26] Given that it is common practice to soak dentures in water overnight, this may be an inadvertent source of contamination, and some form of disinfectant such as hypochlorite for nonmetal containing prostheses, should be included.[27]

CONCLUSION

This study has shown that dentures are a reservoir for respiratory pathogens in the oral cavity, thus increasing the risk of developing AP. This study used a robust method of sampling the denture microflora and characterizing it using culture-independent techniques. We have shown a high prevalence of putative respiratory pathogens on the dentures of ambulatory adults, a finding that could explain the source of infection in some cases of AP. Adoption of routine oral hygiene practices including mechanical cleaning, and the use of antiseptic cleansing agents could help to reduce the risk of respiratory

infection among the elderly population.[28] Further detailed microbiological investigations using next-generation sequencing will further aid our understanding of the risks associated with ono-compliance of denture cleanser regimens.

REFERENCES

1. Guzmán JM, Pawliczko A, Beales S, et al: Ageing in the Twenty-First Century: A Celebration and A Challenge. United Nations Population Fund (UNFPA), New York, and Help Age International, London, 2012.

2. Farquharson D, Butcher JP, Culshaw S: Periodontitis, Porphyromonas, and the pathogenesis of rheumatoid arthritis. *Mucosal Immunol* 2012;5:112–120.

3. Pizzo G, Guiglia R, Lo Russo L, et al: Dentistry and internal medicine: from the focal infection theory to the periodontal medicine concept. *Eur J Intern Med* 2010;21:496–502.

4. Coulthwaite L, Verran J: Potential pathogenic aspects of denture plaque. *Br J Biomed Sci* 2007;64:180–189.

5. Shulman JD, Beach MM, Rivera-Hidalgo F: The prevalence of oral mucosal lesions in US adults: data from the Third National Health and Nutrition Examination Survey, 1988–1994. *J Am Dent Assoc* 2004;135:1279–1286.

6. Guest JF, Morris A: Community-acquired pneumonia: the annual cost to the National Health Service in the UK. *Eur Respir J* 1997;10:1530–1534.

7. Gleeson K, Eggli DF, Maxwell SL: Quantitative aspiration during sleep in normal subjects. *Chest* 1997;111:1266–1272.

8. El-Solh AA: Association between pneumonia and oral care in nursing home residents. *Lung* 2011;189:173–180.

9. Sumi Y, Miura H, Michiwaki Y, et al: Colonization of dental plaque by respiratory pathogens in dependent elderly. *Arch Gerontol Geriatr* 2007;44:119–124.

10. Inaba H, Amano A: Roles of oral bacteria in cardiovascular diseases–from molecular mechanisms to clinical cases: implication of periodontal diseases in development of systemic diseases. *J Pharmacol Sci* 2010;113:103–109.

11. Newton A: Denture sore mouth: a possible aetiology. *Br Dent J* 1962;112:357–360.

12. Andrews T, Steen C: A review of oral preventative strategies to reduce ventilator-associated pneumonia. *Nurs Crit Care* 2013;18:116–122.

13. Iinuma T, Arai Y, Abe Y, et al: Denture wearing during sleep doubles the risk of pneumonia in the very elderly. *J Dent Res* 2015;94:28S–36S.

14. Sumi Y, Miura H, Sunakawa M, et al: Colonization of denture plaque by respiratory pathogens in dependent elderly. *Gerodontology* 2002;19:25–29.

15. Abe S, Ishihara K, Okuda K: Prevalence of potential respiratory pathogens in the mouths of elderly patients and effects of professional oral care. *Arch Gerontol Geriatr* 2001;32:45–55.

16. Zuanazzi D, Souto R, Mattos MB, et al: Prevalence of potential bacterial respiratory pathogens in the oral cavity of hospitalized individuals. *Arch Oral Biol* 2010;55:21–28.

17. Przybylowska D, Mierzwińska-Nastalska E, Swoboda-Kopeć E, et al: Potential respiratory pathogens colonisation of the denture plaque of patients with chronic obstructive pulmonary disease. *Gerodontology* 2014. doi:10.1111/ger.12156.

18. Paranhos HF, Silva-Lovato CH, deSouza RF, et al: Effect of three methods for cleaning dentures on biofilms formed *in vitro* on acrylic resin. *J Prosthodont* 2009;18:427–431.

19. Budtz-Jorgensen E, Stenderup A, Grabowski M: An epidemiologic study of yeasts in elderly denture wearers. *Community Dent Oral Epidemiol* 1975;3:115–119.

20. Bassim CW, Gibson G, Ward T, et al: Modification of the risk of mortality from pneumonia with oral hygiene care. *J Am Geriatr Soc* 2008;56:1601–1607.

21. vander Maarel-Wierink CD, Vanobbergen JN, et al: Oral health care and aspiration pneumonia in frail older people: a systematic literature review. *Gerodontology* 2013;30:3–9.

22. Smith AJ, Robertson D, Tang MK, et al: Staphylococcus aureus in the oral cavity: a three-year retrospective analysis of clinical laboratory data. *Br Dent J* 2003;195:701–703; discussion 694.

23. Smith K, Robertson DP, Lappin DF, et al: Commercial mouthwashes are ineffective against oral MRSA biofilms. *Oral Surg Oral Med Oral Pathol Oral Radiol* 2013;115:624–629.

24. Lynch JP, 3rd, Zhanel GG: Escalation of antimicrobial resistance among *Streptococcus pneumoniae*: implications for therapy. *Semin Respir Crit Care Med* 2005;26:575–616.

25. Tumbarello M, DePascale G, Trecarichi EM, et al: Clinical outcomes of *Pseudomonas aeruginosa* pneumonia in intensive care unit patients. *Intensive Care Med* 2013;39:682–692.

26. Oostdijk EA, deSmet AM, Blok HE, et al: Ecological effects of selective decontamination on resistant gram-negative bacterial colonization. *Am J Respir Crit Care Med* 2010;181:452–457.

27. Loveday HP, Wilson JA, Kerr K, et al: Association between healthcare water systems and Pseudomonas aeruginosa infections: a rapid systematic review. *J Hosp Infect* 2014;86:7–15.

28. Ramage G, Zalewska A, Cameron DA, et al: A comparative *in vitro* study of two denture cleaning techniques as an effective strategy for inhibiting *Candida albicans* biofilms on denture surfaces and reducing inflammation. *J Prosthodont* 2012;21:516–522.

PART II

ORAL HEALTH, BIOFILMS, AND DENTURE STOMATITIS

9

BIOFILMS IN THE EDENTULOUS ORAL CAVITY

AMIT SACHDEO, BDS, MS, DMSC,[1] ANNE D. HAFFAJEE, BDS,[2] AND SIGMUND S. SOCRANSKY, DDS[2]

[1]Department of Prosthodontics, Tufts University-School of Dental Medicine, Boston, MA
[2]Department of Periodontology, The Forsyth Institute, Boston, MA

Keywords

Complete dentures; biofilm; microbiota; edentulous; DNA–DNA hybridization; checkerboard

Correspondence

Dr. Amit Sachdeo, Department of Prosthodontics, Tufts University–School of Dental Medicine, One Kneeland St., Boston, MA 02111. E-mail: amit.sachdeo@tufts.edu

This research received the following support, grants, and awards: NIDCR grant DE14368; American College of Prosthodontists (ACP)/P&G Research Fellowship in Complete Denture Prosthodontics; Academy of Prosthodontics Foundation Research Grant; Greater New York Academy of Prosthodontics (GNYAP) Research Award; ACP/ESPE Research Fellowship in Geriatric Prosthodontics; Northeastern Gnathological Society's Granger-Pruden Award.

This study was also awarded first place in the table clinic competition at the 2005 ACP Annual Session in Los Angeles, CA.

Accepted December 12, 2007

Published in *Journal of Prosthodontics* 2008; Vol. 17, Issue 5, pp. 348–56

doi: 10.1111/j.1532-849X.2008.00301.x

ABSTRACT

Purpose: The oral cavity presents numerous surfaces for microbial colonization. These surfaces produce biofilms of differing complexities unique to each individual. Several studies have looked at biofilms in dentate patients. There has been limited research regarding biofilms on dentures or soft tissues of edentulous patients. The purpose of the present investigation was to provide meaningful data describing microbial ecological relationships in the oral cavity of edentulous patients and to evaluate the microbiota on hard and soft tissue surfaces and saliva in edentulous patients wearing complete dentures.

Materials and Methods: Sixty-one edentulous subjects with complete maxillary and mandibular dentures were recruited. "Supragingival" biofilm samples were taken from 28 denture teeth for each subject. Biofilm samples were also taken from the dorsal, lateral, and ventral surfaces of the tongue, floor of mouth, buccal mucosa, hard palate, vestibule/lip, "attached gingiva," and saliva. Samples were individually analyzed for their content of 41 bacterial species using checkerboard DNA–DNA hybridization. Levels and proportions of each species were determined for every sample location. Results: Periodontal pathogens such as *Aggregatibacter actinomycetemcomitans* and *Porphyromonas gingivalis* were clearly present in the samples from the edentulous subjects. Microbial profiles in samples from the soft tissue surfaces differed among site locations. Samples from the dorsum of the tongue exhibited the highest bacterial counts followed by the "attached gingiva" and the lateral surfaces of the tongue, while the lowest mean counts were found in samples from the

Journal of Prosthodontics on Complete and Removable Dentures, First Edition. Edited by Jonathan P. Wiens, Jennifer Wiens Priebe, and Donald A. Curtis.
© 2018 American College of Prosthodontists. Published 2018 by John Wiley & Sons, Inc.

buccal mucosa and labial vestibules. Using cluster analysis of the proportions of the test species, three clusters were formed. The first cluster comprised saliva, supragingival plaque, and the lateral and dorsal surfaces of the tongue. The second cluster comprised the other six soft tissue surfaces. Species on the denture palate formed a third cluster.

Conclusions: One of the major findings in this study was the detection of periodontal pathogens, *A. actinomycetemcomitans* and *P. gingivalis*, in the edentulous subjects, as these species were thought to disappear after removal of all natural teeth. This finding has implications regarding future dental treatment and the general health of individuals. Distinct patterns of microbial colonization were seen on the different soft tissue surfaces. Thus, this investigation provided the first step in defining the organisms that are associated with edentulous patients on both soft (mucosa) and hard surfaces (denture). The study also provided meaningful data that described microbial ecological relationships in the oral cavity of edentulous subjects. The authors believe that this study is the first comprehensive assessment of the microbiota in the complete denture-wearing subject.

There has been some controversy over the number of current and future edentulous patients worldwide. Several studies have suggested that fluoridation and changing demographics are leading to the falling rate of edentulism.[1,2] Other authors have indicated that edentulism is on the rise.[3–5]

In 1994, Lang[3] reported that the number of edentulous persons over 65 years of age in need of complete dentures in the United States and Canada appeared to be decreasing as a percent of the total population; however, he also stated that the total number of patients needing these services by the year 2030 will be almost the same as it is today. A survey by Cates in 1989[5] showed that the geriatric population in the United States was increasing and was expected to continue to rise through the 21st century. Despite changing demographics, treating complete denture geriatric patients is expected to be a large part of dental care well into the next century.[3–7]

Douglass et al[4,8] concluded that the adult population within the United States in need of complete dentures would increase from 33.6 million in 1991 to 37.9 million in 2020. They emphasized the need for complete denture prosthodontic training in dental education, as a sizable minority of the patient population will continue to need complete denture services, despite the previous assumption of declining rates of edentulism. Part of the process to optimize treatment of edentulous patients is the need to understand the microbiota present not only on mucosal surfaces, but also on the surfaces of prostheses.

The oral cavity presents numerous surfaces for microbial colonization. These surfaces are colonized by biofilms of differing microbial complexity unique to each individual.[9] Several studies have described biofilms in dentulous patients,[10–12] but there have been relatively few studies of the microbiota of the mucous membranes or saliva in edentulous subjects and even fewer looking at the microbiota on complete dentures. Studies of the edentulous oral cavity of infants prior to tooth eruption have suggested that *Prevotella melaninogenica* was the most frequently isolated anaerobic species found in 70% of infants.[13] Other common anaerobes detected in edentulous infants included *Fusobacterium nucleatum, Veillonella* species, and non-pigmented *Prevotella*. The source of the anaerobes appeared to be the mother, because there was a correlation between maternal salivary concentration and the infant's colonization by these species, particularly *P. melaninogenica*.[14]

At the other end of the age spectrum, the microbiota of 51 edentulous subjects (mean age 74 years) with complete dentures was studied using culture techniques.[15] Biofilm samples taken from the intaglio (tissue) surfaces of the dentures as well as the palate, buccal mucosa, dorsum of the tongue, and saliva were analyzed using nonselective and selective media techniques. "Black-pigmented *Bacteroides*" were found in 96% of subjects, while yeasts were found in 49% of subjects. *Streptococcus mutans* was found in 84% of saliva samples; 92% of the samples yielded lactobacilli.

Data in the literature have suggested that species such as *S. mutans* required hard surfaces for sustained colonization,[16–19] even though they might be detected in dentate subjects at low levels on the soft tissues.[20,21] It has also been shown that *S. mutans* essentially disappeared from the oral cavity when all the teeth were extracted and reappeared if hard surfaces were provided in the form of dentures.[16–19] Other investigators have stated that *Aggregatibacter actinomycetemcomitans* and *Porphyromonas gingivalis* disappeared from the oral cavity after extraction of all teeth and did not reappear even when hard surfaces such as dentures were provided.[22,23] These species have also been reported to have a strong association to various systemic diseases in the dentate population.[24–31]

These data are intriguing in that they suggest that teeth are essential for colonization of species such as *A. actinomycetemcomitans* and *P. gingivalis*. Further, hard surfaces appear essential for the colonization of *S. mutans*. Theilade and Budtz-Jorgensen[32] examined the predominant cultivable microbiota on removable dentures in subjects with denture-induced stomatitis. They suggested that the gingival crevice as well as the fluid passing through the gingival crevice might be essential for the colonization of most Gram negative rods, including common species such as *F. nucleatum, Prevotella intermedia*, and *Prevotella nigrescens*. The data from studies examining the oral microbiota in edentulous patients are fragmentary, often derived from small number of samples and/or patients, using techniques that are not able to detect low number of organisms and a wide spectrum of bacterial taxa.

The purpose of the present investigation was to examine the microbiota of biofilms that form on dentures and the oral soft tissues and in the saliva of edentulous, denture-wearing subjects using checkerboard DNA–DNA hybridization.[33] This technique is used to determine sequence similarity between DNAs of different origin and the amount of sequence repetition within one DNA. It is a useful tool for the enumeration of bacterial species in large samples of microbiologically complex systems.[33–35]

MATERIALS AND METHODS

Subject Population

The subject population consisted of 61 edentulous subjects (54% male, 46% female) who used complete maxillary and mandibular dentures on a daily basis. The baseline characteristics of these subjects are presented in Table 1. Subjects of any racial/ethnic group were accepted for study as long as they were in good general health.

To be included in the study, subjects had to be over 20 years of age, have been edentulous for at least 1 year and worn complete maxillary and mandibular dentures on a daily basis.

Subjects who had received antibiotic therapy in the 3 months prior to the start of the study or who had any oral lesions (e.g., candidiasis, ulcerations, leukoplakia, oral cancer) or a systemic condition that required antibiotic coverage for routine dental procedures (e.g., heart conditions, joint replacements) were excluded from the study.

TABLE 1　Demographic features of the subjects

Mean age in years (± SD)	59.6 (± 11.3)
% Males (N)	54 (33)
% Females (N)	46 (28)
% Current smokers (N)	43 (26)
% White* (N)	64 (39)
% African-American (N)	34 (21)
% Asian (N)	2(1)

N denotes the actual number of subjects.
*1 subject in the White group reported being Hispanic.

Soft Tissue Samples

Microbial samples were taken from eight separate oral soft tissue locations in each subject using MasterAmp™ buccal swab brushes (Epicentre Technologies, Madison, WI). Four hundred and eighty-eight samples were obtained by gently stroking each site in an area large enough to yield sufficient number of microorganisms for DNA probe analysis. The samples were collected from three areas of the tongue: one from the dorsum of the tongue, one from the ventral surface, and one sample from both the lateral surfaces of the tongue. This was done by first taking a sample from the left lateral surface of the tongue and then using the same swab to take a sample from the right lateral surface. Similarly, there was one sample for both the left and right buccal mucosa and the maxillary and mandibular labial vestibules, respectively. Microbial samples were also taken from the floor of the mouth, hard palate, and the maxillary anterior "attached gingiva" (fixed keratinized tissue). The samples were placed in separate tubes containing 0.15 ml Tris EDTA (TE) buffer (10 mM Tris-HCL, 0.1 mM EDTA, pH 7.6), and 0.15 ml 0.5 M NaOH was added.

Denture Samples

Twenty-eight separate microbial samples were taken from the dentures of each subject while the dentures were in the mouth. Each sample was obtained using separate sterile curettes from the mesio-buccal surface of every denture tooth. The samples were placed in separate tubes containing 0.15 ml of TE buffer and processed as described for the soft tissue samples. A total of 1708 samples from the denture teeth were collected. An additional sample from the midpoints of the exterior, polished surfaces of each denture hard palate was taken using a MasterAmp™ buccal swab brush. All the dentures had polished exterior surfaces without any rugae.

Saliva Samples

Each subject provided a sample of whole unstimulated saliva by expectorating into a sterile tube. A total of 61 samples were collected. A 0.2-ml sample of whole saliva was mixed with 0.15-ml sterile, filtered TE buffer. A 0.2-ml sample of this mixture was transferred to a new tube, and 0.15 ml of 0.5-M NaOH was added. The samples were processed as described for the soft tissue and denture samples.

Microbial Analysis of the Samples

All samples were analyzed using checkerboard DNA–DNA hybridization to determine the levels of 41 bacterial species presented in Table 2.[33] In brief, the samples were placed in separate Eppendorf tubes containing 0.15-ml TE (10 mM TrisHCl, 1 mM EDTA, pH 7.6), and 0.15 ml of 0.5-M NaOH was added to each tube. The samples were lysed, and the DNA placed in lanes on nylon membranes using a Minislot

TABLE 2   Species for which DNA probes were prepared for the study

Aggregatibacter actinomycetemcomitans 43718 and 29523	*Actinomyces israelii 12102*
Actinomyces gerencseriae 23840	*Actinomyces odontolyticus 17929*
Actinomyces naeslundii genospecies 1 12104	*Campylobacter gracilis 33236*
Actinomyces naeslundi genospecies 2 43146	*Campylobacter showae 51146*
Campylobacter rectus 33238	*Capnocytophaga ochracea 33596*
Capnocytophaga gingivalis 33624	*Eikenella corrodens 23834*
Capnocytophaga sputigena 33612	*Eubacterium saburreum 33271*
Eubacterium nodatum 33099	*Fusobacterium nucleatum ss polymorphum 10953*
Fusobacterium nucleatum ss nucleatum 25586	*Fusobacterium periodonticum 33693*
Fusobacterium nucleatum ss vincentii 49256	*Leptotrichia buccalis 14201*
Gemella morbilliorum 27824	*Peptostreptococcus micros 33270*
Neisseria mucosa 19696	*Prevotella intermedia 25611*
Porphyromonas gingivalis 33277	*Prevotella nigrescens 33563*
Prevotella melaninogenica 25845	*Selenomonas noxia 43541*
Propionibacterium acnes 11827 and 11828	*Streptococcus constellatus 27823*
Streptococcus anginosus 33397	*Streptococcus intermedius 27335*
Streptococcus gordonii 10558	*Streptococcus mutans 25175*
Streptococcus mitis 49456	*Streptococcus sanguinis 10556*
Streptococcus oralis 35037	*Treponema denticola B1*
Tannerella forsythia 43037	*Veillonella parvula 10790*
Treponema socranskii S1	

All strains were obtained from the American Type Culture Collection (ATCC, Manassas, VA), except *Treponema denticola B1* and *Treponema socranskii S1*, which were obtained from The Forsyth Institute (Boston, MA).

device (Immunetics, Cambridge, MA). After fixation of the DNA to the membranes, the membranes were placed in a Miniblotter 45 (Immunetics) with the lanes of DNA at 90° to the lanes of the device. Digoxigenin-labeled whole genomic DNA probes to 41 bacterial species were hybridized in individual lanes of the Miniblotter. After hybridization, the membranes were washed and then incubated with anti-digoxigenin antibody conjugated with alkaline phosphatase. Signals were detected using AttoPhos substrate (Amersham Life Science, Arlington Heights, IL) and were read using a Storm Fluorimager (Molecular Dynamics, Sunnyvale, CA), a computer-linked instrument that read the intensity of the fluorescence signals resulting from the probe-target hybridization. Two lanes in each run contained standards at concentrations of 10^5 and 10^6 cells of each species. The sensitivity of the assay was adjusted to permit detection of 10^4 cells of a given species by adjusting the concentration of each DNA probe. Signals were evaluated using the Storm Fluorimager and converted to absolute counts by comparison with the standards on the same membrane. Failure to detect a signal was recorded as zero.

Data Evaluation

Microbiological data available for each of the 61 subjects were the counts of 41 test species in "supragingival" biofilm samples taken from the mesial aspect of each denture tooth in each subject. The counts for each species from 28 "supragingival" sites were averaged within each subject and then averaged across subjects. In a similar fashion, the percentage

of the total DNA probe count was determined for each species at each site in each subject and averaged within and then across each subject. The mean values for each species were depicted graphically as "microbial profiles" ordered according to the microbial complexes.[34]

Counts and proportions of 41 test species were available for one sample per subject from each of the following oral surfaces: tongue dorsum, tongue lateral, tongue ventral, floor of mouth, buccal, hard palate, vestibule/lip, attached gingiva, and the exterior surface of the denture hard palate as well as the counts and proportions of each species in a sample of unstimulated saliva. The counts for each species were averaged across subjects for each intraoral location. Significance of difference in counts or proportions of each species among intraoral locations were determined using the Friedman test and adjusted for multiple comparisons.[36]

Cluster analysis was performed on the mean proportions of the 41 species in samples from eight soft tissue surfaces, saliva, denture teeth and the exterior surfaces of the hard palate of the dentures. Similarities were computed using the chord coefficient[37] and sorted using an average unweighted linkage sort.[38]

RESULTS

Microbiota of Denture Biofilm Samples

Figure 1 presents the mean counts ($\times 10^5$) and mean proportions of the 41 test species in the biofilm samples from the

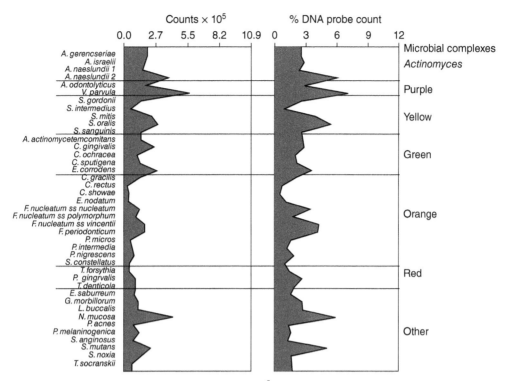

FIGURE 1 Microbial profiles of mean counts ($\times 10^5$) and mean% DNA probe counts of 41 bacterial species in 61 edentulous subjects. Counts for each species were averaged separately across up to 28 sites in each subject and then across subjects. Similarly, the proportion that each species comprised of the total DNA probe count was determined at each site, and then averaged within and then across subjects. The species were ordered according to the complexes described by Socransky et al.[34]

denture teeth of 61 edentulous subjects. Mean counts of the *Actinomyces* species, *V. parvula*, *Streptococcus* species, with the exception of *S. intermedius*, *C. gingivalis*, *E. corrodens*, *N. mucosa*, and *S. mutans* were quite high, while mean counts of many of the orange complex species and the entire red complex species were relatively low. The mean proportions followed a similar pattern. A striking feature was the presence of the periodontal pathogens, *A. actinomycetemcomitans* and *P. gingivalis*.

Microbiota of Soft Tissue and Saliva Samples in Edentulous Subjects

Figure 2 presents the mean total DNA probe counts for saliva samples, eight soft tissue surfaces and the polished, and exterior surface of the denture palates. Samples from the dorsal surfaces of the tongue exhibited the highest bacterial counts, followed by the "attached gingiva" (fixed keratinized tissue) and the lateral surfaces of the tongue. The lowest mean counts were found in samples from the buccal surfaces and the labial vestibules. Mean proportions of 31 of the test species differed significantly among sample locations, with the exception of *A. naeslundii* genospecies 2, *S. gordonii*, *S. sanguinis*, *C. ochracea*, *F. nucleatum ss polymorphum*, *F.*

periodonticum, S. constellatus, L. buccalis, N. mucosa, and *S. mutans* (Fig 3). The pattern of colonization differed among species. For example, *S. mitis* and *S. oralis* were found in lower proportions in saliva, the dorsal and lateral tongue surfaces, and the denture hard palates when compared to their proportions on the other soft tissue surfaces. *P. melaninogenica* was found in the highest proportions on the dorsal surfaces of the tongue. *A. odontolyticus*, *C. sputigena*, and *G. morbillorum* were detected in the highest proportions on the polished surfaces of the denture palates.

Comparison of the Microbiota of the Tongue Dorsum, Hard Palate, and Polished (exterior) Denture Palate

Figure 4 presents the mean total DNA probe counts in samples from the dorsal surfaces of the tongue, hard palate, and the polished (exterior) surfaces of the denture palate for the 61 edentulous subjects. The total DNA probe count was highest on the dorsal surfaces of the tongue and lowest in samples from the hard palates when comparing the three groups. The total DNA probe count for the polished, exterior surfaces of the denture palates was higher than that seen on the subjects' hard palates. When comparing the three surfaces for the 41 bacterial species, 40 species showed a significant

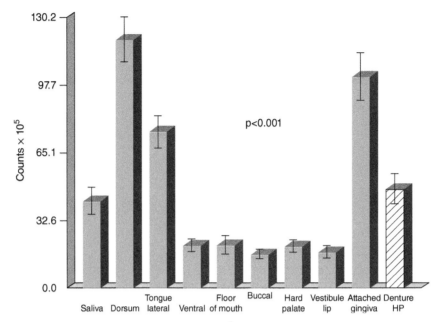

FIGURE 2 Mean total DNA probe counts ($\times 10^5$, $\pm$ SD) in samples of saliva, eight soft tissue surfaces, and the denture hard palate from 61 edentulous subjects. Total counts were averaged across subjects for each sample location separately. Significant differences among sample locations were sought using the Kruskal–Wallis test and adjusted for multiple comparisons.[36]

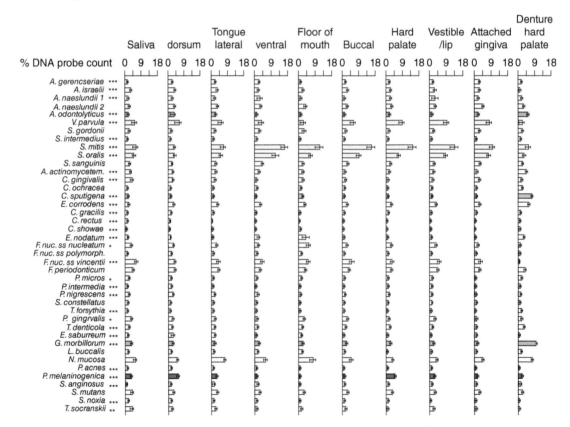

FIGURE 3 Mean% DNA probe counts ($\pm$ SD) of 41 species in samples of saliva, eight soft tissue surfaces, and the denture hard palate from 61 edentulous subjects. The proportion that each species comprised of the total DNA probe count was computed and averaged across subjects for each sample location separately. Significant differences among sample locations was sought using the Kruskal–Wallis test and adjusted for multiple comparisons: $*p < 0.05$; $**p < 0.01$; $***p < 0.001$. The colored bars represent species that were markedly different among sample locations.

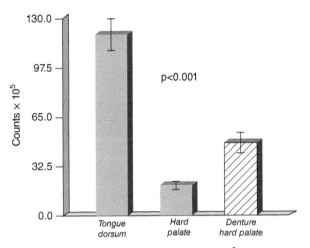

FIGURE 4 Mean total DNA probe counts ($\times10^5$, $\pm$ SD) in samples from the tongue dorsum, hard palate, and the exterior surface of the denture hard palate from 61 edentulous subjects. Total counts were averaged across subjects for each sample location separately. Significant differences among sample locations were sought using the Kruskal–Wallis test and adjusted for multiple comparisons.

difference among the three groups with p-values <0.001 (Fig 5). The exception was *S. mitis*, which was found in high levels in all three locations. Significant differences in mean proportions were observed for 21 of the test species.

Cluster analysis was employed to group the mean microbial profiles of the sample locations. The technique employed the minimum similarity coefficient and an average unweighted linkage sort using the mean species proportions of samples from saliva, the eight oral soft tissue locations, and the denture palatal surfaces (Fig 6). Two clusters were formed with >85% similarity consisting of the dorsal and lateral surfaces of the tongue, supragingival plaque, and saliva (cluster 1); and the "attached gingiva" (fixed keratinized tissue), hard palates, labial vestibules, buccal vestibules, ventral surfaces of the tongue, and floor of the mouth (cluster 2). The polished (exterior) surfaces of the denture palates did not cluster with the other sample locations.

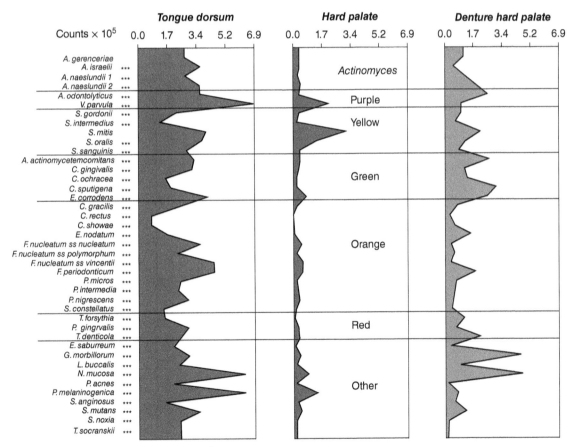

FIGURE 5 Mean counts ($\times10^5$) of 41 species in samples from the tongue dorsum, hard palate, and the exterior surface of the denture hard palate from 61 edentulous subjects. Counts were averaged across subjects for each sample location separately. Significant differences among sample locations were sought using the Kruskal–Wallis test and adjusted for multiple comparisons: ***$p < 0.001$.

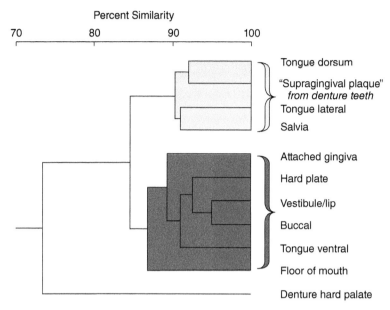

FIGURE 6   Dendrogram of a cluster analysis of the mean species proportions in samples from saliva, eight oral soft tissue surfaces, the denture teeth, and the exterior of the denture hard palate in 61 edentulous subjects. A minimum similarity coefficient and an average unweighted linkage sort were employed. Two clusters were formed at >85% similarity. The exterior surface of the denture hard palate did not cluster with the other sample locations.

DISCUSSION

This study presents cross-sectional data of the microbiota of dentures, oral soft tissues, and saliva of 61 edentulous subjects wearing both maxillary and mandibular complete dentures. All subjects in this investigation had been edentulous for at least 1 year. The "supragingival" plaque composition of the biofilms that formed on eight soft tissue surfaces, polished palatal surfaces (external) of the dentures, denture teeth, and the microbiota of saliva samples were examined between the 61 subjects and then for different intraoral locations within the same subject.

The 41 test species examined in the current investigation were those often found in studies of plaque and soft tissue biofilms in dentate subjects.[10,35] These species were also found in the "supragingival" plaque samples and soft tissue biofilm samples of the edentulous subjects. The results from the current investigation are significant in that much of the recent research has concentrated on the oral health of dentate patients, including examination of the association between oral disease and systemic health. Given the results of the current investigation, it may be important to provide the denture-wearing population care and follow-up similar to their non-denture-wearing counterparts.

The composition of the microbiota of different soft tissue surfaces, saliva, and the polished (exterior) surfaces of the denture palates was examined for 41 test species. On average, the test species could be found in samples from all locations, although there were marked differences among surfaces in the

microbiota with significant differences detected for 31 species. The highest mean total counts and counts of most species were detected on the dorsal surfaces of the tongue. The "attached gingiva" (fixed keratinized tissue), which represented the anterior ridges of edentulous maxillae, harbored the second highest mean counts, while the lowest counts were found on buccal mucosal surfaces and the labial vestibules.

Cluster analysis of the mean microbial profiles of the samples demonstrated that the microbiota of the lateral and dorsal surfaces of the tongue and saliva were similar to one another; however, they were different from the microbial profiles of the remaining six surfaces. This is similar to the findings in dentate subjects of Mager et al,[10] who found the proportions of bacterial species differed markedly on different intraoral surfaces and that the microbiota of saliva was most similar to that of the dorsal and lateral surfaces of the tongue. The microbiotas of the soft tissues resembled each other more than the microbiotas that colonized the teeth both above and below the gingival margin.

An important finding of the current investigation was that the periodontal pathogens *A. actinomycetemcomitans* and *P. gingivalis* were found in both the supragingival and soft tissue samples of the edentulous subjects. This finding is in contrast to reports in the literature that suggested that these species disappeared from the oral cavity after extraction of all teeth and did not reappear even when hard surfaces, such as complete dentures, were provided.[22,23] Furthermore, several investigators have reported a strong association between these periodontal pathogens and various systemic diseases,[24–31] although only biofilms in dentulous subjects were examined. The results of the current study suggest that complete denture patients may also be at risk for systemic disease from these two periodontal pathogens if they gain access to the circulation via trauma or pathology of the oral mucosa.

An interesting comparison was that of the microbiota of the tongue dorsum and the outer polished surface of the denture palates. It might be expected that the levels and types of bacteria seen on the dorsum of the tongue would be similar to those found on the palatal surfaces (polished, external) of complete dentures; however, in the cluster analysis of the microbiota, the microbiota of the denture palate did not cluster with that of any of the other surfaces. The effect of the different types of surfaces for initial attachment is the probable cause for such a difference in the levels and types of species on the two surfaces. A larger number of bacteria will likely adhere to the tongue due to papillae providing an increased surface area and possibly a more consistent moist environment. The highly polished external surface of the denture palates appeared to minimize colonization, leading to fewer microbes.

There were certain limitations associated with this study. One limitation was that probes to only 41 microbial species were employed. While this is far greater than any previous study, it is recognized that a substantial portion of the microbiota may not be represented. It has been suggested that over 700 species, many of which are uncultivable, can colonize the oral cavity;[9] however, the 41 probes used in this study have been shown to account for about 50% to 55% of the biomass in biofilm samples from dentate subjects.[35] Additional probes that should be considered in future denture studies would be *Candida albicans* and *S. salivarius*.

One might also argue that the microbiota seen in the denture-wearing subjects in this study could be attributed to the presence of "hard-tissue," in the form of complete dentures. It would be interesting to examine the composition of biofilms on the soft tissues of subjects with no natural teeth remaining and no hard-tissue replacements present in the form of either complete dentures or dental implants.

With a rise in the size of the elderly population, one can now also expect an increase in complete-denture patients, and therefore, it is critical for oral healthcare providers to pay equal attention to the dental needs of edentulous patients. This investigation provided an extensive examination of the microbiota of a limited number of edentulous, denture-wearing subjects. It is hoped that these data could have an impact on oral healthcare in complete denture patients.

CONCLUSIONS

The results of this study demonstrated that the periodontal pathogens *A. actinomycetemcomitans* and *P. gingivalis*, which were thought to be eliminated with the extraction of all natural teeth, were seen in significant numbers in the edentulous subjects. Microbial profiles differed according to the specific surfaces for colonization. The microbiota of the denture teeth, lateral and dorsal surfaces of the tongue, and saliva were similar to one another, and differed from the microbiota of the other six soft tissue surfaces and denture hard palates, which formed distinct cluster groups.

When comparing the mean total DNA probe counts among the dorsal surfaces of the tongue, denture palates, and the subjects' palates, the highest mean counts were found on the tongue dorsum, followed by the polished (exterior) surface of the denture palate, and were lowest on the hard palate.

REFERENCES

1. Cutress TW, Hunter PB: Past, present, and future trends in dental health and the dental system in New Zealand. *N Z Dent J* 1992;88:2–9.
2. Mojon P, Thomason JM, Walls AW: The impact of falling rates of edentulism. *Int J Prosthodont* 2004;17:434–440.
3. Lang BR: A review of traditional therapies in complete dentures. *J Prosthet Dent* 1994;72:538–542.
4. Douglass CW, Shih A, Ostry L: Will there be a need for complete dentures in the United States in 2020? *J Prosthet Dent* 2002;87:5–8.
5. Cates N: Trends in long-term care for the elderly. *Health Matrix* 1988–1989;6:50–57.
6. Redford M, Drury, TF, Kingman A, et al: Denture use and the technical quality of dental prostheses among persons 18–74 years of age: United States, 1988–1991. *J Dent Res* 1996;75:714–725.
7. Ettinger RL, Jakobsen J: Denture treatment needs of an overdenture population. *Int J Prosthodont* 1997;10:355–365.
8. Douglass CW, Gammon MD, Atwood DA: Need and effective demand for prosthodontic treatment. *J Prosthet Dent* 1988;59:94–104.
9. Aas JA, Paster BJ, Stokes LN, et al: Defining the normal bacterial flora of the oral cavity. *J Clin Microbiol* 2005;43:5721–5732.
10. Mager DL, Ximinez-Fyvie LA, Haffajee AD, et al: Distribution of selected bacterial species on intraoral surfaces. *J Clin Periodontol* 2003;30:644–654.
11. Socransky SS, Manganiello AD, Propas D, et al: Bacteriological studies of developing supragingival dental plaque. *J Periodont Res* 1977;12:90–106.
12. Li J, Helmerhorst EJ, Leone CW, et al: Identification of early microbial colonizers in human dental biofilm. *J Appl Microbiol* 2004;97:1311–1318.
13. Kononen E, Asikainen S, Jousimies-Somer H: The early colonization of gram-negative anaerobic bacteria in edentulous infants. *Oral Microbiol Immunol* 1992;7:28–31.

14. Kononen E, Jousimies-Somer H, Asikainen S: Relationship between oral gram-negative anaerobic becteria in saliva of the mother and the colonization of her edentulous infant. *Oral Microbiol Immunol* 1992;7:273–276.

15. Kononen E, Asikainen S, Alaluusua S, et al: Are certain oral pathogens part of normal oral flora in denture-wearing edentulous subjects? *Oral Microbiol Immunol* 1991;6:119–122.

16. Carlsson J, Soderholm G, Almfeldt I: Prevalence of *Streptococcus sanguis* and *Streptococcus mutans* in the mouth of persons wearing full dentures. *Arch Oral Biol* 1969;14:243–249.

17. Emilson CG, Thorselius I: Prevalence of mutans streptococci and lactobacilli in elderly Swedish individuals. *Scand J Dent Res* 1988;96:14–21.

18. Loesche WJ: The role of *Streptococcus mutans* in human dental decay. *Microbiol Rev* 1986;50:353–380.

19. Theilade E, Budtz-Jorgensen E, Theilade J: Predominant cultivable microflora of plaque on removable dentures in patients with healthy oral mucosa. *Arch Oral Biol* 1983;28:675–680.

20. Eger T, Zoller L, Muller HP, et al: Potential diagnostic value of sampling oral mucosal surfaces for Actinobacillus actinomycetemcomitans in young adults. *Eur J Oral Sci* 1996;104:112–117.

21. Frisken KW, Tagg JR, Orr MB: Suspected periodontopathic microorganisms and their oral habitats in young children. *Oral Microbiol Immunol* 1987;2:60–64.

22. Danser MM, van Winkelhoff AJ, de Graaff J, et al: Putative periodontal pathogens colonizing oral mucous membranes in denture-wearing subjects with a past history of periodontitis. *J Clin Periodontol* 1995;22:854–859.

23. Danser MM, van Winkelhoff AJ, van der Velden U: Periodontal bacteria colonizing oral mucous membranes in edentulous patients wearing dental implants. *J Periodontol* 1997;68:209–216.

24. Scannapieco FA, Bush RB, Paju S: Periodontal disease as a risk factor for adverse pregnancy outcomes. A systematic review. *Ann Periodontol* 2003;8:70–78.

25. Scannapieco FA, Bush RB, Paju S: Associations between periodontal disease and risk for nosocomial bacterial pneumonia and chronic obstructive pulmonary disease. A systematic review. *Ann Periodontol* 2003;8:54–69.

26. Scannapieco FA, Bush RB, Paju S: Associations between periodontal disease and risk for atherosclerosis, cardiovascular disease, and stroke. A systematic review. *Ann Periodontol* 2003;8:38–53.

27. Scannapieco FA, Rethman MP: The relationship between periodontal diseases and respiratory diseases. *Dent Today* 2003;22:79–83.

28. Campus G, Salem A, Uzzau S, et al: Diabetes and periodontal disease: a case-control study. *J Periodontol* 2005;76:418–425.

29. Cueto A, Mesa F, Bravo M, et al: Periodontitis as risk factor for acute myocardial infarction. A case control study of Spanish adults. *J Periodontal Res* 2005;40:36–42.

30. Moliterno LF, Monteiro B, Figueredo CM, et al: Association between periodontitis and low birth weight: a case-control study. *J Clin Periodontol* 2005;32:886–890.

31. Li X, Kolltveit KM, Tronstad L, et al: Systemic diseases caused by oral infection. *Clin Microbiol Rev* 2000;13:547 558.

32. Theilade E, Budtz-Jorgensen E: Predominant cultivable microflora of plaque on removable dentures in patients with denture-induced stomatitis. *Oral Microbiol Immunol* 1988;3:8–13.

33. Socransky SS, Smith C, Martin L, et al: "Checkerboard" DNA–DNA hybridization. *Biotechniques* 1994;17:788–792.

34. Socransky SS, Haffajee AD, Cugini MA, et al: Microbial complexes in subgingival plaque. *J Clin Periodontol* 1998;25:134–144.

35. Socransky SS, Haffajee AD: *Periodontal microbial ecology. Periodontology 2000* 2005;38:135–187.

36. Socransky SS, Haffajee AD, Smith C, et al: Relation of counts of microbial species to clinical status at the sampled site. *J Clin Periodontol* 1991;18:766–775.

37. Ludwig JA, Reynolds JF: *Statistical Ecology.* New York, NY, Wiley, 1988.

38. Sneath PH, Sokal RR: *Numerical Taxonomy–The Principles and Practice of Numerical Classification.* San Francisco, CA, W. H. Freeman, 1973.

10

EPIDEMIOLOGY AND ETIOLOGY OF DENTURE STOMATITIS

LINDA GENDREAU, DDS, AND ZVI G. LOEWY, PHD
GlaxoSmithKline Consumer Healthcare, Parsippany, NJ

Keywords
Stomatitis; biofilm; denture; epidemiology; etiology; Candida.

Correspondence
Zvi G. Loewy, GlaxoSmithKline, 1500 Littleton Road, Parsippany, NJ 07054. E-mail: zvi.g.loewy@gsk.com

Presented at the Annual Session of the American College of Prosthodontists in Orlando, FL, November 5, 1997.

Funded by The American College of Prosthodontists.

Accepted July 20, 2010

Published in *Journal of Prosthodontics* 2011; Vol. 20, Issue 4, pp. 251–60

doi: 10.1111/j.1532-849X.2011.00698.x

ABSTRACT

Denture stomatitis, a common disorder affecting denture wearers, is characterized as inflammation and erythema of the oral mucosal areas covered by the denture. Despite its commonality, the etiology of denture stomatitis is not completely understood. A search of the literature was conducted in the PubMed electronic database (through November 2009) to identify relevant articles for inclusion in a review updating information on the epidemiology and etiology of denture stomatitis and the potential role of denture materials in this disorder. Epidemiological studies report prevalence of denture stomatitis among denture wearers to range from 15% to over 70%. Studies have been conducted among various population samples, and this appears to influence prevalence rates. In general, where reported, incidence of denture stomatitis is higher among elderly denture users and among women. Etiological factors include poor denture hygiene, continual and nighttime wearing of removable dentures, accumulation of denture plaque, and bacterial and yeast contamination of denture surface. In addition, poor-fitting dentures can increase mucosal trauma. All of these factors appear to increase the ability of *Candida albicans* to colonize both the denture and oral mucosal surfaces, where it acts as an opportunistic pathogen. Antifungal treatment can eradicate *C. albicans* contamination and relieve stomatitis symptoms, but unless dentures are decontaminated and their cleanliness maintained, stomatitis will recur when antifungal therapy is discontinued. New developments related to denture materials are focusing on means to reduce development of adherent biofilms. These may have value in reducing

Denture stomatitis is a very common disorder affecting denture wearers. It is characterized as inflammation and erythema of the oral mucosal areas covered by the denture.[1–3] Several studies suggest that up to two-thirds or more of individuals who wear removable complete dentures can suffer from denture stomatitis.[3–6] Despite its frequency, denture stomatitis is most often asymptomatic; only a minority of sufferers experience pain, itching, or burning sensation, and the disorder is primarily diagnosed during examination as presence of inflammation or swelling of mucosal tissues covered by the denture.[2,7]

Despite its commonality, the etiology of denture stomatitis is poorly understood. Associations of denture stomatitis have been reported with mucosal trauma due to poor denture fit, increasing age of the denture user, increased age of dentures, bacterial and fungal (primarily *Candida*) infection, and poor denture hygiene;[1,4,5,8] however, no clear cause-and-effect relationships have been demonstrated for most associated etiologic factors. Indeed, the current thinking is that the etiology of denture stomatitis is multifactorial. In many incidences it likely includes a pathogenic response to *Candida* infection, and primarily infection with *C. albicans*.[5–7]

While access to dental care is improving, and persons are retaining their natural dentition for longer periods of their lives, the occurrence of edentulousness remains significant, especially among the elderly. The need for long-term use of dentures will remain for the foreseeable future, and as a consequence, a sizable at-risk population for denture stomatitis will remain.[9] This review provides an update on the epidemiology and etiology of denture stomatitis and the potential role of denture materials in this disorder. As denture matrices differ in the ability of oral bacteria and yeast to form biofilms and colonize them, they may reflect greater or lesser susceptibility for occurrence of denture stomatitis.

METHODS

Articles were identified by a search of the PubMed electronic literature database. Articles listed in the PubMed database through November 2009 are included. Search terms included "denture stomatitis" and "denture sore mouth" associated with terms related to epidemiology, etiology, and treatment. The search was limited to studies in humans and those published in English.

Titles and abstracts of identified articles were reviewed by this study's authors (LG, ZGL), and relevant articles

bacterial and yeast colonization, and could lead to reductions in denture stomatitis with appropriate denture hygiene.

obtained. Data related to epidemiology and etiology were extracted and summarized for this review. Additional articles addressing the potential impact of denture materials on denture stomatitis were reviewed and summarized.

RESULTS AND DISCUSSION

Epidemiology

Table 1 summarizes studies evaluating the prevalence of denture stomatitis. Prevalence rates, as prevalence among denture wearers only, are reported, as this is the at-risk population for denture stomatitis. Individuals wearing complete versus partial dentures, or combinations of complete and partial dentures were not separated into classes, as many of the articles did not provide this information. Several studies categorized denture stomatitis by severity, which was generally assessed using scales developed by Newton[10] or Budtz-Jorgensen and Bertram.[11]

Several studies reported denture stomatitis prevalence based on general population surveys. NHANES III (3rd National Health & Nutrition Examination Survey), surveyed a representative U.S. population sample. The study included 33,994 individuals, of whom 17,235 underwent dental examination and 3450 had at least one removable denture.[12,13] In the United States, about 20% of adults wear removable dentures. The prevalence of denture stomatitis among denture users reported in the NHANES III study was 28% (Table 1), with prevalence rates of 35% and 18% among persons wearing removable complete maxillary and mandibular dentures, respectively. National and regional population-based studies conducted in Denmark, Slovenia, Spain, and Turkey reported prevalence of denture stomatitis among denture wearers of 65%, 14.7%, 19.6%, and 18.5%, respectively.[14,15–17] The high incidence of denture stomatitis observed in the Danish study was associated with poor denture hygiene and a high prevalence of associated *Candida* infection in an elderly population.[14] The study from Turkey involved dental exams in 765 randomly selected residents of the Kartal region of Istanbul. Twenty-six percent of this study population wore removable dentures, and the incidence of denture stomatitis was quite low (18.5%).[15] Two population-based studies have been conducted in Finland, one a national sample[18] and the other an age-stratified sample of home-living elderly residents in Helsinki.[19] The studies reported a prevalence of denture stomatitis of 48% and 35%,

TABLE 1 Epidemiology of denture stomatitis

Study population	Age	# Denture users	Subjects with denture stomatitis (DS)			
			Method used to diagnose denture stomatitis	# with DS	DS prevalence	Ref
Random U.S. population sample participating in NHANES III study conducted in 1988 to 1994.	59.2 ± 0.5 yr	3450 57.7% M 42.3% F	Standardized oral examination conducted by trained dentists. DS was graded according to the Newton severity scale.	963	28%	12
Random sample of 10% of residents age >65 yr from 3 communities in Denmark	Mean 74.5 yr (range 65 to 92)	463	In-home examination by one investigator. Method used for DS diagnosis not stated	291	65%	14
Age-stratified, random sample among home-living residents of Helsinki, Finland (Helsinki Aging Study, 1989 to 91)	76, 81, and 86 yr	260 63 M 197 F	Examinations conducted at Univ of Helsinki, Inst. of Dentistry). DS not defined, lesions reported as inflammation, papillary hyperplasia, & fibrotic hyperplasia	91 17 M 74 F	35% 27% M 37.6% F	18
Third German Oral Health Study (DMS III), 1997. Random, age-stratified population-based sample	Young cohort: range 34 to 44 yr Older cohort: range 65 to 74 yr	655[b] 47.3% M 52.7% F 1367[b] 44.7% M 55.3% F	Standardized dental examinations with DS diagnosed using WHO guidelines	NR[c]	2.5% in young cohort 18.3% in older cohort	3
Representative sample of denture wearers from 1984 Finland oral health survey	NR[c]	3875 37.3% M 62.7% F	Regionally conducted oral examinations. Method to assess DS not reported	1860 626 M 1230 F	48% 43.2% M 50.6% F	19
Representative, population-based sample of adults in Istanbul, Turkey	35.6 ± 26.6 yr[a]	178	At-home oral examination using WHO guidelines to diagnose oral lesions	33 14 M 19 F	18.5%	15
Population-based, age-stratified sample of adult residents of Orvieto, Spain	54.3 ± 13.5 yr[a]	102	Oral examination to identify oral lesions. Method to characterize DS not specified.	24 9 M 15 F	19.6%	16
Random, age-stratified population-based sample from Ljubljana, Slovenia	Range 25 to 75 yr[a]	163 78 M 85 F	Dental examination	24 9 M 15 F	14.7% 11.5% M 17.7% F	17
Population sample of elderly residents (> 65 yrs) of Santiago, Chile stratified by age, gender, and socioeconomic status	65 to 74 yr[a] (n = 560) ≥75 yr[a] (n = 329)[a]	574 179 M 395 F	WHO diagnostic criteria for oral lesions graded by a single examiner	198 45 M 153 F	34.5% 25.1% M 38.7% F	20
Nursing-home and long-term care facility residents in Denmark	Range 64 ≥ 85 yr	582	Oral examinations conducted by one investigator at institutions. Method used to diagnose DS not indicated.	197	33.9%	21
Elderly full denture wearers in Istanbul, Turkey attending a university denture clinic		70	DS scored with using Budtz-Jorgensen 4-point scale	31	44%	22

(continued)

TABLE 1 (*Continued*)

Study population	Age	# Denture users	Subjects with denture stomatitis (DS)		
			Method used to diagnose denture stomatitis	# with DS	DS prevalence	Ref
Patients at the Laasko long-term care facility (Helsinki, Finland)	83.3 ± 8.1 yr[a]	106 25 M 81 F	Examinations conducted by single investigator; method to characterize DS not specified.		25%	23
Residents from 22 randomly selected nursing homes in Avon, UK	84.5 ± 8.3 yr[a] (range 42 to 102 yr)	331	Clinical examination conducted by single investigator at nursing homes; DS graded using Budtz-Jorgensen scale.	110	33.2%	24
Entire institutionalized population of Taubate, Brazil	74.9 ± 12.9 yr[a] (only 66% knew their age)	201	Clinical examination at nursing homes. Method to characterize DS not specified	108	54%	25
Geriatric residents of a long-term care facility (Val Fleuri, Belgium)	85.6 ± 6.9 yr[a] range 66 to 101 yr	146	Clinical examination conducted by single investigator at nursing homes; DS graded using Budtz-Jorgensen scale	104	71%	26
Elderly residents of a long-term care facility in Edmonton Canada	83.4 ± 17.6 yr[a]	38	Oral examination conducted by 1 of 2 previously calibrated clinicians. DS graded using Newton criteria	13	34.2%	27
Population-based sample of elderly community-dwelling and nursing home residents in Greece	Mean age 78 yr[a] range 65 to 99	222	DS graded using Newton criteria	33	14.9%	28
Elderly complete denture wearers living in retirement homes in southern Brazil	66.7 ± 10.2 yr	59 24 M 35 F	Examination conducted by expert in stomatology with DS graded per Newton classification	26 11 M 15F	44.1% 45.8%0 M 42.9% F	29
Residents, age > 60 from 2 rural communities in Brazil	NR[c]	146	Examination conducted by one investigator at local dental clinic. Method used to characterized DS not indicated		58.2%	30
Edentulous referral patients treated (1976 to 1983) at dental clinic of Univ of BC, Vancouver, BC, Canada	Range 24 to 90 yr	200 24% M 76% F	Chart review. Method to characterize DS stomatitis not reported.	ND	17%	31
Edentulous patients wearing dental protheses examined at a prosthodontic clinic in Mexico	Mean 67 yr	105 43 M 62 F	Examination at clinic. Method to characterize DS not specified.	50 21 M 29 F	47.6% 48.8% M 46.8% F	32
Denture wearers seeking treatment at a university dental clinic in Brazil	62 ± 12.8 yr	236 25% M 75% F	Sequential patients seeking dental care at clinic. Method to characterize DS not specified.	ND	42.4%	33
Consecutive denture patents seeking dental treatment at clinic of medical school in Istanbul, Turkey	Mean 65 yr range 45 to 81 yr	234	Patient questionnaire and clinical examination; method to characterize DS not specified.	130	55.5%	34

Study population	Age	n	Method to characterize denture stomatitis	n	Prevalence	Ref
Patients attending 2 prosthodontic clinics in Jordan for denture replacement or adjustment	65 ± 10.1 yr range 18 to 100 yr	321 203 M 118 F	Method to characterize denture stomatitis not specified	94 45 M 49 F	29% 22.2% M 41.5% F	35
Complete denture wearers, over age 60 seen at dental clinic at a medical school in central Turkey for replacement or adjustment of dentures	65.7 ± 2.7 yr range 60 to 85 yr	310 159 M 151 F	Clinical examination with DS identified and categorized per Newton classification	111 56 M 55 F	35.8% 35.2% M 36.4% F	36
Complete denture wearers seen at a university dental clinic in Glasgow, Scotland for denture replacement	Mean 73 yr range 49 to 89 yr	37	Clinical examination. DS classified per Newton classification	26	70.3%	37
Otherwise healthy subjects with complete dentures consulting university dental clinic (Ataturk Univ, Turkey)	range 36 to 82 yr	70 39 M 31 F	Clinical examination with DS diagnosed and classified per Budtz-Jorgensen scale	49 30 M 19 F	70% 76.9% M 61.3% F	38
Outpatients seen at prosthodontic clinic of the Univ of Montreal for replacement of complete maxillary or maxillary and mandibular dentures	Mean 64.5 yr	40 11 M 29 F	Oral examination performed by a single investigator with confirmatory diagnosis. DS classified per Newton typing.	31	77.5%	39
Follow-up to clinical trial evaluating complete dentures (n=76) and mandibular implant overdentures (n=97) after 1 year	72.1 ± 4.4 yr	173 80 M 93 F	Oral examination conducted by 2 calibrated examiners. DS diagnosed by Newton classification.	110 48 M 62 F	63.6% 60.0% M 66.7% F	40
Otherwise healthy patients seen at university prosthodontic clinic in Bilbao, Spain	Mean 65.1 yr[a] range 40 to 87 yr	100	Oral examination with DS diagnosed using Newton classification	45	45%	41
Patients attending prosthodontic clinic of the Jordan Univ. of Science & Technology	Mean 59 and 54 yr for M and F range 39 to 100	300 175 M 125 F	Oral examination to assess presence of DS. DS categorized using Newton classification	157 89 M 68 F	52% 50.9% M 54.4% F	42

[a] Age only given for total study population;
[b] total population (no value given for denture wearers);
[c] NR, Not Reported; DS, denture stomatitis.

respectively. The representative national population-based survey conducted in Finland in 1984 included 7190 adults, of whom 3856 wore removable dentures, suggesting that almost 44% of adults in Finland had dentures.[18] A national populationbased survey conducted in Germany in 1997, the Third German Oral Health Study, reported denture stomatitis prevalence in the general population (not exclusively denture wearers) to be 2.5% and 18.3% in cohorts aged 34 to 44 and 65 to 74 years, respectively.[3]

Over a dozen studies have evaluated denture stomatitis prevalence exclusively among elderly populations, reporting prevalence ranging from 15% to 71%.[14,18,20–30] The studies assessed elderly living in both community and in nursing-home or long-term care facility settings. A 1987 publication by Vigild reported a 34% prevalence of denture stomatitis among elderly denture wearers living in nursing homes and long-term care facilities in Denmark.[21] This is about one-half the rate of stomatitis reported in a 1975 study conducted among community-dwelling elderly Danes by Budtz-Jorgensen et al[14] Two studies have evaluated denture stomatitis among elderly residents of Finland, reporting prevalence rates of 35% and 25% among home-living and institutionalized denture wearers, respectively.[18,23] Studies conducted in South America reported a prevalence of denture stomatitis of 34.5%, 58.2%, and 54% among elderly community residents in Santiago, Chile, elderly denture wearers in a rural community in Brazil, and elderly patients in Brazilian long-term care facilities, respectively.[20,25,30]

Several studies reporting prevalence of denture stomatitis focused on denture wearers visiting dental or prosthetic clinics for treatment, adjustment, or replacement of dentures. The studies included sites in Canada (three studies), Mexico, Brazil, Turkey (three studies), Jordan (two studies), Scotland, and Spain.[31–42] This group of studies mostly involved single sites. To reduce inter-patient variability, the designs usually involved a single investigator at each site conducting examinations and diagnosing and categorizing denture stomatitis. Denture stomatitis prevalence ranged from 17% to over 77%, with eight of the twelve studies reporting prevalence of 45% or more. The size of the individual studies varied, and this may have impacted the outcomes; the prevalence of stomatitis in six studies evaluating 200 or more denture wearers was 17% to 55.5%,[31,33–36,42] while in four studies involving 100 or fewer subjects, prevalence ranged from 45% to 77.5%.[37–39,41]

A number of studies (Table 1) either report, or allow calculation of, denture stomatitis prevalence in men and women. The two population-based studies conducted in Finland reported a higher percentage of denture users to be female, and a higher prevalence rate of denture stomatitis among women.[18,19] A similar pattern was observed for a study conducted in Slovenia.[17] The other population-based studies did not provide adequate information to determine gender-associated prevalence for this disorder. Similar to the observations among elderly denture wearers in Finland, a study of elderly Chilean denture wearers reported increased prevalence of stomatitis among women (38.7%) versus men (25.1%). In contrast, a survey of elderly Brazilians living in retirement homes failed to show a significant association between gender and stomatitis prevalence.[21,30] Several studies surveying the prevalence of denture stomatitis among patients visiting dental and prosthodontic clinics have also assessed gender relationships; however, results from these surveys are inconsistent, with three, two, and one of these clinic-based surveys reporting no association of stomatitis with gender, a higher prevalence among women, and a higher prevalence among men, respectively.[32,35,36,38,40,42]

While a large number of studies have reported prevalence of denture stomatitis, there are issues and potential concerns regarding study designs. The US NHANES, German DMSIII, and the oral health survey conducted in Finland are clearly studies conducted in representative population-based samples;[3,12,19] however, several other studies, while claiming to be population-based, enrolled subjects from more limited populations, and the ability to extrapolate data from these studies to a broader, representative national population is questionable. In addition, while most studies used questionnaires to retrieve information regarding denture care, none include the actual questionnaires in the publication. This limits the ability to compare outcomes between studies and to reproduce studies by reusing or adapting questionnaires. It should be noted that characterizing denture stomatitis relies on different grading scores. While scores proposed by Newton[10] and Budtz-Jorgensen and Bertram[11] are quite similar (grades obtained from either scale can be inter-polated to the other), some studies do not report having used standardized scales for grading or characterizing severity of stomatitis.

Etiological Associations

The epidemiology studies discussed above identify several factors associated with denture stomatitis. Demographic factors include increasing age of denture wearers, female gender, smoking, and concurrent illnesses that compromise immune function. Factors related to denture use itself include poor-fitting dentures, which exacerbate oral mucosal trauma and irritation, increasing age of the denture, use of maxillary versus mandibular dentures, lack of appropriate denture care and hygiene, the presence of pathogenic microbial infection (primarily *Candida*), and continual wearing of dentures. These factors have been considered in prior reviews.[1,2,4,5,12,43] Past reviews also suggest a potential role of contact allergy from denture materials in denture stomatitis. While an allergic response may have been a significant contributory factor in denture stomatitis in the past, use of modern denture materials have virtually eliminated allergic response as a significant risk factor in denture stomatitis.

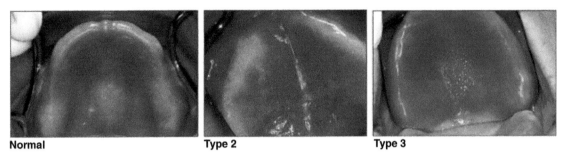

Normal   **Type 2**   **Type 3**

FIGURE 1   Denture stomatitis clinical photographs based on Newton classification (courtesy of Professor Steven Offenbacher).

The current view is that the etiology of denture stomatitis is multifactorial, and has a number of associative factors rather than a single cause.[2] Poor denture hygiene, pathogenic *Candida* infection, and continual wearing of dentures appear to be the predominant associated etiological factors for denture stomatitis and represent likely targets for interventions using a combination of pharmacological therapy provided by healthcare professionals and improved denture hygiene by denture users. This review discusses several etiological factors, including associations of denture stomatitis with denture-induced trauma and denture hygiene.

Association of Denture Stomatitis with Denture-Induced Trauma   Budtz-Jorgensen and Bertram[11] reported an association of simple localized inflammation, a level of palatal inflammation similar to Newton's Type I, with poor denture fit and related irritation and trauma. Poorly fitting dentures have been reported by others to be associated with higher risk for denture stomatitis.[21] More extensive forms of stomatitis that manifested with granular inflammation were found to be more strongly associated with poor hygiene and *Candida* infection.[11] Several epidemiological studies have reported the relative incidence of Type I compared to Type II and III denture stomatitis, and suggest localized inflammation to be present in about one-half of individuals with this disorder (Fig 1).[15,17,24,27,37-39] A recent study by Emami et al[40] tested

the hypothesis that increased occlusal pressure can contribute to mucosal trauma in denture stomatitis. These authors compared the incidence of denture stomatitis among 173 elderly edentulous patients who randomly received new conventional maxillary and mandibular dentures (n = 76) with those receiving two-implant mandibular overdentures (n = 97), which provided improved stability and fit and reduced occlusal pressure. After 1 year, the overall incidence of dentures stomatitis was 64%, with severity approximately equally divided among Newton's Type I and Type II; however, patients with conventional dentures were significantly more likely to have denture stomatitis than those with mandibular overdentures (OR: 4.52; 95% CI: 2.24–9.14; $p < 0.0001$). There were no differences in cleanliness or how subjects wore dentures between the groups. Improved stability appeared to reduce risk for stomatitis.

Association of Denture Hygiene with Denture Stomatitis   Poor denture hygiene is clearly accepted as a critical risk factor for denture stomatitis (Fig 2). As summarized later, numerous studies demonstrate a clear association between poor denture hygiene and increased risk for and prevalence of denture stomatitis.[11,22,24,31,33-35,44-47] These studies report that many denture wearers attempt to maintain denture hygiene only by brushing dentures, as one would brush natural dentition; however, this is inadequate for maintaining

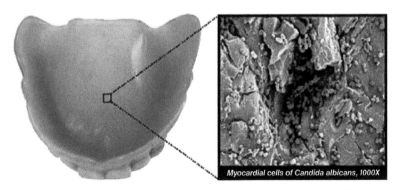

Myocardial cells of Candida albicans, 1000X

FIGURE 2   Microscopic representation of attached microbial cells on the surface of a denture.

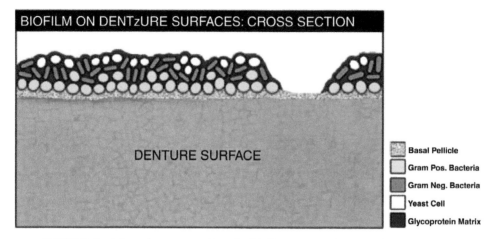

FIGURE 3   Schematic representation of a biofilm cross section on a denture surface.

proper denture hygiene, and other methods, such as use of commercial disinfectant solutions, or soaking dentures in dilute sodium hypochlorite, are required as part of daily and routine denture maintenance. Not removing dentures at night while sleeping has also been associated with poor hygiene and increased risk for developing denture stomatitis.[11,23,31,33–35,44,46,47] In addition to poor hygiene, constant denture wearing maintains relatively anaerobic and low-pH conditions between the denture base and the mucosa, which can promote opportunistic overgrowth of pathogenic yeasts, such as *Candida*.

Budtz-Jorgensen and Bertram reported poor denture hygiene to be associated with increased denture and oral mucosal colonization with *Candida*, greater mucosal trauma, and increased severity of inflammation among 58 stomatitis patients (mean age 57.7 years) who had used full dentures for an average of 26.8 years.[11] Several other studies comparing adult denture wearers with and without denture stomatitis report stomatitis to be significantly associated with poor denture cleanliness.[22,31,34,44]

Inadequately cleaned dentures rapidly develop an adherent biofilm and accumulate pathogenic denture plaque. Biofilm and plaque contain bacteria and yeasts that reside on the denture surfaces and can also colonize the oral mucosa (Fig 3). The biofilm and yeast contaminants have a role in oral inflammation in denture stomatitis.[48,49] The microbial ecology of the biofilm is complex. A recent study that identified bacterial and yeast contaminants from swabs of denture biofilms reported 82 bacterial phylotypes and three fungal species. While many bacteria were common to biofilms from both healthy individuals and denture stomatitis patients, the study identified 26 and 32 bacterial phylotypes unique to healthy subjects and those with stomatitis. Of fungal species, *C. albicans* was the only fungal species found in the denture biofilms of stomatitis patients; it was also present in healthy subjects, but these subjects had other *Candida* species present (Fig 4).[48]

While poor denture hygiene can increase the risk for denture stomatitis, maintaining hygiene has been shown to prevent recurrence. Following successful therapeutic treatment of *Candida*-associated denture stomatitis, 18 of 22 patients were reported to maintain remission for 3 years through stringent denture hygiene.[45]

An association between poor denture hygiene and denture stomatitis is clear. Unfortunately, the majority of persons who wear dentures are elderly and many may have impairments that make proper cleansing and care of their dentures difficult. In addition, since proper cleaning requires dentures to be removed, persons who report that they continually wear their dentures, especially persons who wear their dentures overnight, cannot practice adequate hygienic maintenance. For cleaning, brushing dentures alone, or washing them with water is not adequate to prevent formation of the surface biofilm. Proper cleaning should include removing dentures and soaking them in a commercial disinfectant solution, or diluted sodium hypochlorite. Using ultrasonic cleaning is an alternative cleansing approach.[50] Two studies have reported success using a microwave to disinfect dentures as a treatment for *Candida-associated* denture stomatitis. Both studies reported that the microwaving regimen reduced *Candida* on dentures, and the study by Neppelenbroek et al reported this

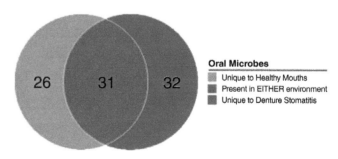

FIGURE 4   Oral microbe distribution cataloged by state of health.

to be effective for treating denture stomatitis, and to have a low rate of recurrence over a 3-month follow-up period.[51,52]

Association of Candida Infection with Denture Stomatitis

Candida and *C. albicans* are often found on the dentures and oral mucosa of individuals without any signs of denture stomatitis.[53,54] The role of *Candida*, and specifically *C. albicans*, in development of denture stomatitis is associated with pathogenic overgrowth of *Candida* on denture surfaces and the oral mucosa, and is widely accepted as a leading etiological factor in this disorder. A quantitative presence of *Candida* has been found to be associated with denture stomatitis disease manifestation.[55] In their 1970 publication, Budtz-Jorgensen and Bertram reported a significant association between inflammation and yeast colonization in patients with denture stomatitis,[11] and this association has been confirmed in subsequent studies.[22,32,37,38,44,56–58]

It is possible that the etiological role in denture stomatitis occurs in combination with other factors, especially poor denture hygiene and continuous wearing of dentures.[1,2,5,6,11,14,22,37,43,49] As reviewed by Odds,[53] while *C. albicans* is a normal commensal organism, it can become pathogenic in situations that predispose individuals to infection. While most *Candida*-related lesions are acute events, chronic lesions almost always occur on the soft palate and are associated with wearing dentures, where *C. albicans* is the most prevalent Candidial species. Other common oral *Candida* species include *C. glabrata*, *C. krusei*, *C. parapsilosis*, and *C. tropicalis*. These species, however, are present with lower prevalence than *C. albicans* and have not been shown to have an increased prevalence or a pathological role in denture stomatitis.

C. albicans can grow either as mycelial or hyphal forms. A greater presence of *C. albicans* hyphae has been reported in patients with denture stomatitis. This has led to the hypothesis that *C. albicans* in this form has greater pathological activity.[5,14] It has also been hypothesized that the hyphal form of *C. albicans* can better adhere to and penetrate fissures on denture surfaces and is thus more invasive to the oral mucosa (Fig 5).[5,6] Song et al[59] recently characterized yeast isolates from patients with denture stomatitis; *C. albicans* was the predominant species. The authors noted that yeasts that colonized the dentures and mucosa of stomatitis patients formed colonies with diverse morphologies, while the same yeast species when present in healthy denture wearers formed colonies with smooth morphology.[59] Bilhan et al reported a significantly higher presence of *C. albicans* hyphae among patients with denture stomatitis compared to healthy denture users without palatal inflammation.[60] Emami et al reported a significant association between abundance of myceliated colonies of *C. albicans* with increased severity of denture stomatis.[39] While changes in *C. albicans* morphology have been associated with the presence, and perhaps severity, of denture stomatitis, no variant strains of this yeast

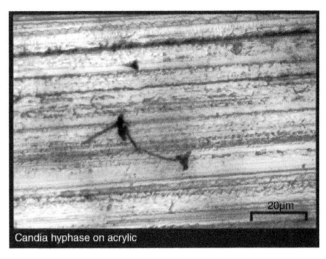

FIGURE 5 Photomicrograph of *Candida* hyphae on an acrylic surface (courtesy of Professor J. Verran and Sarah L. Jackson).

having unique virulence factors or pathogenic associations for denture stomatitis have been identified to date.[61,62]

The effectiveness of antifungal therapy in the treatment of denture stomatitis directly supports an etiological role of *Candida* infection in this disorder, and has been reviewed by Lombardi andBudtz-Jorgensen.[63] Double-blind, placebo-controlled studies have reported that treatment with either oral fluconazole (50 mg/day for 14 days) or topical miconazole (2% gel applied to denture fitting surface three times daily for 14 days) significantly reduced the presence of yeasts on oral mucosa and reduced inflammation in denture stomatitis.[64,65] In a controlled trial in patients with denture stomatitis who did not change their normal denture hygiene practices, 2 weeks of daily treatment with nystatin powder (~215,000 IU/day) applied to the maxillary denture fitting surface significantly reduced yeast colonization and palatal inflammation compared to no treatment.[66] DePaola et al[67] and Schwartz et al,[68] respectively, reported nystatin, used either in an oral rinse in combination with a denture soaking solution (oral rinse: 1,000,000 U twice daily plus daily overnight [6 hours] soaking in a nystatin solution for 28 days), or as an oral rinse alone (same dose and regimen), significantly reduced yeast colonization and resolved inflammation in denture stomatitis. A controlled trial reported 14 days treatment with amphotericin B (10 mg) administered as an oral dissolving lozenge, soaking dentures in 0.2% chlorhexidine solution, or the combination of the two treatments significantly and equivalently reduced erythema in denture stomatitis; however, recurrence of inflammation to near baseline severity occurred within 14 days of stopping treatment.[69] Uncontrolled trials have reported capsule and liquid formulations of itraconazole (100 mg b.i.d. for 15 days), fluconazole alone (50 mg orally for 14 days), or in combination with chlorhexidine applied to the denture fitting surface twice daily for 2 weeks, and amphotericin (40 mg oral dissolving lozenges 4 times daily + topical cream applied to the denture fitting surface) all to be efficacious for treating denture stomatitis.[70–73] In general, all studies indicated the various treatments to be well tolerated.

Clearly, antifungal therapy is effective in the acute treatment of inflammation associated with denture stomatitis, and this is considered supportive of the pathogenic role of *Candida* infection in this disorder; however, unless there is an associated improvement in denture cleanliness and reduction of *Candida* contamination on denture surfaces, the effectiveness of antifungal treatment is limited, and rapid recurrence of denture stomatitis can often occur within a short period of time after stopping treatment. For example, Chandra et al reported 16- to >128-fold reductions in the potency of amphotericin, nystatin, chlorhexidine, and fluconazole for inhibiting growth of *C. albicans* grown on denture adherent biofilms in vitro, versus their effects on *C albicans* grown in simple culture.[74] Hence, the rapid recurrence of denture stomatitis that can occur after stopping antifungal treatment likely reflects recontamination by residual yeast that are present on the denture surfaces and which are relatively unaffected or resistant to the treatment.

Role of Denture Materials in Denture Stomatitis

Dentures themselves have a role in promoting the development of stomatitis. A primary role is the ability of bacteria and yeast to colonize denture materials, forming a biofilm. Biofilms adhere to denture surfaces, forming the plaque deposit, which provides a source of continued exposure of the mucosa to the organisms contained within this biofilm. In vitro studies have shown that microorganisms within the biofilm appear to have resistance to antifungal and antimicrobial treatment, though the mechanism for this is not fully understood.[6] Whether a decrease in antimicrobial potency represents the biofilm functioning as a simple diffusion barrier, or whether there is a more complex interaction, has not been adequately studied. Therefore, effective decontamination of dentures is a required, and likely separate, treatment approach from that of treating mucosal inflammation and infection in the effective management of denture stomatitis.

The association of poor denture cleanliness with denture stomatitis was shown by Pires et al[75] who achieved significant clinical improvement with denture replacement. Among 39 subjects wearing full dentures and having denture stomatitis, over 80% had poor or deficient denture hygiene, and 100% had *C. albicans* colonization of their dentures and oral mucosa. Denture stomatitis had resolved in almost two-thirds of these subjects 6 months after receiving new dentures and practicing improved hygiene. Replacement also improved denture hygiene within the study group. At the 6-month evaluation, all patients had good (absence of plaque) or regular (removable plaque on inner denture surface only) hygiene, compared to the majority having poor/inadequate hygiene at entry.[75] A similar association was reported by

Webb et al in a study conducted in nursing home patients who had poor denture hygiene and denture stomatitis.[51] Subjects were randomized to maintain their usual hygiene procedures, or had their dentures cleaned daily with overnight soaking in sodium hypochlorite solution or microwaving. Relative to the control group, both cleaning techniques reduced bacteria and *Candida* colonization of dentures ~100-fold, reduced *Candida* counts on the palate, and resulted in significant clinical improvement in denture stomatitis.

Several studies have reported electron microscopic analyses of denture plaque. Twenty-three patients with denture stomatitis evaluated in three studies, of which only one included a control group of seven healthy denture wearers, reported plaque to consist of an electron-dense basal pellicle directly on the denture surface, above which was an opaque layer containing Gram-positive and -negative bacteria and yeast cells, reported to be *C. albicans*. In the single controlled study, with the exception of the presence of *C. albicans*, there were no differences in the appearance of plaque between subjects with and without stomatitis.[76–78]

Ramage et al also used scanning electron microscopy to demonstrate the propensity of *Candida* biofilms to adhere along imperfections and cracks on denture surfaces.[6] Filamentous cell forms of *Candida* were shown to become deeply embedded within surface deformities, and this was hypothesized to at least in part be responsible for the resistance of the *Candida* biofilm to antifungal treatment. Von Fraunhofer and Loewy reviewed factors involved in microbial attachment and colonization of denture surfaces, confirming that surface cracks and surface roughness facilitate attachment of microorganisms and development of the biofilm.[79] Furthermore, these authors noted that prolonged brushing of denture acrylic resin with a toothbrush and abrasive dentrifices can create surface scratches that can enhance bacterial attachment and biofilm growth. Denture soft lining materials can also develop increased surface roughness as they age on the denture surface, and a recent study confirms that this enhances attachment and colonization of these materials with *C. albicans*.[80] Finally, surface hydrophobicity has been shown to selectively increase the ability of hyphal forms of *C. albicans* to colonize denture surfaces, and in vitro studies have shown that decreasing surface hydrophobicity by using hydrophilic coating materials can decrease the ability of *C. albicans*, but not other yeasts, to attach and colonize the denture material surface. This may offer an interesting direction for future development of denture materials that can resist development of biofilms leading to denture stomatitis.[81]

Preventing development of the biofilm on dentures is indicated as the best approach for maintaining denture hygiene. Satisfactory denture sanitization using commercial denture cleansers offers a safe and effective approach for biofilm removal;[79] however, the high prevalence of denture stomatitis among denture wearers, and its association with lack of proper denture hygiene, suggests that only a minority of denture wearers actually practice stringent cleaning of their prostheses. The need to continually maintain proper hygiene, and for denture wearers to have regular follow-up appointments, and perhaps regular professional cleansing of their dentures, seems appropriate to help prevent or treat and prevent relapse of denture stomatitis. The review by Von Fraunhofer and Loewy[79] suggests that modifying denture materials to provide a relatively anionic surface, or using coatings that can prevent bacterial attachment may offer future means for reducing biofilm development.

CONCLUSIONS

Denture stomatitis affects a large percentage of persons wearing removable complete dentures. It has a multifactorial etiology. Key factors that can dramatically increase the risk of denture stomatitis are poor denture fit, poor denture hygiene, and colonization of the denture surface and oral mucosa, primarily mucosa in contact with denture fitting surfaces, with *C. albicans*. Poor denture care and hygienic maintenance leads to rapid establishment of a biofilm and accumulation of denture plaque. Since this provides the means for denture colonization by *Candida* strains, the correlation between lack of hygiene and propensity for Candida infection is clear. Denture materials themselves can contribute to the risk for denture stomatitis, as areas of surface roughness and the hydrophobicity of denture surfaces can promote attachment of microorganisms and development of the biofilm.

It is important to reduce risk for development of denture stomatitis. Good quality prostheses coupled with clear instructions to denture wearers by dentists and prosthodontists on the importance of diligent maintenance and use of a daily cleaning regimen are required. Denture wearers must take it on themselves to be diligent and practice appropriate denture hygiene.

Additionally, denture wearers should remove their dentures at night. Routine follow-up visits to assess that the prostheses maintain proper fit and function, and that users are maintaining denture hygiene is of extreme importance in reducing risk for developing stomatitis. Finally, treatment of stomatitis appears to rely on stringent cleaning or replacement of dentures, together with appropriate antifungal therapy.

ACKNOWLEDGMENTS

The authors thank Dr. Kenneth Mandel and Paul Grech for contributing to this manuscript.

REFERENCES

1. Arendorf TM, Walker DM: Denture stomatitis: a review. *J Oral Rehabil* 1987;14:217–227.
2. Wilson J: The aetiology, diagnosis and management of denture stomatitis. *Br Dent J* 1998;185:380–384.
3. Reichart PA: Oral mucosal lesions in a representative cross-sectional study of aging Germans. *Community Dent Oral Epidemol* 2000;28:390–398.
4. Budtz-Jorgensen E: Clinical aspects of *Candida* infection in denture wearers. *J Am Dent Assoc* 1978;96:474–477.
5. Webb BC, Thomas CJ, Willcox MDP, et al: *Candida*-associated denture stomatitis. Aetiology and management: a review. Part I. Factors influencing distribution of *Candida* species in the oral cavity. *Aust Dent J* 1998;43:45–50.
6. Ramage G, Tomsett K, Wickers BL, et al: Denture stomatitis: a role for *Candida* biofilms. *Oral Surg Oral Med Oral Pathol Oral Radiol Endod* 2004;98:53–59.
7. Budtz-Jorgensen E: The significance of *Candida albicans* in denture stomatitis. *Scand J Dent Res* 1974;82:151–190.
8. Jeganathan S, Lin CC: Denture stomatitis—a review of the aetiology, diagnosis and management. *Aust Dent J* 1992;37:107–114.
9. Petersen PE, Yamamoto T: Improving the oral health of older people: the approach of the WHO Global Oral Health Programme. *Community Dent Oral Epidemiol* 2005;33:81–92.
10. Newton AV: Denture sore mouth. A possible etiology. *Br Dent J* 1962;112:357–360.
11. Budtz-Jorgensen E, Bertram U: Denture stomatitis. I. The etiology in relation to trauma and infection. *Acta Odontol Scand* 1970;28:71–92.
12. Shulman JD, Rivera-Hidalgo F, Beach MM: Risk factors associated with denture stomatitis in the United States. *J Oral Pathol Med* 2005;34:340–346.
13. Shulman JD, Beach MM, Rivera-Hidalgo F: The prevalence of oral mucosal lesions in U.S. adults. Data from the third National Health and Nutrition Examination Survey, 1988–1994. *J Am Dent Assoc* 2004;135:1279–1286.
14. Budtz-Jorgensen E, Stenderup A, Grabowski M: An epidemiologic study of yeasts in elderly denture wearers. *Community Dent Oral Epidemiol* 1975;3:115–119.
15. Mumcu G, Cimilli H, Sur H, et al: Prevalence and distribution of oral lesions: a cross-sectional study in Turkey. *Oral Dis* 2005;11:81–87.
16. Vallejo MJG, Diaz-Canel AIM, Martin JMG, et al: Risk factors for oral soft tissue lesions in an adult Spanish population. *Community Dent Oral Epidemiol* 2002;30:277–285.
17. Kovac-Kavcic M, Skaleric U: The prevalence of oral mucosal lesions in a population in Ljubljana, Slovenia. *J Oral Pathol Med* 2000;28:331–335.
18. Nevalainen MJ, Nahri TO, Ainamo A: Oral mucosal lesions and oral hygiene habits in the home-living elderly. *J Oral Rehabil* 1997;24:332–337.
19. Mikkonen M, Nyyssonen V, Paunio I, et al: Oral hygiene, dental visits and age of denture for prevalence of denture

stomatitis. *Community Dent Oral Epidemiol* 1984;12:402–405.

20. Espinoza I, Rojas R, Aranda W, et al: Prevalence of oral mucosal lesions in elderly people in Santiago, Chile. *J Oral Pathol Med* 2003;32:571–575.

21. Vigild M: Oral mucosal lesions among institutionalized elderly in Denmark. *Community Dent Oral Epidemiol* 1987;15:309–313.

22. Kulak-Ozkan Y, Kazazoglu E, Arikan A: Oral hygiene habits, denture cleanliness, presence of yeasts, and stomatitis in elderly people. *J Oral Rehabil* 2002;29:300–304.

23. Peltola P, Vehkalahti MM, Wuolijoki-Saaristo K: Oral health and treatment needs of the long-term hospitalised elderly. *Gerodontology* 2004;21:93–99.

24. Frenkel H, Harvey I, Newcombe RG: Oral health care among nursing home residents in Avon. *Gerodontology* 2000;17:33–38.

25. Marchini L, Vieira PC, Bossan TP, et al: Self-reported oral hygiene habits among institutionalised elderly and their relationship to the condition of oral tissues in Taubate, Brazil. *Gerodontology* 2006;23:33–37.

26. Budtz-Jorgensen E, Mojon P, Bannon-Clement JM, et al: Oral candidosis in long-term hospital care: comparison of edentulous and dentate subjects. *Oral Dis* 1996;2:285–290.

27. Kuc IM, Samaranayake LP, van Heyst EN: Oral health and microflora in an institutionalized elderly population in Canada. *Int Dent J* 1999;49:33–40.

28. Triantos D: Intra-oral findings and general health conditions among institutionalized and non-institutionalized elderly in Greece. *J Oral Pathol Med* 2005;34:577–582.

29. Thiele MC, Carvalho AP, Grusky LC, et al: The role of candidal histolytic enzymes on denture-induced stomatitis in patients living in retirement homes. *Gerodontology* 2008;25:229–236.

30. Freitas JB, Gomez RS, de Abreu MHNG, et al: Relationship between the use of full dentures and mucosal alterations among elderly Brazilians. *J Oral Rehabil* 2008;35:370–374.

31. Dorey JL, Blasberg B, MacEntee MI, et al: Oral mucosal disorders in denture wearers. *J Prosthet Dent* 1985;53:210–213.

32. Monroy TB, Maldonado VM, Martinez FF, et al: *Candida albicans*, Staphylococcus aureus and Streptococcus mutans colonization in patients wearing dental prosthesis. *Oral Med Pathol* 2005;10:E27–E39.

33. Marchini L, Tamashiro E, Nascimento DFF, et al: Self-reported denture hygiene of a sample of edentulous attendees at a University dental clinic and the relationship to the condition of the oral tissues. *Gerodontology* 2004;21:226–228.

34. Dikbas I, Koksai T, Calikkocaoglu S: Investigation of the cleanliness of dentures in a university hospital. *Int J Prosthodont* 2006;19:294–298.

35. Khasawneh S, Al-Wahadni A: Control of denture plaque and mucosal inflammation in denture wearers. *J Ir Dent Assoc* 2002;48:132–138.

36. Baran I, Nalcaci R: Self-reported denture hygiene habits and oral tissue conditions of complete denture wearers. *Arch Gerontol Geriatr* 2009;49:237–241.

37. Coco BJ, Bagg J, Cross LJ, et al: Mixed *Candida albicans* and *Candida glabrata* populations associated with the pathogenesis of denture stomatitis. *Oral Microbiol Immunol* 2008;23:377–383.

38. Dagistan S, Esin Aktas A, Cgalayan F, et al: Differential diagnosis of denture-induced stomatitis, *Candida*, and their variations in patients using complete denture: a clinical and mycological study. *Mycoses* 2008;52:266–271.

39. Emami E, Sequin J, Rompre PH, et al: The relationship of myceliated colonies of *Candida albicans* with denture stomatitis: an in vivo/in vitro study. *Int J Prosthodont* 2007;20:514–520.

40. Emami E, de Grandmont P, Rompre PH, et al: Favoring trauma as an etiological factor in denture stomatitis. *J Dent Res* 2008;87:440–444.

41. Marcos-Arias C, Lopez Vicente J, Sahand IH, et al: Isolation of *Candida dubleniensis* in denture stomatitis. *Arch Oral Biol* 2009;54:127–131.

42. Al-Dwairi ZN: Prevalence and risk factors associated with denture-related stomatitis in healthy subjects attending a dental teaching hospital in North Jordan. *J Ir Dent Assoc* 2007;54:80–83.

43. Webb BC, Thomas CJ, Willcox MDP, et al: *Candida*-associated denture stomatitis. Aetiology and management. A review. Part 2. Oral diseases caused by Candida species. *Aust Dent J* 1998;43:160–166.

44. Kulak Y, Arikan A: Aetiology of denture stomatitis. *J Marmara Univ Dent Fac* 1993;1:307–314.

45. Cross LJ, Williams DW, Sweeney CP, et al: Evaluation of the recurrence of denture stomatitis and *Candida* colonization in a small group of patients who received itraconazole. *Oral Surg Oral Med Oral Pathol Oral Radiol Endod* 2004;97:351–358.

46. Jeganathan S, Payne JA, Thean HPY: Denture stomatitis in an elderly edentulous Asian population. *J Oral Rehabil* 1997;24:468–472.

47. Schou L, Wight C, Cumming C: Oral hygiene habits, denture plaque, presence of yeasts and stomatitis in institutionalized elderly in Lothian, Scotland. *Dent Oral Epidemiol* 1987;15:85–89.

48. Campos MS, Marchini L, Bernardes LAS, et al: Biofilm microbial communities of denture stomatitis. *Oral Microbiol Immunol* 2008;23:419–424.

49. Coulthwaite L, Verran J: Potential pathogenic aspects of denture plaque. *Br J Biomed Sci* 2007;64:180–189.

50. Shay K: Denture hygiene: a review and update. *J Contemp Dent Pract* 2000;1:1–8.

51. Webb BC, Thomas CJ, Whittle T: A 2-year study of *Candida*-associated denture stomatitis treatment in aged care subjects. *Gerodontology* 2005;22:168–176.

52. Neppelenbroek KH, Pavarina AC, Polomari DM, et al: Effectiveness of microwave disinfection of complete dentures on the treatment of Candida-related denture stomatitis. *J Oral Rehabil* 2008;35:836–846.

53. Odds FC: Mycology in oral pathology. *Acta Stomatolog Belg* 1997;94:75–80.

54. Abbeele AV, de Meel H, Ahariz M, et al: Denture contamination by yeasts in the elderly. *Gerodontology* 2008;25:222–228.

55. Webb BC, Thomas CJ, Willcox MDP, et al: *Candida*-associated denture stomatitis. Aetiology and management: a review. Part 3. Treatment of oral candiosis. *Aust Dent J* 1998;43:244–249.

56. Nanetti A, Stancari F, Ferri M, et al: Relationship between *Candida albicans* and denture stomatitis: a clinical and microbiological study. *Microbiologica* 1993;16:287–292.

57. Dar-Odeh NS, Shehabi AA: Oral candiosis in patients with removable dentures. *Mycoses* 2003;46:187–191.

58. Figueiral MH, Azul A, Pinto E, et al: Denture-related stomatitis: identification of aetiological and predisposing factors—a large cohort. *J Oral Rehabil* 2007;48:448–455.

59. Song X, Sun J, Store G, et al: Colony morphologies, species, and biotypes of yeasts from thrush and denture stomatitis. *Acta Odontol Scand* 2009;67:248–255.

60. Bilhan H, Sulun T, Erkose, G, et al: The role of *Candida albicans* hyphae and *Lactobacillus* in denture-related stomatitis. *Clin Oral Invest* 2009;13:363–368.

61. Pinto E, Ribeiro IC, Ferreira NJ, et al: Correlation between enzyme production, germ tube formation and susceptibility to fluconazole in *Candida* species isolated from patients with denture-related stomatitis and control individuals. *J Oral Pathol Med* 2008;37:587–592.

62. Costa F, Manaia CM, Figueiral MH, et al: Genotypic analysis of *Candida albicans* isolates obtained from removable prosthesis wearers. *Lett Appl Microbiol* 2008;46:445–449.

63. Lombardi T, Budtz-Jorgensen E: Treatment of denture-induced stomatitis: a review. *Eur J Prosthodont Res Dent* 1993;2:17–22.

64. Budtz-Jorgensen E, Holmstrup P, Krogh P: Fluconazole in the treatment of *Candida*-associated denture stomatitis. *Antimicrob Agents Chemother* 1988;32:1859–1863.

65. Watson CJ, Walker DM, Bates JF, et al: The efficacy of topical miconazole in the treatment of denture stomatitis. *Br Dent J* 1982;152:403–406.

66. Bergendal T, Isaccson G: Effect of nystatin in the treatment of denture stomatitis. *Scand J Dent Res* 1980;88:446–454.

67. DePaola LG, Minah GE, Leupold RJ, et al: The effect of antiseptic mouthrinses on oral microbial flora and denture stomatitis. *Clin Prevent Dent* 1986;8:3–8.

68. Schwartz IS, Young JM, Berrong JM: The effect of Listeiine antiseptic on denture microbial flora and denture stomatitis. *Int J Prosthodont* 1988;1:153–158.

69. Olsen I: Denture stomatitis. The clinical effects of chlorhexidine and amphotericin B. *Acta Odontol Scand* 1975;33:47–52.

70. Cross LJ, Bagg J, Aitchison TC: Efficacy of the cyclodextrin liquid preparation of intraconazole in treatment of denture stomatitis: comparison with itraconazole capsules. *Antimicrob Agents Chemother* 2000;44:425–427.

71. Bissell V, Felix DH, Wray D: Comparative trial of fluconazole and amphotericin in the treatment of denture stomatitis. *Oral Surg Oral Med Oral Pathol Oral Radiol Endodon* 1993;76:35–39.

72. Martin-Manzuelos E, Aller AI, Romero MJ, et al: Response to fluconazole and itraconazole of *Candida* spp. in denture stomatitis. *Mycoses* 1996;40:283–289.

73. Arikan A, Kulak Y, Kadir T: Comparison of different treatment methods for localized and generalized simple denture stomatits. *J Oral Rehabil* 1995;22:365–369.

74. Chandra J, Mukherjee PK, Leidich SD, et al: Antifungal resistance of Candidal biofilms formed on denture acrylic *in vitro*. *J Dent Res* 2001;80:903–908.

75. Pires FR, Santos EBD, Bonan PRF, et al: Denture stomatitis and salivary *Candida* in Brazilian edentulous patients. *J Oral Rehabil* 2002;29:1115–1119.

76. Theilade J, Budtz-Jorgensen E: Electron microscopic study of denture plaque. *J Biol Buccale* 1980;8:287–297.

77. Frank RM, Steuer P: Transmission electron microscopy of plaque accumulations in denture stomatitis. *J Prosthet Dent* 1985;53:115–124.

78. Walter B, Frank RM: Ultrastructural relationship of denture surfaces, plaque and oral mucosa in denture stomatitis. *J Biol Buccale* 1985;13:145–166.

79. von Fraunhofer JA, Loewy ZG: Factors involved in microbial colonization of oral prostheses. *Gen Dent* 2009;57:136–143.

80. Tari BF, Nalbant D, Dogruman Al F, et al: Surface roughness and adherence of *Candida albicans* on soft lining materials as influenced by accelerated aging. *J Contemp Dent Pract* 2007;8:18–25.

81. Yoshijima Y, Murakami K, Kayama S, et al: Effect of substrate surface hydrophobicity on the adherence of yeast and hyphal *Candida*. *Mycoses* 2010;53:221–226.

11

CLINICAL AND HISTOLOGICAL FINDINGS OF DENTURE STOMATITIS AS RELATED TO INTRAORAL COLONIZATION PATTERNS OF *CANDIDA ALBICANS*, SALIVARY FLOW, AND DRY MOUTH

Sandra Altarawneh, DDS, MS,[1] Sompop Bencharit, DDS, MS, PHD, FACP,[1] Luisito Mendoza, DDS,[2] Alice Curran, DMD, MS,[3] David Barrow,[4] Silvana Barros, DDS, PHD,[2] John Preisser, PHD,[5] Zvi G. Loewy, PHD,[6] Linda Gendreau, DDS, MS,[7] and Steven Offenbacher, DDS, PHD, MMSC[2]

[1]Department of Prosthdontics, University of North Carolina School of Dentistry, Chapel Hill, NC
[2]Department of Periodontology, University of North Carolina School of Dentistry, Chapel Hill, NC
[3]Department of Diagnostic Sciences & General Dentistry, University of North Carolina School of Dentistry, Chapel Hill, NC
[4]Department of Dental Research, University of North Carolina School of Dentistry, Chapel Hill, NC
[5]Department of Biostatistics, University of North Carolina School of Dentistry, Chapel Hill, NC
[6]Department of Pharmaceutical & Biomedical Sciences, Touro College of Pharmacy, New York, NY
[7]GlaxoSmithKline, Parsippany, NJ

Keywords
C. albicans; denture; hyposalivation; stomatitis; exfoliative cytology

Correspondence
Sandra Altarawneh, Department of Prosthodontics, University of North Carolina School of Dentistry, 330 Brauer Hall, CB# 7450, Chapel Hill, NC 27599. E-mail: altaraws@dentistry.unc.edu

This work was supported by NIH research grants UL-1-RR025746 and R21HL092338, GSK Consumer Healthcare, and the American College of Prosthodontists Educational Fund.

The funder had no role in manuscript preparation or submission of the manuscript; however, Authors ZGL and LG are, respectively, former and current employees of GSK, one of the funders.

Accepted March 24, 2012

Published in *Journal of Prosthodontics* 2013; Vol. 22, pp. 13–22

doi: 10.1111/j.1532-849X.2012.00906.x

ABSTRACT

Purpose: Multifactorial etiological factors contribute to denture stomatitis (DS), a type of oral candidiasis; however, unlike other oral candidiasis, DS can occur in a healthy person wearing a denture. In this study, we therefore attempt to explore the association between candida, denture, and mucosal tissue using (1) exfoliative cytology, (2) the candidal levels present in saliva, on mucosal tissues and on denture surfaces, and (3) the salivary flow rate and xerostomic symptoms.

Materials and Methods: A cross-sectional study enrolled 32 edentulous participants, 17 without DS as controls and 15 with DS (Newton's classification type II and III). Participants with systemic or other known oral conditions were excluded. Participants completed a xerostomia questionnaire, and salivary flow rates were measured. Samples of unstimulated whole saliva (UWS) and stimulated whole saliva (SWS) were collected. UWS was used for fungal culturing. Periodic acid-Schiff (PAS) stain and quantitative exfoliative cytology were performed on samples from affected and unaffected mucosa from each participant. Levels of Candida species (*albicans* and non-*albicans*) were determined in salivary samples (expressed as colony-forming units, CFU), as well as from swab samples obtained from denture fitting surfaces, in addition to affected and unaffected mucosa.

Results: There were no significant differences in salivary flow rates, mucosal wetness, or frequency of reported dry mouth comparing participants with and without DS. Exfoliative cytology of mucosal smears demonstrated significantly higher ($p = 0.02$) inflammatory cell counts in DS patients, as compared with smears of healthy denture-wearers. *Candida albicans* was significantly more prevalent in saliva ($p = 0.03$) and on denture surfaces ($p = 0.002$) of DS participants, whereas mucosal candidal counts and the presence of cytological hyphae did not show significant difference comparing DS to healthy participants.

Conclusions: In this investigation, we presented a unique group of healthy edentulous patients. This population may reflect the general DS population without systemic or other oral diseases. The prominent etiological factor for DS in this population is the presence of candida in denture and saliva. We found that other factors such as saliva flow/xerostomia, fitting of the denture, and the presence of candida in the mucosa, are less important in this population. Therefore, DS treatments in healthy patients should first focus on sanitization of an existing denture and/or fabrication of a new denture.

Multiple etiological factors contribute to denture stomatitis (DS).[1–6] These factors include (1) microorganisms such as Candida organisms (in particular *Candida albicans)* and gram-negative anaerobes; (2) impaired salivary flow and salivary gland function; (3) trauma from ill-fitting dentures; (4) poor denture and oral hygiene; and (5) impaired immune response secondary to systemic conditions.[5,7–18] Certain strains of Candida, specifically hyphal-forming *C. albicans* clonal types, are more commonly found in candidal infections in DS patients. These virulent strains are capable of epithelial binding, disruption of epithelial integrity, and invasion.[19–24] Besides Candida, antibiotics have been reported to be effective in some refractory DS cases to provide resolution. This suggests that anaerobic pathogens may potentially play a role in some DS circumstances.[13–16] Thus, Candida and gram-negative anaerobes may function together in the pathogenesis of DS.

Impaired salivary flow or altered salivary protein and inorganic composition, often but not always associated xerostomia, have been suggested to lead to a shift in the oral microbiome composition that favors fungal overgrowth. Note that a patient's report of "dry mouth" does not always reflect the reduction of salivary flow or alteration of salivary composition.[25,26] Salivary secretory IgA level is a critical modulator of microbial aggregation, microbial clearance, and surface adherence.[25,26] Thus, impaired sIgA has been attributed to microbial overgrowth.[27–29] The relation between salivary flow and viscosity has been suggested to also potentially play a role in DS by altering the epithelial resistance to candidal binding and invasion.

DS is often associated with ill-fitting dentures associated with atrophic osseous ridge anatomy.[5–7] It is unclear whether the inflammatory state of DS induces ridge resorption resulting in a loose and easily displaced denture, or whether the trauma associated with the denture (e.g., through poor tissue adaptation, clenching or inadequate interridge space) can provide a mechanical stress that induces mucosal inflammation and bone resorption via poor tissue perfusion, necrosis, or trauma. Nonetheless, the denture can serve as a habitat for high-density biofilm, which can harbor high levels of bacteria and yeasts, especially in patients with poor oral hygiene, poor denture hygiene, or wearing dentures overnight.[7,17,18] Thus, the denture itself is believed to serve as both traumatic inducer and a reservoir for triggering a local microbial infection-mediated inflammatory response.

Current and past literature reveals that patients with compromised immunity due to a systemic condition, such as diabetes, are prone to refractory DS as well as other forms of oral candidiasis.[7–12] Overgrowth of Candida in DS is a common finding and can be a precursor to oropharyngeal and esophageal candidiasis, which can become a life-threatening disseminating infection among HIV/AIDS patients or in those with other immunocompromised conditions, especially those associated with T-cell functional deficits.[22–24]

Although several studies have been done to examine these etiologic factors of DS, most focus on only one or a few factors. Moreover, a large body of literature on DS presents results that overlap between DS patients with other forms of oral candidiasis. Note that healthy individuals without dentures will not have any oral candidiasis. On the contrary, healthy denture wearers often present with DS. It is plausible that in the general denture-wearing population, some etiological factors may play a larger role than others. For example, healthy denture wearers would have little problem from systemic and local immunity or from xerostomia or impaired salivary function. The interaction between candida and the denture mediated with normal saliva is perhaps the most prominent DS etiological factor in healthy denture wearers.

To reflect healthy denture wearers with limited influence from systemic conditions and other factors besides DS that contribute to oral candidiasis, we decided to conduct an exploratory cross-sectional investigation. Our goal was to examine the association between clinical signs of DS (measuring the severity of stomatitis with the Newton Classification[30] and the denture fit using the Kapur index[31]) and candidal overgrowth by examining (1) the exfoliative cytology, (2) the candidal levels present in saliva, on mucosal tissues, and on denture surfaces, and (3) salivary flow rate and xerostomic symptoms. We believe that the overall healthy status of the patient population provides a unique cohort for studying the etiology of DS, reflecting the majority of the denture-wearing population.

MATERIALS AND METHODS

Study Design, Participants, and Sample Size Estimates

This was a single-center, case control study design intended to collect biological samples from participants with and without DS, specifically with mucosal lesions (Newton's Classification type II or type III).[30] The following biological markers were obtained: (1) gene expression profiles as determined by Affymetrix (Affymetrix Inc., Santa Clara, CA) arrays obtained using tissue biopsy samples, (2) exfoliative cytology was performed on mucosal surfaces to examine for the presence or absence of C. albicans infection as determined by periodic acid-Schiff (PAS) cytology, (3) the presence or absence and relative level of C. albicans on mucosal and denture surfaces was determined using cultivable methods, (4) tissue and denture surfaces were sampled to measure the presence, absence, and levels of 18 dental biofilm organisms by deoxyribonucleic acid-deoxyribonucleic acid (DNA-DNA) checkerboard and cultured

for C. albicans, (5) the rate of salivary flow and the levels of selected proinflammatory cytokines in saliva were measured, and (6) C-reactive protein levels were measured in the serum.

This was an exploratory study, and a targeted sample size of 30 (15 patients per group) was determined to provide 80% power with two-sided $\alpha = 0.05$ significance tests to detect changes in means from continuous variables between diseased and nondiseased patients that are 1.06 times the standard deviation of the variable. The sample size was considered sufficient as effect sizes such as this, or larger, are common for levels of dental biofilm organisms and proinflammatory cytokines.[7,17,22] To allow for an 8% to 10% possible drop-out rate, 32 patients were enrolled to ensure that 30 (15 participants per group) completed the study. In this report, we limit the analyses to the clinical findings, the cytology, and the cultivable data.

The study protocol was approved by the UNC Institutional Review Board (IRB), No. 07–2014. A total of 32 edentulous patients were enrolled according to the inclusion and exclusion criteria listed in Appendix A. The control group (n = 17) had no signs or symptoms of DS, and the diseased group (n = 15) presented with type II (n = 8) or III (n = 7) DS (Newton's classification).[30] This level of DS includes the moderate (type II) and severe (type III) forms. Representative clinical appearance of cases and controls appear in Figure 1. All enrolled participants completed the two-visit study. For all parameters of interest, there was no apparent gradient progressing from health to type II to type III; therefore, type II and type III remained grouped as a single DS diseased group, as initially intended.

Demographics

The mean age of the 32 participants was 64.8. The healthy group was comprised of 14 women, 3 men, 11 Caucasians, and 6 African Americans. The stomatitis group was comprised of 9 women, 6 men, 9 Caucasians, 3 African Americans, and 3 Asians. There were no significant differences in age, race, or gender in the DS and Healthy groups. Baseline characteristics and Kapur index results are included in Table 1 and show no significant differences between groups.

Clinical Evaluation of Dentures (Kapur Index)

A qualified examiner (prosthodontist) assessed the fit of the maxillary and mandibular dentures (if present) using the Kapur Index[31] as follows:

Retention:

3: good—maximum resistance to vertical pull and sufficient lateral force.

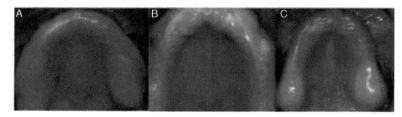

FIGURE 1   Clinical photographs of (A) a control patient, (B) Newton classification II stomatitis, and (C) Newton classification III stomatitis.

TABLE 1   Demographics and baseline characteristics of the participants

	Control (n = 17)	DS (n = 15)
Age (mean ± SD)	66.2 ± 9.7	63.2 ± 8.83
Gender		
Male	3 (17.6%)	6 (40%)
Female	14 (82.4%)	9 (60%)
Race		
Caucasian	11 (64.7%)	9 (60%)
African American	6 (35.3%)	3 (20%)
Asian		3 (20%)
Kapur Index of max. Denture (mean ± SD)	3.56 ± 1.46	3.00 ± 1.57

2: moderate—moderate resistance to vertical pull and little or no resistance to lateral force.

1: minimum—slight resistance to vertical pull and little or no resistance to lateral force.

0: no retention—denture displaces itself.

Stability:

2: sufficient—demonstrates slight or no rocking on its supporting structures under pressure.

1: some—demonstrates moderate rocking on its supporting structures under pressure.

0: no stability—demonstrates extreme rocking on its supporting structures under pressure.

Because not all of the patients had a mandibular denture, mean values for the total scores of retention and stability for the maxillary denture were calculated.

Clinically poor denture = sum score <3

Clinically fair denture = sum score 3 to 4.

Clinically good denture = sum score >4.

Unpaired T-test was performed to assess statistical differences between means of scores of the maxillary dentures for DS and healthy groups.

Unstimulated Saliva Collection

Patients were instructed to remove their dentures and refrain from eating, drinking, smoking, brushing their teeth, or chewing gum for 15 minutes before salivary collections. All collections were performed between 9:00 and 11:00 AM. Participants were instructed to swallow to clear the mouth of any accumulated saliva, and whole unstimulated saliva was allowed to pool in a sterile polypropylene graduated collection vial for 5 minutes. A fraction of the sample was sent immediately to the microbiology lab for rapid processing to prevent overgrowth of the Candida species. Samples were aliquoted into Eppendorf tubes, centrifuged for 10 minutes at 3000 g, and the supernatant stored at −80 °C for proteomic and cytokine analysis.

Stimulated Saliva Collection

Patients were instructed to place their dentures back before collection began. Stimulated whole saliva was quantified using a modification of the Saxon test,[32] where each participant was asked to chew on a folded strip of paraffin for 2 minutes after swallowing to clear the mouth of the accumulated saliva. The collected saliva was then quantified as milliliters of saliva generated per minute (mL/min) and recorded on the CRF. Participants found to have a resting (unstimulated) saliva rate of less than 0.01 mL/min and stimulated salivary rate of less than 0.10 mL/min were characterized as having hyposalivation.[33,34]

Xerostomia Questionnaire

Patients were asked to complete the xerostomia questionnaire (see Appendix B) after the salivary collection. This questionnaire is derived from the validated questionnaire from the Dental ARIC study as described by Beck et al.[35] ANOVA (items no 3, 13, and 14) and Spearman correlations (items no 5 to 12) by regression analysis were used to analyze relationships between salivary flow rates and patient-reported symptoms of dry mouth.

Mucosal Wetness

Patients were instructed to swallow, and sialopaper was placed on the midline of the anterior third of the dorsum of the tongue for 5 seconds. Sialopaper was then transferred to Periotron (Model 6000) (Ora Flow Inc. Plainview, NY) for reading. After reading, the sialopaper was discarded. Measurement was done twice. The *T*-test was used to determine differences between the means of readings comparing groups.

Exfoliative Examination

Smears were taken from the affected palatal mucosa and unaffected palatal mucosa for the stomatitis group, and only one sample from the palatal mucosa for the control group. Samples were taken from the buccal vestibular area and dorsum of the tongue as well. Participants with dry mouth (xerostomia) were instructed to rinse with a small amount of water before collection of the sample. Selected areas were wiped firmly, using a wooden tongue blade, until a visible accumulation of oral fluids was present. Accumulated samples were transferred to a clean glass slide until a thin coat was visible when the slide was held against light. Slides were then sprayed with Cytofix/Cytoperm (Becton, Dickinson and Company, Franklin Lakes, NJ) with one or two swipes from a distance of about 1 foot and allowed to dry for 10 minutes.

When adequate samples could not be collected using this procedure, the sampling steps outlined above were repeated in a different area of the palatal mucosa, until an adequate sample was collected. These samples were used for cytology and PAS identification of fungal forms. The following scoring system was used for the PAS-cytology assessments:

  0: inadequate cell sample
  1: benign smear
  2: bacteria only
  3: benign inflammatory smear
  4: bacteria plus inflammatory cells
  5: fungal spores
  6: fungal organisms

Culture

BBL CultureSwab (Becton, Dickinson and Company) was used to swab the denture and the mucosal surface, with a total of three swabs for the diseased group (from the denture, mucosal surface of affected area, and unaffected area), and two swabs for the control group (from the denture and the mucosal surface). Samples obtained from swabbing were cultured on Sabouraud Dextrose agar containing quemicetine succinate. Samples were spiral plated to Sabouraud's dextrose plates to obtain a quantitative value of colony-forming units per milliliter (CFU/mL). Samples were also plated on a total aerobic plate to compute the percentage of total aerobic recoverable CFU on a nonselective medium to allow for identification of both *albicans* and non-*albicans* Candida.

Candida colonies were counted after 48 hours, and the patients classified according to the number of CFU as follows: negative (CFU/mL = 0), carrier (CFU/mL < 400), and positive (CFU/mL > 400). A fraction of the UWS was sampled in Sabouraud Dextrose agar containing quemicetine succinate. Candida colonies were counted after 48 hours, and the patients classified in the same way as for the BBL culture swabs.

Mucosal Biopsy

At the end of the appointment, patients were anesthetized, and 4 mm punch biopsies were collected from the palate. In healthy patients, the biopsy was taken from the posterior ridge area. All patients were followed up 1-week postsurgery. In DS participants, two punch biopsies were taken: a diseased sample from the palatal area that was the most severe clinical area, and a second biopsy from a relatively less-affected area of inflammation, sampling the palatal site that was most normal in appearance. All biopsies extended to the periosteum and included a full-thickness mucosal sample from periosteum to keratinized epithelium.

RESULTS

Salivary Flow Rates

There was no significant difference in the rate of stimulated or unstimulated salivary flow comparing healthy individuals to DS patients (Table 2).

Xerostomia Symptoms

There was no significant difference in the frequency of reported dry mouth comparing DS to control patients; however, among all patients there were significant associations

TABLE 2   Flow rate of unstimulated and stimulated whole saliva in control and DS participants

Participants	Salivary flow (ml/min)	
	UWS (mean ± SD)	SWS (mean ± SD)
Control (n = 17)	0.5 ± 0.23	1.43 ± 0.57
DS type II (n = 8)	0.5 ± 0.15	1.14 ± 0.43
DS type III (n = 7)	0.55 ± 0.23	1.34 ± 0.57
p Value (ANOVA)	0.84	0.46
DS combined (n = 15)	0.53 ± 0.19	1.23 ± 0.5
p Value (unpaired *t*-test)	0.71	0.31

UWS = unstimulated whole saliva collected for 5 minutes; SWS = stimulated whole saliva collected by chewing folded strip of paraffin for 2 minutes; Hyposalivation = unstimulated saliva rate of less than 0.01 mL/min, and stimulated saliva rate of less than 0.10 mL/min.

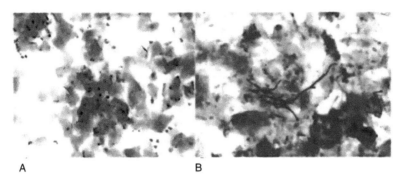

FIGURE 2   PAS exfoliative cytology representative slides. (A) A healthy control benign smear; oral cytologic smear of palatal mucosa showing typical squamous cells and scattered chronic inflammatory cells (10x), (B) DS fungal hyphae; oral cytologic smear from palatal mucosa showing candidal hyphae. (40x).

between symptomology and flow and wetness measures. A significant correlation was found between unstimulated salivary flow rate and perceived "Rate the dryness of your tongue" ($r^2 = 0.36$, $p = 0.0405$). There was also a significant association between stimulated salivary flow rate and "Rate the level of your thirst" ($r^2 = 0.51$, $p = 0.0028$). All other correlations were not significant and were in the range of (-0.23 to 0.10). For questions number 3, 13, and 14, there were no significant associations between the reported symptoms and the flow rate of both unstimulated and stimulated saliva.

Cytology

According to the cytology results of the palatal mucosal swabs (Fig 2, Table 3), it was noticed that type II and type III DS are associated with higher scores reflecting inflammatory cells, bacteria, and fungal morphotypes. Inflammatory cells in the palatal mucosa showed a significant difference ($p = 0.02$) between DS and control participants. It is noteworthy that fungal forms were often found in control participants. There was no statistically significant difference in the cytology of the vestibular and tongue swabs comparing DS type II or type III to health; however, the vestibular area and the tongue as well as the palate had a trend for more prevalent fungal forms in DS patients.

Cultivable *C. albicans* Levels in Saliva and on Denture and Mucosal Surfaces

In the saliva, *C. albicans* was detected in 80% (12/15) of the DS participants, but only 41.2% (7/17) of the control participants ($p = 0.03$, Chi-square). There was no greater detection rate of *C. albicans* in severe (type III) DS as compared to mild (type II) DS. In the dentures, *C. albicans* was present in 73.2% of dentures sampled from DS participants and only in 11.8% of dentures sampled from healthy individuals ($p = 0.002$), Chi Square. In the mucosal swabs there was

no significant difference in *C. albicans* counts between diseased and healthy mucosa ($p = 0.2$). There was a high degree of concordance between the presence of *C. albicans* in the saliva versus that detectible on the denture ($r^2 = 0.31$, $p = 0.0007$). *C. albicans* prevalence by location comparing saliva versus healthy mucosa was not significant ($p = 0.059$), nor was it significant when compared to diseased mucosa ($p = 0.79$). Among participants with detectible *C. albicans*, the level (CFU) of *C. albicans* within the saliva tended to be higher among DS participants, compared to healthy controls (Fig 3). When *C. albicans* was present, the mean salivary level of log CFU was 5.03 in DS and 4.4 in health. This difference (0.63) indicates that the mean level was 4.3-fold higher in the saliva of participants with DS when detected (Fig 3). Non-*albicans* Candida was also significantly detected, especially in DS patients. Table 4 shows the prevalence of both *C. albicans* and non-*albicans* in all patients.

DISCUSSION

Role of Saliva

In healthy denture wearers without a systemic condition, saliva is known to be an important etiological factor in the development of DS. In this study, there was no difference in the frequency of reported dry mouth, or in the rate of stimulated or unstimulated salivary flow comparing control individuals to DS patients. Note also that most of the participant-reported symptoms of dry mouth did not correlate with saliva flow. Only three questions (of 14) in the xerostomia questionnaires had any statistical significance. Torres et al[9] found that 67.9% of the individuals with xerostomia were colonized by *Candida* spp.; however, the difference between these patients and those without xerostomia was not statistically significant. Närhi et al[8] found significantly higher counts of yeasts in individuals with salivary flow rates below normal. According to Pereira-Cenci et al[36] patients with low

TABLE 3   **PAS exfoliative cytology results for palatal and vestibular area and tongue**

	Palatal area			Vestibular area and tongue		
	Healthy	Diseased	*p* Value	Healthy	Diseased	*p* Value
Adequate (Yes)	12(44.4%)	15(55.6%)		17(53.1%)	15(46.9%)	
(No)	5(100.0%)	0(0.0%)	0.02			
Bacteria (Yes)	6(40.0%)	9(60.0%)		12(46.2%)	14(53.9%)	
(No)	11(64.7%)	6(35.3%)	0.16	5(83.3%)	1(16.7%)	0.10
Inflammatory cells (Yes)	0(0.0%)	4(100.0%)		3(37.5%)	5(62.5%)	
(No)	17(60.7%)	11(39.3%)	0.02*	14(58.3%)	10(41.7%)	0.31
Fungal spores (Yes)	5(35.7%)	9(64.3%)		12(46.2%)	14(53.9%)	
(No)	12(66.7%)	6(33.3%)	0.08	5(83.3%)	1(16.7%)	0.10
Fungal hyphae (Yes)	4(40.0%)	6(60.0%)		7(43.8%)	9(56.3%)	
(No)	13(59.1%)	9(40.9%)	0.32	10(62.5%)	6(37.5%)	0.29
Atypical cells (Yes)	0(0.0%)	1(100.0%)				
(No)	17(54.8%)	14(45.2%)	0.28	17(53.1%)	15(46.9%)	
Score						
Inadequate cell sample	6(100.0%)	0(0.0%)				
Benign smear	4(57.1%)	3(42.9%)		4(100.0%)	0(0.0%)	
Bacteria only	2(50.0%)	2(50.0%)		1(50.0%)	1(50.0%)	
Benign inflammatory cells	0(0.0%)	1(100.0%)				
Bacteria plus inflammatory cells						
Fungal spores	1(25.0%)	3(75.0%)		5(50.0%)	5(50.0%)	
Fungal organisms	4(40.0%)	6(60.0%)	0.13	7(46.6%)	8(53.3%)	0.28
Score dichotomized (fungal)	5(35.7%)	9(64.3%)		12(48.0%)	13(52.0%)	
No fungal	12(66.7%)	6(33.3%)	0.08	5(83.3%)	1(16.7%)	0.12

*Statistically significant (*p* < 0.05)

or impaired salivary flow and/or composition presented higher Candida species counts when compared with saliva from patients with normal salivary flow. Hibino et al[37] reported that both stimulated and unstimulated salivary flow rates of the noncarriers were higher than the carriers, although the difference was not statistically significant.

In their study to determine risk factors associated with oral candidiasis onset and chronic maintenance, Campisi et al[38]

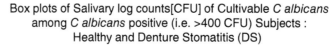

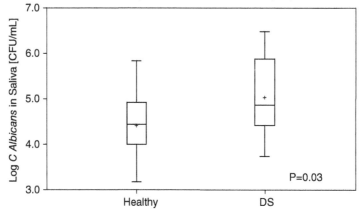

FIGURE 3   Mean log *C. albicans* counts in saliva among DS and control participants. The boxplot indicates the log CFU *C. albicans*/mL of saliva. The plot shows median, upper, and lower 25th percentile range (box boundaries) and range as outer markings. The plus sign shows the mean log values.

TABLE 4 Prevalence of detectable *C. albicans* and non-*albicans* in saliva, denture, and mucosal surfaces for control and DS participants. The table indicates the number of patients positive for Candida [*albicans* and *non-albicans*] and the percent positive within the disease category. The *p* values are chi-square statistics between the control and the DS groups.

	Saliva (N = 32)		Denture (N = 32)		Unaffected mucosa (N = 32)		Affected mucosa (N = 15)	
	C. albicans	Non-*albicans*	*C. albicans*	Non-*albicans*	*C. albicans*	Non-*albicans*	*C. albicans*	Non-*albicans*
Control (N = 17)	7(41.2%)	7(41.2%)	2(11.8%)	8(47.1%)	1(5.9%)	7(41.18%)		
DS type II (N = 8)	7(87.5%)	0(0.00)	6(75.0%)	0(0.00%)	2(25.0%)	2(25.0%)	2(25.0%)	3(37.5%)
DS type III (N = 7)	5(71.4%)	0(0.00)	5(71.4%)	2(28.6%)	2(28.6%)	4(57.1%)	4(57.1%)	3(42.9%)
Total (N,%)	19(59.4%)	7(21.9%)	13(40.6%)	10(31.3%)	5(15.6%)	13(40.6%)	6(40.0%)	6(40.0%)
p Values	0.03*	0.02*	0.002*	0.06*	0.27	0.45	0.20	0.83

*Statistically significant ($p < 0.05$)

found both denture wearing and xerostomia to be local risk factors according to their analysis. The sample size in our study is too small to refute or resolve any of these conflicting findings. Our results, however, suggest that at least in healthy denture wearers, DS can develop with normal saliva flow. One key issue is that the typical assessments of salivary function from a physiological perspective (e.g., salivary flow rate, mucosal wetness, xerostomia symptoms) may not be associated with the antifungal capacity of the saliva. Clearly, future studies intending to examine the role of salivary immunoglobulins (e.g., sIgA) and specific antifungal components, such as lactoferrin, histatin-5, lysozyme, and histidine-rich polypeptides in recoverable yeast counts, in addition to physiological assessments, would be informative.

Denture Fitting

In this study, the fit of the dentures did not appear to be a strong contributing factor for DS in healthy denture wearers. There was no statistical difference in Kapur index between DS and control subjects (Table 1); however, it is important to point out that the average Kapur index for the control patients was in the middle of the fair range, whereas the average index for the DS patients was at the cutoff between the fair to poor range. The small sample size limits our interpretation of the contribution of denture fit to DS in healthy patients, and it is possible that this factor may be statistically significant in a larger sample size.

Role of Candida

In this study, *C. albicans* was approximately twice as likely to be present in the saliva of DS patients (80%) as compared to control patients (35.3%); however, there was no clear trend for the CFU levels of salivary *C. albicans* to show a gradient of higher numbers associated with the transition from type II to type III DS. When *C. albicans* was detected in healthy or DS participants, the level within the saliva was found to be 4.3-fold higher among DS participants.

A strong relationship between DS and the presence of Candida in saliva has been reported previously.[39,40] On the other hand, patients with Candida in saliva may not develop DS.[41] This is in agreement with our findings. Since the frequency of detection of *C. albicans* is lower on the denture (11.8%) than in the saliva (41.2%) of healthy patients, it would appear that saliva and/or mucosa represents the reservoir of infectious agent in these healthy individuals and that the denture is less frequently colonized with *C. albicans*. According to Pires et al,[42] the clinical resolution of DS was not related to the levels of Candida in saliva and, furthermore, a decrease of Candida counts in saliva usually is not followed by clinical improvement of DS.

In our study, there was a significant difference in the prevalence of detectible *C. albicans* counts from denture surface between DS and control participants ($p = 0.03$). *C. albicans* was 20.6-fold more likely to be cultured from the denture in DS patients than in healthy ones (i.e., 11/15 vs. 2/17; Table 4). If we examine the levels of *C. albicans* cultured from dentures there was a nonsignificant trend for higher denture counts among those with DS. Grouping the denture counts for healthy patients into three categories as no growth, [1+, 2+], and [3+, 4+] resulted in a distribution of 41.2%, 47.1%, and 11.7%, respectively. Similarly for DS samples the distribution was 26.7%, 40%, and 33.3% ($p = 0.18$), suggesting the trend toward higher denture counts of *C. albicans* in DS participants. The notion that greater numbers of Candida spp. were recovered from smears prepared from the fitting surfaces of the dentures than from those on the palatal mucosa has been known since the 1970s.[43,44] It has been shown that *C. albicans* colonies were recovered more frequently from the tissue fitting surface of the acrylic resin denture than from the corresponding palatal mucosa in DS patients.[40] However, according to Radford et al,[45] it is difficult to attribute the etiology of the condition entirely to the presence of *C. albicans* in denture plaque, as they found in their review that methods of sample collection accounted for individual variation, since palatal imprints yielded 55% of participants with yeast present, denture plaque sampling 80%, and saliva sampling 95%. Interestingly, in our study we found a high degree of concordance between the presence of C. *albicans* in the saliva versus that detectible on the denture ($r^2 = 0.31$, $p = 0.0007$). It was also noticed that nonalbicans species are more prevalent in control patients, especially upon comparing prevalence in the unaffected mucosa in these individuals; however, whether non-*albicans* presence in patient's saliva or mucosa is associated with any protective effect cannot be concluded from this small cohort.

Exfoliative Cytology Findings in DS

Reports have been variable on whether the inflammation associated with DS is secondary to denture trauma or if it is simply a result of candidal infection. According to Barbeau et al,[1] the presence of yeasts on the denture in denture-related stomatitis is probably linked to extensive inflammation. Considering the hypothesis that inflammation could be present before Candida colonization, this could explain the variable results in the treatment of denture-related stomatitis with antifungal treatment alone.[1]

According to Edgerton and Levine,[46] stomatitis pathogenesis can occur through two separate mechanisms. They state, "Alterations in the composition of pellicle formed in stomatitis conditions, such as degradation of pellicle components, may directly promote colonization of C. *albicans* on 'stomatitis' pellicle. Alternatively, C. *albicans* may be a secondary colonizer or may require bacterial cell products to stimulate adhesion, as has been shown with in vitro studies of *Streptococcus mutans* and C. *albicans*.[47] In this case, altered pellicle deposition in the disease process may initially enhance adhesion of other bacteria, which would subsequently promote adhesion of Candida."[48]

Ritchie et al[48] found that bacteria, leukocytes, and yeast hyphae could be detected in all patients even when cultures were negative. Examination of PAS-stained smears prepared from denture scrapings showed higher numbers of yeast cells in DS patients by Budtz-Jorgensen et al[13] as well; however, in our study, the presence of hyphae, as determined from the PAS smear from tissue was not pathognomic for disease.

CONCLUSIONS

The overall healthy status of the patient population in this study provides a unique cohort for the study of three important DS etiological factors including candida, denture, and saliva. DS in healthy patients appears to have a unique pathogenesis different from other oral candidiasis. We selected participants to limit the influence of systemic conditions and others (e.g., medications) that may compromise immunity and saliva factors. In this study, we confirm that DS is perhaps a result of the denture acting as a reservoir of candidal organism. Normal saliva in healthy patients appears to be the medium for candidal organisms' movement between the denture and tissue, but plays a limited role in DS development. Denture fitting and xerostomic factors are perhaps not primary factors, at least in this same sample size, healthy, denture-wearing population. The results also suggest that unlike other oral candidiasis, there is no association between the fungal presence in the tissue and the clinical symptoms of DS. Therefore, treatments for DS should first focus on sanitization of an existing denture or fabrication of a new denture, rather than antifungal treatment in healthy denture wearers.

ACKNOWLEDGMENT

The authors thank C. R. Mack for proofreading this manuscript.

APPENDIX A: Inclusion and exclusion criteria

Inclusion criteria	Exclusion criteria
1. At least 45 years of age	1. Less than 45 years of age
2. Men or women without menses for 12 consecutive months or who have had a complete hysterectomy	2. Have chronic disease with oral manifestations other than denture/mucosal stomatitis
3. Wear complete maxillary denture (overdentures, implant-retained or tooth-retained dentures acceptable) without daily use of denture adhesive	3. Have gross oral pathology
	4. Have overt denture abrasion associated with symptoms
	5. Participants with clinically significant organic diseases, including impaired renal function, bleeding disorder, or any condition requiring antibiotic premedication for dental visits
4. Must have read, understood, and signed an informed consent form	6. Participants with active infectious diseases such as hepatitis, HIV, or tuberculosis
5. Must understand and be willing to comply with all study procedures and restrictions	7. Participants who are immunosuppressed because of medications or condition
	8. Participants who have used antibiotics or antifungals for any medical or dental condition within 1 month before screening
6. Must be in good general health; diabetics included	9. Participants using ongoing medications initiated less than 3 months before enrollment
7. Must have type II or type III denture stomatitis for denture stomatitis group	10. Participants with a known or suspected intolerance to local oral anesthesia
	11. Participants who have participated in another clinical study or have taken an investigational drug within 30 days of screening
8. Must have no signs of denture stomatitis for control group	12. Participants who have used tobacco products within 6 months of screening
	13. Employees of the sponsor or the investigator or members of their immediate family
	14. Participants who have previously participated in this study
	15. Postmenopausal women on hormone replacement therapy

APPENDIX B: Xerostomia questionnaire

- Do you have any difficulties in swallowing any foods? (yes/no)
- Does your mouth feel dry when eating a meal? (yes/no)
- Do you sip liquids to aid in swallowing food? (yes/no)
- Does the amount of saliva in your mouth seem to be too little, too much, or you don't notice it?
- Rate the difficulty you experience in speaking because of dryness in your mouth. (1–10 scale).
- Rate the difficulty you experience in swallowing because of dryness in your mouth. (1–10 scale).
- Rate how much saliva is in your mouth. (1–10 scale).
- Rate the dryness of your mouth. (1–10 scale).
- Rate the dryness of your throat. (1–10 scale).
- Rate the dryness of your lips. (1–10 scale).
- Rate the dryness of your tongue. (1–10 scale).
- Rate the level of your thirst. (1–10 scale).
- Dryness of lips (present or absent).
- Dryness of buccal mucosa/cheek areas (present or absent).

REFERENCES

1. Barbeau J, Seguin J, Goulet JP, et al: Reassessing the presence of *Candida albicans* in denture-related stomatitis. *Oral Surg Oral Med Oral Pathol Oral Radiol Endod* 2003;95:51–59.
2. Budtz-Jorgensen E: Etiology, pathogenesis, therapy, and prophylaxis of oral yeast infections. *Acta Odontol Scand* 1990;48:61–69.
3. Cumming CG, Wight C, Blackwell CL, et al: Denture stomatitis in the elderly. *Oral Microbiol Immunol* 1990;5:82–85.
4. Glass RT, Belobraydic KA: Dilemma of denture contamination. *J Okla Dent Assoc* 1990;81:30–33.
5. Webb BC, Thomas CJ, Willcox MD, et al: Candida-associated denture stomatitis. Aetiology and management: a review. Part 1. Factors influencing distribution of Candida species in the oral cavity. *Aust Dent J* 1998;43:45–50.
6. Webb BC, Thomas CJ, Willcox MD, et al: Candida-associated denture stomatitis. Aetiology and management: a review. Part 2. Oral diseases caused by Candida species. *Aust Dent J* 1998;43:160–166.
7. Ramage G, Tomsett K, Wickes BL, et al: Denture stomatitis: a role for Candida biofilms. *Oral Surg Oral Med Oral Pathol Oral Radiol Endod* 2004;98:53–59.
8. Narhi TO, Ainamo A, Meurman JH: Salivary yeasts, saliva, and oral mucosa in the elderly. *J Dent Res* 1993;72:1009–1014.

9. Torres SR, Peixoto CB, Caldas DM, et al: Clinical aspects of Candida species carriage in saliva of xerotomic subjects. *Med Mycol* 2003;41:411–415.

10. Jeganathan S, Lin CC: Denture stomatitis—a review of the aetiology, diagnosis and management. *Aust Dent J* 1992;37:107–114.

11. Gendreau L, Loewy ZG: Epidemiology and etiology of denture stomatitis. *J Prosthodont* 2011;20:251–260.

12. Cross LJ, Williams DW, Sweeney CP, et al: Evaluation of the recurrence of denture stomatitis and Candida colonization in a small group of patients who received itraconazole. *Oral Surg Oral Med Oral Pathol Oral Radiol Endod* 2004;97:351–358.

13. Budtz-Jorgensen E, Theilade E, Theilade J: Quantitative relationship between yeast and bacteria in denture-induced stomatitis. *Scand J Dent Res* 1983;91:134–142.

14. Koopmans AS, Kippuw N, de Graaff J: Bacterial involvement in denture-induced stomatitis. *J Dent Res* 1988;67:1246–1250.

15. Pesci-Bardon C, Fosse T, Madinier I, et al: In vitro new dialysis protocol to assay the antiseptic properties of a quaternary ammonium compound polymerized with denture acrylic resin. *Lett Appl Microbiol* 2004;39:226–231.

16. Redding S, Bhatt B, Rawls HR, et al: Inhibition of *Candida albicans* biofilm formation on denture material. *Oral Surg Oral Med Oral Pathol Oral Radiol Endod* 2009;107:669–672.

17. Sachdeo A, Haffajee AD, Socransky SS: Biofilms in the edentulous oral cavity. *J Prosthodont* 2008;17:348–356.

18. Coco BJ, Bagg J, Cross LJ, et al: Mixed *Candida albicans* and *Candida glabrata* populations associated with the pathogenesis of denture stomatitis. *Oral Microbiol Immunol* 2008;23:377–383.

19. Salerno C, Pascale M, Contaldo M, et al: Candida-associated denture stomatitis. *Med Oral Patol Oral Cir Bucal* 2011;16:e139–143.

20. Dahlen G, Blomquist S, Carlen A: A retrospective study on the microbiology in patients with oral complaints and oral mucosal lesions. *Oral Dis* 2009;15:265–272.

21. Bilhan H, Sulun T, Erkose G, et al: The role of *Candida albicans* hyphae and Lactobacillus in denture-related stomatitis. *Clin Oral Investig* 2009;13:363–368.

22. Leigh JE, Steele C, Wormley F, et al: Salivary cytokine profiles in the immunocompetent individual with Candida-associated denture stomatitis. *Oral Microbiol Immunol* 2002;17:311–314.

23. Nikawa H, Jin C, Makihira S, et al: Susceptibility of *Candida albicans* isolates from the oral cavities of HIV-positive patients to histatin-5. *J Prosthet Dent* 2002;88:263–267.

24. Rodriguez-Archilla A, Urquia M, Cutando A, et al: Denture stomatitis: quantification of interleukin-2 production by mononuclear blood cells cultured with *Candida albicans*. *J Prosthet Dent* 1996;75:426–431.

25. Higuchi Y, Ansai T, Awano S, et al: Salivary levels of hyaluronic acid in female patients with dry mouth compared with age-matched controls: a pilot study. *Biomed Res* 2009;30:63–68.

26. Wolff M, Kleinberg I: Oral mucosal wetness in hypo- and normosalivators. *Arch Oral Biol* 1998;43:455–462.

27. Fukushima C, Matsuse H, Saeki S, et al: Salivary IgA and oral candidiasis in asthmatic patients treated with inhaled corticosteroid. *J Asthma* 2005;42:601–604.

28. Hagewald S, Bernimoulin JP, Kottgen E, et al: Salivary IgA subclasses and bacteria-reactive IgA in patients with aggressive periodontitis. *J Periodontal Res* 2002;37:333–339.

29. Tanida T, Okamoto T, Okamoto A, et al: Decreased excretion of antimicrobial proteins and peptides in saliva of patients with oral candidiasis. *J Oral Pathol Med* 2003;32:586–594.

30. Newton AV: Denture sore mouth. A possible etiology. *Br Dent J* 1962;112:357–360.

31. Kapur KK: A clinical evaluation of denture adhesives. *J Prosthet Dent* 1967;18:550–558.

32. Kohler PF, Winter ME: A quantitative test for xerostomia. The Saxon test, an oral equivalent of the Schirmer test. *Arthritis Rheum* 1985;28:1128–1132.

33. Bergdahl M, Bergdahl J: Low unstimulated salivary flow and subjective oral dryness: association with medication, anxiety, depression, and stress. *J Dent Res* 2000;79:1652–1658.

34. Bergdahl M: Salivary flow and oral complaints in adult dental patients. *Community Dent Oral Epidemiol* 2000;28:59–66.

35. Beck JD, Elter JR, Heiss G, et al: Relationship of periodontal disease to carotid artery intima-media wall thickness: the atherosclerosis risk in communities (ARIC) study. *Arterioscler Thromb Vasc Biol* 2001;21:1816–1822.

36. Pereira-Cenci T, Del Bel Cury AA, Crielaard W, et al: Development of Candida-associated denture stomatitis: new insights. *J Appl Oral Sci* 2008;16:86–94.

37. Hibino K, Samaranayake LP, Hagg U, et al: The role of salivary factors in persistent oral carriage of Candida in humans. *Arch Oral Biol* 2009;54:678–683.

38. Campisi G, Panzarella V, Matranga D, et al: Risk factors of oral candidosis: a twofold approach of study by fuzzy logic and traditional statistic. *Arch Oral Biol* 2008;53:388–397.

39. Berdicevsky I, Ben-Aryeh H, Szargel R, et al: Oral candida of asymptomatic denture wearers. *Int J Oral Surg* 1980;9:113–115.

40. Webb BC, Thomas CJ, Willcox MD, et al: Candida-associated denture stomatitis. Aetiology and management: a review. Part 3. Treatment of oral candidosis. *Aust Dent J* 1998;43:244–249.

41. Wilson J: The aetiology, diagnosis and management of denture stomatitis. *Br Dent J* 1998;185:380–384.

42. Pires FR, Santos EB, Bonan PR, et al: Denture stomatitis and salivary Candida in Brazilian edentulous patients. *J Oral Rehabil* 2002;29:1115–1119.

43. Davenport JC: The oral distribution of candida in denture stomatitis. *Br Dent J* 1970;129:151–156.

44. Lamfon H, Al-Karaawi Z, McCullough M, et al: Composition of in vitro denture plaque biofilms and susceptibility to antifungals. *FEMS Microbiol Lett* 2005;242:345–351.

45. Radford DR, Challacombe SJ, Walter JD: Denture plaque and adherence of *Candida albicans* to denture-base materials in vivo and in vitro. *Crit Rev Oral Biol Med* 1999;10:99–116.

46. Edgerton M, Levine MJ: Characterization of acquired denture pellicle from healthy and stomatitis patients. *J Prosthet Dent* 1992;68:683–691.

47. Branting C, Sund ML, Linder LE: The influence of Streptococcus mutans on adhesion of *Candida albicans* to acrylic surfaces in vitro. *Arch Oral Biol* 1989;34:347–353.

48. Ritchie GM, Fletcher AM, Main DM, et al: The etiology, exfoliative cytology, and treatment of denture stomatitis. *J Prosthet Dent* 1969;22:185–200.

12

THE EFFECT OF A DENTURE ADHESIVE ON THE COLONIZATION OF *CANDIDA* SPECIES IN VIVO

Eunghwan Kim, dds, ms,[1] Carl F. Driscoll, dmd, facp,[2] and Glenn E. Minah, dds, phd[3]

[1]*Former Resident, Advanced Education Program in Prosthodontics*
[2]*Associate Professor, Director, Advanced Education Program in Prosthodontics*
[3]*Professor, Department of Oral and Craniofacial Biological Science*

Keywords

Denture; denture adhesive; saliva; denture stomatitis; ill-fitting denture

Correspondence

Dr. Carl F. Driscoll, Room 3 D 08, Restorative Department, Baltimore College of Dental Surgery, University of Maryland, 666 West Baltimore Street, Baltimore, MD 21021. E-mail: CFD001@dental.umaryland.edu.

From the Baltimore College of Dental Surgery, University of Maryland, Baltimore, MD.

Accepted April 2, 2003

Published in *Journal of Prosthodontics* 2003; Vol. 12, Issue 3, pp. 187–91

doi:10.1016/S1059-941X(03)00050-0

ABSTRACT

Purpose: The purpose of this study was to evaluate the effect of a single denture adhesive on oral quantities of *Candida* species in vivo by determination of absolute and proportional counts of *Candida* species on dentures and in saliva of individuals who used this denture adhesive for a period of 14 days.

Materials and Methods: Samples were collected from saliva and maxillary dentures of 12 patients who wore existing dentures without adhesives for 2 weeks, then wore dentures with adhesive (Poly Grip Free; Glaxo Smith Kline, U.K.) for 2 weeks. Periodically, maxillary dentures were sampled by adding saline to the intaglio surface, dispersing by sonication and removing aliquots for culturing. These aliquots and saliva were diluted and plated in duplicate on bismuth sulfite, glycerine, and glucose yeast agar (Biggy) for recovery of *Candida* and on trypticase soy agar for total viable counts (TVC) of the microbiota. After 72 hours of incubation at 37 °C in air with 10% CO_2, colony-forming units were enumerated. in each individual, absolute counts of *Candida* and TVC, and proportional counts of *Candida* relative to TVC were compared and statistically evaluated during the periods of no adhesive use (control) and adhesive use (test).

Results: There were no statistically significant differences between the test and control periods for recovery of total *Candida* or TVC in saliva or on dentures, or the percent of *Candida* relative to TVC in saliva or on dentures.

Conclusion: Within the limitations of this study, the data suggested that the denture adhesive tested did not significantly alter the denture microbiota during the 14-day trial period.

Of the 20% of the adult population in the United States who wear removable prostheses, at least 22% use denture adhesives.[1,2] Between 1996 and 1997, 55 million units of denture adhesives were sold in the United States.[3] Potential benefits of denture adhesives are reported to be (1) improved chewing ability, (2) increased denture stability, (3) improved comfort and confidence, (4) reduced food collection under dentures, (5) alleviation of denture "sore spots," (6) improved mastication, (7) use in denture postinsertion care, and (8) use in patients with various medical or oral conditions including denture stomatitis.[4–6]

The question of what effect denture adhesive may have on the oral microflora is especially important in those patients with denture stomatitis, which may involve a microbial component. Denture stomatitis has been associated with *Candida albicans*, which colonize and commonly reside on acrylic surfaces of dentures, especially on the intaglio surface of the maxillary denture.[7,8] Denture stomatitis is also associated with denture trauma, which may be alleviated to some extent by using a soft lining material or denture adhesive.[6] Relining of dentures with soft liners is generally preferred over using a denture adhesive for retention and stability, especially with an immediate or transitional prosthesis.[9] Unsealed soft liners, however, showed increased colonization of *Candida* compared with those sealed with an acrylic varnish, implying that porosity of soft liners may result in the amplified yeast loads.[10]

The soft lining material has been reported to increase *Candida* species populations, owing in part to its porosity,[11,12] but its potential to support or inhibit microbial growth is not fully understood. This question has been examined in vitro by Bartels,[14] Stafford and Russell,[15] and Makihira et al,[16] and in vivo by Scher et al.[17] Bartels[14] and Stafford and Russell[15] found no inhibitory effects on oral bacteria, represented as saliva samples or pure cultures of *Candida* species. Stafford and Russell[15] did, however, demonstrate that a medium made of denture adhesive powder and 1% sucrose could support growth of *Streptococcus mitis* and *Candida albicans*, but not *Neisseria pharynges*. Makihira et al,[16] on the other hand, found 2 of 6 brands of denture adhesive to be inhibitory to *Candida albicans* and 1 brand to be inhibitory to *Candida tropicalis*, which they attributed in part to the low pH of the denture adhesives. In an in vivo investigation, Scher et al[17] reported that denture stomatitis was decreased with denture adhesives with reduction of *Candida albicans*, regardless of whether or not amphotericin had been incorporated into the denture adhesive. It was concluded that the denture adhesives had no positive effects on the growth of *Candida* species and that reduction of *Candida* species was probably related to improvement of the inflammatory conditions.

The purpose of the present study was to determine the in vivo effect on the denture microbiota of a commonly used denture adhesive in denture patients during a 14-day period of customary use by comparing absolute and proportional counts of *Candida* species on dentures and in saliva of individuals who used this denture adhesive. Our primary interest was the denture population at the University of Maryland Dental School that was supplied with the Poly Grip Free (Glaxo Smith Kline, U.K.) adhesive, and thus we focused our efforts on that single brand. A broad survey of other popular brands may be of interest despite the difficulty in obtaining formulas from manufacturers. Ellis et al[18] analyzed the constituents of several adhesives by infrared spectroscopy, and found that all contained mild antimicrobials, ingredients that swell in the presence of moisture, and additives that affect such properties as flavoring or surface tension.

MATERIALS AND METHODS

A group of 12 healthy subjects (4 males and 8 females: average age, 68.6; range, 65 to 76) were selected from a population of patients who had been wearing maxillary complete dentures, independent of the type of the opposing arch, for at least 6 months without denture adhesive. All of the subjects were in good general health, had no significant medical history, and had not received antibiotics for the previous 6 weeks. Age and gender were not selection criteria.

All subjects received intraoral and extraoral examinations. There were no abnormal findings of the tongue, palate, cheek, floor of the mouth, or nasopharyngeal area. All subjects were screened for the presence of *Candida* species in saliva. Only subjects positive for *Candida* species were included in this study. Of 13 screened subjects, only 1 subject was negative for *Candida* species. Saliva was sampled because it is easy to collect and represents a general indicator of oral colonization by *Candida*.

Dentures of selected participants were evaluated for stability and retention[19] and were found to be clinically adequate, with no signs of palatal inflammation. Most of the dentures were fabricated by the University of Maryland Postgraduate Prosthodontic Program and had not been relined before the study began. Before selection, each subject signed a consent form approved by the Institutional Review Board of the University of Maryland at Baltimore, which included a questionnaire to determine his or her comprehension of the experimental procedures.

A 2-mL specimen of saliva was collected by having the subject expectorate into a sterile cup. Saliva was cultivated on days 0, 7, 14, 21, and 28 for the presence of *Candida* species and total bacteria. Cultivation of the same microbial categories on the patient's dentures was conducted on days 0, 14, and 28. Sampling was conducted at either 10:00 A.M. or 2:00 P.M., and attempts were made to reschedule individuals at the same time for subsequent sample collection. Specimens were placed in enclosed plastic containers for transport to the laboratory and were processed for cultivation within 1 hour of collection. Subjects were encouraged to clean dentures daily and received instruction on using a denture brush (John O. Butler, Chicago, IL). Only water, with no denture cleansers or soap, was allowed during the testing period. For the first 2 weeks, subjects did not use any denture adhesive. Starting on day 14, each subject applied the denture adhesive (Poly Grip Free denture adhesive cream) to the maxillary denture twice a day for an additional 2 weeks. On days 0, 14 (after sampling), and 28 (after sampling), each denture was cleansed using the soft denture brush with water and then thoroughly rinsed with water.

Microbial sampling of dentures first entailed dispersal of the denture biofilm by sonication for 2 minutes (Kontes Cell-Disruptor, Kontes, Hazelwood, NJ) with a solution of 5.0 mL of 0.85% sterile sodium chloride solution (normal saline) that was placed in the intaglio of the maxillary denture. A 0.1-mL aliquot was then removed by micropipette and serially diluted to 10^{-5} by 10-fold dilution in normal sterilized saline. Cultivation procedures were similar to those used by Olan-Rodriquez et al.[10] Appropriate dilutions were plated in duplicate on trypticase soy agar (TSA; Difco, Detroit, MI), a nonselective medium for determination of total viable counts (TVC), and on bismuth sulfite, glycine, glucose yeast extract agar (Biggy; Difco, Detroit, MI) for recovery of *Candida* species. Several species of *Candida* could be tentatively identified on the latter medium by colony morphology. After 72 hours of incubation in air containing 10.0% CO_2 at 37 °C, total colony-forming (TCF) units on all countable agar plates were enumerated using a stereomicroscope (American Optical, Buffalo, NY) and colony-counting device (American Optical).

Saliva was diluted, plated, and cultured using the same dilution procedures, media, and cultivation technique as for the denture sample. Initial screening for *Candida* species was conducted by triple-streaking a sterile wire loop sample of saliva on Biggy medium, which was then incubated as previously described.

Microbiological data from a sample of each subject was recorded in tabulated formats as absolute counts of *Candida* species per mL of saline diluent on Biggy plates and TVCs of recoverable oral bacteria per mL of diluent on TSA plates. The percentage of *Candida* species relative to TVC was also recorded.

Data were entered on an Excel computer file, transformed into logarithms of base 10, and analyzed statistically by SPSS by Sigma Stat 2.0 (Jandel, San Rafael, CA). To test for the differences in *Candida* species and total viable counts from dentures or saliva during periods, with (test) or without (control) denture adhesives, a matchedpairs t test was used. The same test was used in comparisons of counts from dentures versus saliva. The effect of denture adhesives on the percentage of *Candida* species was analyzed by the Wilcoxon signed rank test. With a p value of <0.05 considered significant.

RESULTS

Mean absolute counts of *Candida* species in either saliva or dentures during test or control periods are presented in Table 1. In saliva, mean values were similar during test and control periods, and differences were nonsignificant. Denture values for total *Candida* species were higher during the test period, but test versus control comparisons were nonsignificant. *Candida* species were found in significantly greater numbers on dentures than in saliva.

In both denture samples and saliva, mean TVC values were slightly higher during the no-adhesive period, but statistical differences were nonsignificant for both datasets (Table 2). Salivary TVCs were significantly higher than denture TVCs.

Mean values for the proportion of *Candida* species relative to TVC were higher in dentures during the control period compared to the test period, but the differences were not statistically significant (Table 3). Test versus control salivary proportions were nonsignificant. Values for absolute counts of *Candida* species per mL of saliva were considerably lower than counts per mL of denture fluid, and the differences were significant ($p = 0.007$) (Table 4).

TABLE 1   Statistical Analysis of Absolute Counts of *Candida* Species

	N	Mean $\log_{10}$	SD $\log_{10}$	Significance (p value)
Saliva/mL				
Without adhesive	12	3.4	2.0	0.93[*]
With adhesive	12	3.4	1.8	
Denture/mL				
Without adhesive	12	4.3	1.5	0.97[†]
With adhesive	12	4.2	2.1	

[*]Matched-pair t test.
[†]Wilcoxon signed-rank test.

TABLE 2   Statistical analysis of TVC

	N	Mean $\log_{10}$	SD $\log_{10}$	Significance (p value)[*]
Saliva/mL				
Without adhesive	12	7.46	0.40	0.852
With adhesive	12	7.47	0.29	
Denture/mL				
Without adhesive	12	6.98	0.64	0.16
With adhesive	12	7.27	0.49	

[*]Matched-pair t test.

TABLE 3 Statistical Analysis of the Percentage of *Candida* Species Relative to TVC

	N	Mean	SD	Significance (p value)*
Saliva/mL				
Without adhesive	12	0.18	35	0.625
With adhesive	12	0.18	0.29	
Denture/mL				
Without adhesive	12	2.33	4.57	0.37
With adhesive		2.21	4.23	

*Wilcoxon signed-rank test.

DISCUSSION

This present study has demonstrated that using a denture adhesive for 14 days produced no statistically significant increase or decrease of *Candida* or absolute counts of microorganisms in the oral cavity or on denture intaglio surfaces, compared with a similar period without using adhesive. Although the data showed increases or decreases of microorganisms with or without denture adhesives in individual subjects, no general trends were seen. The percentage of *Candida* relative to TVC on dentures showed similar statistical results. All colonies on countable Biggy plates appeared consistent with the morphology of *Candida albicans*, but were not confirmed by more in-depth identification.

Although the present research suggests that denture adhesives may not directly affect oral quantities of *Candida* species or increase total bacteria, researchers have previously assumed that proliferation of microorganisms would be enhanced due to the stickiness of adhesives, or their stagnation if not replaced often. However, regularly removing the adhesive and washing the intaglio surfaces of their dentures before applying a new film may serve to reduce the microbial buildup. In the present study, the numbers of *Candida* and TVC of most subjects showed decreases during the first 2 weeks of the trial (no adhesives). This finding might indicate that subjects were motivated to follow diligent denture care procedures as a result of participation in the study.

Because most of the subjects' dentures had been fabricated within 1–1/2 years, the dentures had proper retention and stability, with adequate fit between the intaglio surfaces of dentures and the tissue surface. This would suggest that the denture adhesive film was thin. Most patients who use denture adhesives, however, do so because of retention and stability problems, implying thicker denture adhesive films than in the present study. This, in addition to inflammatory conditions, may produce different effects on the microbiota. The previous in vivo study of denture adhesives in patients with denture stomatitis by Sher et al,[17] however, found that adhesives were associated with reduced *Candida* levels, due presumably to reduced trauma and thus decreased inflammation of the mucosal tissue.

Clinical implications of *Candida* colonization of denture adhesives may be evident in patients who seek relief from denture stomatitis or who wear transitional prosthesis. If adhesives stimulate *Candida* proliferation, then they could exacerbate tissue inflammation in the case of denture stomatitis.[7,8] Although not directly addressed in the present investigation, it appears that regularly replacing denture adhesive after removing the old adhesive may aid control of the denture biofilm. For this reason, it may be also be advantageous from a microbiological standpoint with immediate or transitional prostheses.

Limitations of the present investigation were the absence of multiple brands of denture adhesives, small study population, and relatively short trial period. Future studies should include longitudinal assessment of yeast proliferation over a longer period. Long-term use of ill-fitting dentures should also be considered, to evaluate the effects of prothesis quality and thereby the film thickness of adhesives. Makihira et al[16] observed differences in pH of *Candida* cultures grown on commercial denture adhesives, all of which exhibited a pH < 6.0 before exposure to *Candida*. It was observed that a pH between 5 and neutral may stimulate *Candida* proliferation, and also may be a risk factor for cementum demineralization. Several denture adhesives had a sufficiently low pH (<3) to potentially inhibit *Candida*. The pH of Poly Grip Free was found to be 5.92 ± 0.36 after hydration but before oral exposure.

In summary, the findings of our study indicate that denture adhesive can be used safely for a short period, if patients are diligent in denture-cleansing procedures.

TABLE 4 Comparison of Absolute Counts of *Candida* Species in Saliva and on Dentures, With and Without Denture Adhesive

	Saliva Mean $\log_{10}$	Saliva SD $\log_{10}$	Denture Mean $\log_{10}$	Denture SD $\log_{10}$	Saliva Versus Denture Significance (p value)*
Without adhesive	3.4	2.0	4.26	1.5	0.007
With adhesive	3.4	1.8	4.20	2.0	0.007

*Matched-pair *t* test.

CONCLUSIONS

Within the confines of this study, the following conclusions can be drawn:

1. The denture adhesive cream (Poly Grip Free) did not affect the colonization of *Candida* species as measured by absolute and proportional counts, or absolute counts of bacteria on the surface of the dentures or in the saliva during a short-term (14-day) study period.

2. Patient hygiene may have been a factor in the lack of significant microbial changes. Daily cleaning of dentures by the subjects or daily replacement of the adhesive may have contributed to the lack of significant microbial changes noted.

REFERENCES

1. Douglas CW, Shin A, Ostry L: Will there be a need for complete dentures in the United States in 2020? *J Prosthet Dent* 2002;87:5–14.
2. Redford M, Drury TF, Kingman A, et al: Denture use and the technical quality of dental prostheses among persons 18–74 years of age: United States, 1988–1991. *J Dent Res* 1996;75: 714–725.
3. Pinto D: *Chain Drug Review*. 1998;20; 46
4. Tarbet WT, Boone M, Schmidt NF: Effect of a denture adhesive on complete denture dislodgement during mastication. *J Prosthet Dent* 1980;44:374–378.
5. Karlsson S, Swartz B: Effect of a denture adhesive on mandibular denture dislodgement. *Quintessence Int* 1990;21:625–627.
6. Adisman K: The use of dental adhesives as an aid to denture treatment. *J Prosthet Dent* 1989;62:711–715.
7. Webb BC, Thomas CJ, Willcox MD, et al: *Candida-associated* denture stomatitis. Aetiology and management: A review. Part 1. Factors influencing distribution of Candida species in the oral cavity. *Aust Dent J* 1998;43:45–50.
8. Radford DR, Challacombe SJ, Walter JD: Denture plaque and adherence of *Candida albicans* to denture-base materials in vivo and in vitro. *Crit Rev Oral Biol Med* 1999;10: 99–116.
9. Slaughter A, Katz RV, Grasso JE: Professional attitudes toward denture adhesives: A Delphi technique survey of academic prosthodontists. *J Prosthet Dent* 1999;82:80–99.
10. Olan-Rodriguez L, Minah GE, Driscoll CF: *Candida albicans* colonization of surface-sealed interim soft liners. *J Prosthodont* 2000;9:184–188.
11. Imai Y, Tamaki Y: Measurement of adsorption of salivary proteins onto soft denture lining materials. *J Prosthet Dent* 1999;82:348–351.
12. Samaranayake LP, MacFarlane TW: An in vitro study of the adherence of *Candida albicans* to acrylic surfaces. *Arch Oral Biol* 1980;25:603–609.
13. Waters MG, Jagger RG: Water absorption of RTV silicone denture soft lining material. *J Dent* 1996;24:105–108.
14. Bartels H: Bacteriological appraisal of adhesive denture powders. *J Dent Res* 1945;24:15–16.
15. Stafford GD, Russell C: Efficiency of denture adhesives and their possible influence on oral microorganisms. *J Dent Res* 1971;50:832–836.
16. Makihira S, Nikawa H, Satonobu SV, et al: Growth of *Candida* species on commercial denture adhesive in vitro. *Int J Prosthodont* 2001;14:48–52.
17. Scher EA, Ritchie GM, Flowers DJ: Antimycotic denture adhesive in treatment of denture stomatitis. *J Prosthet Dent* 1978;40:622–627.
18. Ellis B, El-Nakash S, Lamb DJ: The composition and rheology of denture adhesives. *J Dent* 1980;8:109–118.
19. Olshan AM, Ross NM, Mankodi S, et al: A modified Kapur scale for evaluating denture retention and stability: Methodology study. *Am J Dent* 1992;5:88–90.

13

EFFECT OF CHLORHEXIDINE ON DENTURE BIOFILM ACCUMULATION

Ingrid Machado de Andrade, DDS, PHD,[1] Patricia C. Cruz, DDS, MS,[1] Cláudia H. Silva-Lovato, DDS, PHD,[1] Raphael F. de Souza, DDS, PHD,[1] Maria Cristina Monteiro Souza-Gugelmin, DDS, PHD,[2] AND Helena de Freitas Oliveira Paranhos, DDS, PHD[1]

[1]Department of Dental Materials and Prosthodontics, Ribeirão Preto Dental School, University of São Paulo, Ribeirão Preto, Brazil

[2]Department of Clinical, Toxicological and Bromatological Analysis, Faculty of Pharmaceutical Sciences of Ribeirão Preto, University of São Paulo, Ribeirão Preto, Brazil

Keywords
Complete denture; biofilm; denture cleansers; chlorhexidine; oral hygiene

Correspondence
Helena de Freitas Oliveira Paranhos, Ribeirão Preto Dental School - Dental Materials and Prosthodontics, Av. café, s/n Ribeirão Preto 14040-904, Brazil.
E-mail: helenpar@forp.usp.br

Financial support from the São Paulo Research Foundation (FAPESP; grant no. 2005/55705-2).

Accepted February 14, 2011

Published in *Journal of Prosthodontics* 2012; Vol. 21, Issue 1, pp. 2–6

doi: 10.1111/j.1532-849X.2011.00774.x

ABSTRACT

Purpose: Adequate denture hygiene can prevent and treat infection in edentulous patients, who are frequently elderly and have difficulty brushing their teeth. This study evaluated the efficacy of complete denture biofilm removal using a chlorhexidine solution in two concentrations: 0.12% and 2.0%.
Materials and Methods: Sixty complete denture wearers participated in a trial for 21 days after receiving brushing instructions. They were distributed into three groups, according to the tested solution and regimen (n = 20): (G1) Control (daily overnight soaking in water); (G2) daily immersion at home in 0.12% chlorhexidine for 20 minutes after dinner; and (G3) a single immersion in 2.0% chlorhexidine for 5 minutes at the end of the experimental period, performed by a professional. Biofilm coverage area (%) was quantified on the internal surface of maxillary dentures at baseline and after 21 days. Afterward, the differences between initial and posttreatment results were compared by means of the Kruskal-Wallis test $(a = 0.05)$.
Results: Median values for biofilm coverage area after treatment were: (G1) 36.0%; (G2) 5.3%; and (G3) 1.4%. Differences were significant (KW = 35.25; $p < 0.001$), although G2 and G3 presented similar efficacy in terms of biofilm removal.

Conclusions: Both chlorhexidine-based treatments had a similar ability to remove denture biofilm. Immersion in 0.12% or 2.0% chlorhexidine solutions can be used as an auxiliary method for cleaning complete dentures.

Increasing life expectancy has led to a rising number of elderly people worldwide,[1] resulting in a high prevalence of edentulism and complete denture wearing.[2,3] Several studies have shown that the oral health of denture wearers is precarious.[4–7] Poor hygiene is associated with lack of guidance, the intrinsic characteristics of the denture, and reduced manual dexterity as a consequence of aging.[8]

Poor denture hygiene allows biofilm accumulation, an important stage for the development of several oral and systemic infections.[9,10] The continuous presence of a biofilm formed by bacteria and yeasts is the main etiological factor of denture stomatitis.[11,12] Thus, the indication of denture cleansing is of paramount importance to prevent or treat infections in the edentulous mouth.[13,14]

Denture care products should be able to remove inorganic/organic deposits and stains, be easy to handle, have bactericidal and fungicidal properties, present no toxicity to patients, be compatible with the denture materials, and have a low cost.[15]

However, these requirements are difficult to achieve in a clinical setting. Denture hygiene methods can be classified as mechanical or chemical.[8,16] Brushing is the most widespread mechanical method,[13] with the advantage of being simple, inexpensive, and effective.[8,16] However, patients with low dexterity may find it difficult to perform, and there is a possibility of acrylic resin wear and superficial damage to relining materials. Chemical methods can overcome some of these disadvantages. Chemical denture cleansers are able to dislodge food debris, biofilm, and tobacco stains from prosthodontic surfaces effectively. According to Gornitsky,[17] chemical denture cleansers could be a good choice for the elderly, who require adjunctive measures to clean their dentures. These cleansers are classified according to their composition and mechanism, namely, hypochlorites, peroxides, enzymes, acids, crude drugs, and disinfectants.

Several disinfectants have been suggested for denture disinfection. These products are readily accepted by denture wearers because they are easy to handle, accessible, and have a pleasant odor; however, alterations to prosthetic materials may be a concern when disinfecting agents are used.[11]

Chlorhexidine is one of the most widely used agents in dentistry and has been used as an adjunct in the treatment of oral candidiasis since the 1970s. It is an antiseptic agent with a broad spectrum of antimicrobial activity including *Candida albicans* and other common *non-albican* yeast species.[18,19] The most common preparation for oral use is chlorhexidine gluconate, a water-soluble compound, which has physiological pH and is dissociable, allowing the release of positively charged chlorhexidine[20] to be attracted by negative charges of bacteria.

In a 0.2% concentration, chlorhexidine gluconate has been successfully used as an antiseptic oral rinse in the treatment of denture stomatitis.[18] In a 0.12% concentration, it has been used as an antiseptic mouthwash in periodontal management. The gel in the 2.0% concentration has demonstrated an ability to clean dentinal walls when used during endodontic treatment,[21] while the 2.0% suspension is used as an overnight denture disinfectant.[18]

Given the antimicrobial potential shown by chlorhexidine in several areas of dentistry, the aim of this study was to evaluate the efficacy of 0.12% and 2.0% chlorhexidine solutions as denture cleansers, by conducting a clinical trial to evaluate their biofilm removal capability.

MATERIALS AND METHODS

Patient Selection

After approval by the Institutional Ethics Committee and signature of the informed consent form by the potential participants, 60 patients were selected (17 men and 43 women; age range: 45 to 80 years). They presented good overall health and healthy denture-supporting tissues. The inclusion criteria were that participants should wear maxillary and mandibular complete dentures made of heat-polymerized acrylic resin; the wearing time of the present dentures should range from 5 to 10 years. In addition, an initial biofilm score of 1 or higher should be observed on the internal surface of maxillary dentures, according to an additive index.[22]

Hygiene Methods and Experimental Design

The experimental period lasted 21 days. Before the use of each method, biofilm was eliminated by brushing with a specific brush for complete dentures (Denture, Condor S.A., Santa Catarina, Brazil) and liquid soap (JOB Quimica, Produtos para limpeza Ltda., Monte Alto, Brazil). All participants were instructed to brush their dentures three times a day, after each meal for 2 minutes with tap water, using a specific brush for complete dentures (Bitufo, Itupeva, Brazil). They were also instructed to rinse the oral cavity with tap water after brushing. They were randomly assigned to one of the following hygiene methods (n = 20):

1. Control: Participants were instructed to keep their dentures immersed in water overnight.
2. 0.12% chlorhexidine: Dentures were immersed daily at home in 0.12% chlorhexidine (Faculty of Pharmaceutical Sciences of Ribeirão Preto, University of São Paulo, Ribeirão Preto, Brazil). Immersion was to be carried out for 20 minutes after dinner. Afterward, dentures were rinsed before insertion in the oral cavity. Participants were instructed to keep their dentures immersed in water overnight.
3. 2.0% chlorhexidine: At the end of the experimental period (21 days), a researcher immersed the dentures in 2.0% chlorhexidine (Faculty of Pharmaceutical Sciences of Ribeirão Preto, University of São Paulo) for 5 minutes. Participants were instructed to keep their dentures immersed in water overnight.

Denture Biofilm Coverage Area

The internal surfaces of the maxillary dentures were disclosed with 1% neutral red solution. The surfaces were then photographed with a digital camera and flash (Canon EOS Digital Rebel EF-S 18–55, Canon MR-14 EX, Canon Inc., Tokyo, Japan) with standard film-object distance and exposure time, and the camera fixed on a stand (CS-4 Copy Stand, Testrite Inst. Co., Inc., Newark, NJ). Total surface area and areas corresponding to the stained region were measured using image processing software (Image Tool 3.0). The biofilm percentage was calculated using the ratio between biofilm area multiplied by 100 and total surface area of the internal denture base.[8,23,24] This procedure was performed by a researcher who gave no instructions, delivered no products to patients, and did not handle the dentures. After the use of each method and quantification, the biofilm was eliminated by brushing with a specific brush for complete dentures (Denture) and liquid soap (JOB Quimica).

Data Analysis

The outcome variable for this trial, biofilm coverage area (%), did not show distribution close to normality and had no homogeneous variations. Thus, a nonparametric analysis was used. The Kruskal-Wallis test was used for comparison among the three groups followed by the Dunn multiple comparison test. Analysis was performed at $\alpha = 0.05$ using a software package SPSS 15.0.0 (SPSS Inc., Chicago, IL).

RESULTS

Figure 1 shows a box-plot graph with the biofilm coverage areas after the trial. The control treatment seemed to remove less biofilm than the other methods. The experimental methods presented nearly similar biofilm removal results.

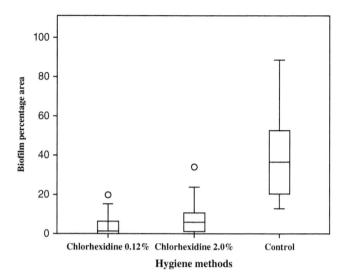

FIGURE 1   Biofilm coverage area for each group following treatment.

TABLE 1   Mean ranks for the treatments and results ofthe Dunn multiple comparison test

Treatment	Mean rank	Grouping*
Control	39.3	A
0.12% chlorhexidine	4.1	B
2.0% chlorhexidine	7.8	B

*Identical upper case letters denote no significant differences between the treatments.

The Kruskal-Wallis test found significant difference among the treatments ($KW = 35.25$; $p < 0.001$). The experimental methods were similar, whereas the control group differed significantly (Table 1). This implies that denture hygiene by means of brushing was improved with the addition of the tested chlorhexidine-based treatments; however, the two experimental regimens (0.12% and 2.0% chlorhexidine) attained similar outcomes.

No adverse effect or stains were observed after the use of any of the chlorhexidine-based treatments, as disclosed by clinical examination. Participants described no complication after using the two experimental regimens, and none complained about the aftertaste associated with the chlorhexidine-based treatments.

DISCUSSION

An important feature of a complete denture cleanser is its capacity to remove biofilm, and this property should be assessed by laboratory and clinical tests.[25] This study evaluated the efficacy of complete biofilm removal from dentures using chlorhexidine solutions of two concentrations: 0.12% and 2.0%. The experimental methods presented similar results, whereas the control group (soaking in water) was significantly different. Immersion in 0.12% or 2.0% chlorhexidine solutions can improve denture hygiene when used as an auxiliary method for cleaning complete dentures.

Chlorhexidine destroys bacteria by breaking their membranes and inducing cytoplasmatic precipitation.[26] It is a cationic molecule capable of interacting with inorganic human dentine particles and also bonds to negatively charged surfaces, such as the bacterial cell wall.[12,20] Although the antimicrobial analysis was not the focus of this study, several studies that have performed antimicrobial analyses are in agreement with these results as regards the effectiveness of chlorhexidine as a denture cleanser.

Lamfon et al,[27] for example, assessed the resistance of C. albicans biofilms to both antifungal and antimicrobial agents in vitro. The minimal inhibitory concentration (MIC) of fluconazole, miconazole, and chlorhexidine for C. albicans was first determined. C. albicans biofilms were found to be highly resistant to fluconazole and miconazole compared with the same cells grown in suspension ($>1024 \times$ MIC). In contrast, chlorhexidine inhibited the growth of C. albicans biofilms at a concentration of up to $8 \times$ MIC. When the susceptibility of biofilms over time was investigated, higher reductions were observed for chlorhexidine and miconazole than fluconazole for biofilms of 2 and 6 hours.

Similarly, Lamfon et al[28] investigated the in vitro composition of denture biofilms and the susceptibility of Candida spp. within these biofilms to antifungal agents. It was observed that exposure to single agents, for example, miconazole, fluconazole, or chlorhexidine did not inhibit the growth of Candida spp. when used in clinically relevant doses. Combinations of miconazole and chlorhexidine, to mimic patient use, did reduce bacterial and candidal growth for several days. Hence, the use of dual therapy appeared to be useful in reducing the number of viable organisms within denture plaque grown in vitro, although resistance to these agents was also evident.

Similarly, Silva-Lovato and Paranhos[23] evaluated the effectiveness of disinfectant solutions (1.0% sodium hypochlorite, 2.0% chlorhexidine digluconate, 2.0% glutaraldehyde, 100% vinegar, sodium perborate-based tabs, and 3.8% sodium perborate) in the disinfection of acrylic resin specimens (n = 10/group) contaminated in vitro by C. albicans, Streptococcus mutans, Staphylococcus aureus, Escherichia coli, or Bacillus subtilis as measured by residual colony-forming units. The acrylic resin specimens were immersed in the disinfectants for 10 minutes. It was concluded that 1.0% sodium hypochlorite, 2.0% glutaraldehyde, 2.0% chlorhexidine, 100% vinegar, and 3.8% sodium perborate are valid alternatives for the disinfection of acrylic resin.

Montagner et al[12] evaluated the antifungal action of different agents on microwavable acrylic resin specimens, which were previously contaminated with C. albicans. They observed that sodium hypochlorite-based solutions and hydrogen peroxide are more efficacious disinfectants against

C. albicans than 2.0% chlorhexidine solution and an effervescent agent. This lack of antimicrobial action of chlorhexidine 2.0% might be justified by the immersion periods used. The authors immersed the specimens in chlorhexidine for 10 minutes. In this study, the dentures were immersed in 2.0% chlorhexidine for 5 minutes, and the results showed that the solution was effective for biofilm removal. The in vivo design of this study and other features could be a reason for this discrepancy.

Pavarina et al[11] also noted the effectiveness of chlorhexidine as a denture cleanser, though they used the chlorhexidine in a different concentration from that adopted in this trial. In their study, the effectiveness of chemical agents (4.0% chlorhexidine gluconate, 1.0% sodium hypochlorite, iodophors, and alkaline peroxide) for cleansing and disinfecting removable dental prostheses was evaluated, and it was concluded that the 4.0% chlorhexidine gluconate, 1.0% sodium hypochlorite, and alkaline peroxide solutions were effective in reducing the growth of the microorganisms in the 10-minute immersion period.

These results with 0.12% chlorhexidine also are in agreement with Barroeta et al's study,[29] which evaluated the efficacy of four chemical agents (2.0% sodium hypochlorite, 5.0% acetic acid, peroxides, 0.12% chlorhexidine) in different immersion times (5, 10, 15, 20 minutes, and 8 hours) and concluded that all disinfectants were effective in eliminating C. albicans after 20 minutes of immersion.

Redding et al[30] determined the in vitro ability of several thinfilm polymer formulations, with and without incorporated antifungal agents, to inhibit C. albicans biofilm growth on denture material. The fungicides incorporated were: (1) 1.0% chlorhexidine diacetate; (2) 1.0% nystatin; or (3) 1.0% amphotericin B. It was concluded that biofilm reduction with chlorhexidine (up to 98%) was significantly greater than all the other formulations tested.

Future studies should compare the antimicrobial effect of the regimens tested in this study, to better understand their effect on denture biofilm. An immediate application of 2.0% chlorhexidine may be much more efficacious than a single application of lower concentrations, but continuous use may result in biofilms with different microbial compositions. Another recommendation is the evaluation of outcome variables such as the health of supporting tissues and presence of denture stomatitis, as well as adverse effects, that is, stains on denture bases and teeth. The latter approach may lead to a definitive clinical guideline; however, it can be inferred that both tested regimens are clinically efficacious, due to their strong effect on the denture biofilm coverage area. Proprietary solutions of 0.12% chlorhexidine can be easily found by patients and are inexpensive; however, the great advantage of 2.0% chlorhexidine is the need of a single application to achieve important biofilm reduction. Based on these results, a discussion with patients about their preferences may be a reasonable approach to controlling denture biofilm.

CONCLUSION

The tested denture cleansing regimens based on 0.12% and 2.0% chlorhexidine solutions were equally efficacious in removing biofilm and were superior to the control method (soaking in water). Both 0.12% and 2.0% chlorhexidine solutions can be used as auxiliary methods of hygiene, contributing to the maintenance of the oral health care of complete denture wearers.

REFERENCES

1. United Nations Population Division. *World Population Prospects: The 2002 Revision.* New York: United Nations, 2003.

2. Colussi CF, Freitas SF, Calvo MCM: Perfil epidemiologico da carie e do uso e necessidade de protese na populacao idosa de Biguacu, Santa Catarina. *Rev Bras Epidemiol* 2004;7:88–97.

3. Moreira RS, Nico LS, Tomita NE, et al: Oral health of Brazilian elderly: a systematic review of epidemiologic status and dental care access. *Cad Saùde Pùblica* 2005;21:1665–1675.

4. Coelho CM, Souza YT, Dare AM: Denture-related oral mucosal lesions in a Brazilian school of dentistry. *J Oral Rehabil* 2004;31:135–139.

5. Kulak-Ozkan Y, Kazazoglu E, Arikan A: Oral hygiene habits, denture cleanliness, presence of yeasts and stomatitis in elderly people. *J Oral Rehabil* 2002;29:300–304.

6. Marchini L, Tamashiro E, Nascimento DFF, et al: Self-reported denture hygiene of a sample of edentulous attendees at a University dental clinic and the relationship to the condition of the oral tissues. *Gerodontology* 2004;21:226–228.

7. Marchini L, Vieira PC, Bossan TP, et al: Self-reported oral hygiene habits among institutionalized elderly and their relationship to the condition of oral tissues in Taubate, Brazil. *Gerodontology* 2006;23:33–37.

8. Paranhos HFO, Silva-Lovato CH, Souza RF, et al: Effects of mechanical and chemical methods on denture biofilm accumulation. *J Oral Rehabil* 2007;34:606–612.

9. Donlan RM: Biofilm formation: a clinically relevant microbiological process. *Clin Infect Dis* 2001;33:1387–1392.

10. Kuhn DM, Chandra J, Mukherjee PK, et al: Comparison of biofilms formed by Candida albicans and Candida parapsilosis on bioprosthetic surfaces. *Infect Immun* 2002;70:878–888.

11. Pavarina AC, Machado AL, Giampaolo ET, et al: Effects of chemical disinfectants on the transverse strength of denture base acrylics resins. *J Oral Rehabil* 2003;30:1085–1089.

12. Montagner H, Montagner F, Braun KO, et al: In vitro antifungal action of different substances over microwave-cured acrylic resins. *J Appl Oral Sci* 2009;17:432–435.

13. Shay K: Denture hygiene: a review and update. *J Contemp Dent Pract* 2000;1:1–8.

14. Pires FR, Santo EB, Bonan PR, et al: Denture stomatitis and salivary *Candida* in Brazilian edentulous patients. *J Oral Rehabil* 2002;29:1115–1119.

15. Jagger DC, Harrison A: Denture cleansing-the best approach. *Br Dent J* 1995;178:413–417.

16. Paranhos HFO, Silva-Lovato CH, Venezian GC, et al: Distribution of biofilm on internal and external surfaces of upper complete dentures: the effect of hygiene instruction. *Gerodontology* 2007;24:162–168.

17. Gornitsky M, Paradis I, Landaverde G, et al: A clinical and microbiological evaluation of denture cleansers for geriatric patients in long-term care institutions. *J Can Dent Assoc* 2002;68:39–45.

18. Ellepola ANB, Samaranayake LP: Oral candidal infections and antimycotics. *Crit Rev Oral Biol Med* 2000;11:172–198.

19. Ellepola ANB, Saramanayake LP: Adjunctive use of chlorhexidine in oral candidoses: a review. *Oral Dis* 2001;7:11–17.

20. Mohammadi Z, Abbott PV: The properties and applications of chlorhexidine in endodontics. *Int Endod J* 2009;42:288–302.

21. Ferraz CC: In vitro assessment of the antimicrobial action and the mechanical ability of chlorhexidine gel as an endodontic irrigant. *J Endod* 2001;27:452–455.

22. Ambjørgensen E, Valderhaug J, Norheim PW, et al: Assessment of an additive index for plaque accumulation on complete maxillary dentures. *Acta Odontol Scand* 1982;40:203–208.

23. Silva-Lovato CH, Paranhos HFO: Efficacy of biofilm disclosing agent and of three brushes in the control of compete denture cleansing. *J Appl Oral Sci* 2006;14:454–459.

24. Salles AES, Macedo LD, Fernandes RAG, et al: Comparative analysis of biofilm levels in complete upper and lower dentures after brushing associated with specific denture paste and neutral soap. *Gerodontology* 2007;24:217–223.

25. Nikawa H, Hamada T, Yamashiro H, et al: A review of in vitro and in vivo methods to evaluate the efficacy of denture cleansers. *Int J Prosthodont* 1999;12:153–159.

26. Gomes BPFA, Vianna ME, Matsumoto CU, et al: Disinfection of gutta-percha cones with chlorhexidine and sodium hypochlorite. *Oral Surg Oral Med Oral Pathol Oral Radiol Endod* 2005;100:512–517.

27. Lamfon H, Porter SR, McCullough M, et al: Susceptibility of Candida albicans biofilms grown in a constant depth film fermentor to chlorhexidine, fluconazole and miconazole: a longitudinal study. *J Antimicrob Chemother* 2004;53:383–385.

28. Lamfon H, Al-Karaawi, McCullough M, et al: Composition of in vitro denture plaque biofilms and susceptibility to antifungals. *FEMS Microbiol Lett* 2005;242:345–351.

29. Barroeta AU, Méndez GR, Lelis AB: Action de agentes quimicos en la eliminacion de Candida albicans sobre prOtesis dentales. *Acta Odontol Venez* 2007;45:172–177.

30. Redding S, Bhatt B, Rawls R, et al: Inhibition of Candida albicans biofilm formation on denture material. *Oral Surg Oral Med Oral Pathol Oral Radiol Endod* 2009;107:669–672.

14

EVIDENCE REGARDING THE TREATMENT OF DENTURE STOMATITIS

ALEXANDRA YARBOROUGH, DDS,[1] LYNDON COOPER, DDS, PHD, FACP,[2] IBRAHIM DUQUM, BDS, MS,[1] GUSTAVO MENDONÇA, DDS, MSC, PHD,[3] KATHLEEN MCGRAW, MA, MLS,[4] AND LISA STONER, DDS, MS[1]

[1]Department of Prosthodontics, University of North Carolina at Chapel Hill School of Dentistry, Chapel Hill, NC
[2]Department of Oral Biology, University of Illinois at Chicago College of Dentistry, Chicago, IL
[3]Division of Prosthodontics, University of Michigan School of Dentistry, Ann Arbor, MI
[4]Health Sciences Library, University of North Carolina, Chapel Hill, NC

Keywords
Denture stomatitis; complete denture; oral fungal infections; *Candida albicans*; systematic review

Correspondence
Alexandra Yarborough, Department of Prosthodontics, UNC Chapel Hill School of Dentistry, 338 Brauer Hall, CB 7450, Chapel Hill, NC 27599. E-mail: abyarbor@email.unc.edu

The authors thank US GlaxoSmithKline for their support. Neither GSK nor the ACP Board of Directors participated in any aspect of this systematic review.

Accepted November 22, 2015

Published in *Journal of Prosthodontics* 2016; Vol. 25, Issue 4, pp. 288–301

doi: 10.1111/jopr.12454

ABSTRACT

Denture stomatitis is a common inflammatory condition affecting the mucosa underlying complete dentures. It is associated with denture microbial biofilm, poor denture hygiene, poor denture quality, and nocturnal denture use. Numerous treatment methodologies have been used to treat stomatitis; however, a gold standard treatment has not been identified. The aim of this systematic review is to report on the current knowledge available in studies representing a range of evidence on the treatment of denture stomatitis.

Denture stomatitis (DS) is the inflammation of the mucosa underlying a complete denture. This inflammatory condition is common, with a reported prevalence of 15% to 70% of denture wearers.[1] It is attributed to several etiologies including poor denture hygiene, poor denture quality, and nocturnal denture use. DS is an inflammatory mucosal disorder associated with a microbial pathogenesis.[2] Fungal infection is implicated by repeated isolation of opportunistic microbes from dentures of DS patients. Specifically, *C. albicans* is frequently implicated in DS.[3] Additionally, *C. glabrata, C. tropicalis*, and other fungi from the *Candida* species have been isolated from DS patients and their dentures.[4] Typically, more than one yeast species can be isolated intraorally.[5]

A prominent etiologic factor for DS is the measured level of *Candida* in the denture and saliva. Other factors, such as denture quality, xerostomia, and the presence of *Candida* in the mucosa, are of lesser importance.[7] The covariables identified in studies of DS and *Candida* infection include poor denture hygiene, poor denture quality, nocturnal denture use, impaired salivary flow, and compromised immunity; however, disagreement remains regarding the significance of these risk factors.[6,7] Understanding the relative roles of these potential risk factors is an important prerequisite for directing the proper management and treatment of this condition.

DS is characterized by several classical signs but few symptoms. It is rarely associated with severe pain or discomfort. It is often associated with angular chelitis.[8] The spectrum of DS is captured by the Newton classification system. This system stratifies the disease as localized inflammation or pinpoint hyperemia (type 1), diffuse erythema associated with the denture-contacting mucosa (type 2), and papillary (granular) hyperplasia of the keratinized mucosa (type 3).[9] The progression of DS without treatment may lead to systemic infection. In immuno-compromised patients, the fungal component of DS can be devastating. Individuals with uncontrolled diabetes, HIV, and nutritional deficits, and organ transplant patients can develop deep tissue infections that can be very difficult to manage.[10] Relapse is common among immunocompromised patients after cessation of fungal agents.[11]

DS is a chronic condition that challenges treatment. Treatments involve local and systemic antifungal therapies, reduction or eradication of denture-related biofilm, laser treatment of the affected mucosa, or combination approaches. This diversity in treatment approaches is evidenced in a recent meta-analysis of the treatment of DS that included 14 studies comparing different modalities of treatment.[13] The authors concluded that there was no difference between various disinfection methods and antifungal treatment when evaluated at the clinical or micro-biological level. Given the breadth of experience reported in management of DS, the diversity of methods and therapeutic targets, a broader assessment of DS treatments is warranted. The aim of this systematic review is to summarize knowledge presented using a range of evidence (beyond randomized clinical trials) on the treatment of denture stomatitis.

MATERIALS AND METHODS

The intent of this review is to aid clinicians in establishing guidelines for the treatment of denture stomatitis. As such, a broad search was conducted, and inclusion criteria were established. These include the following:

1. Human clinical study, or samples taken from human subjects

2. Clinical trials, case series, observational studies (cross-sectional, longitudinal studies), and case control studies that tested/reported interventions to treat denture stomatitis

3. Inclusion of at least ten subjects

4. Investigation to include complete denture prostheses without the use of dental implants in one or both arches

5. Publication not more than 20 years old

6. Publication in peer-reviewed journal

7. Manuscript in English

An electronic search of publications to August 10, 2013 was established using five databases. The databases searched included PubMed, Embase, Google Scholar, ADA Evidence Based Database, and the Cochrane Collaboration Database.

The main search terms used in the databases were as follows: "denture stomatitis," "oral candidiasis," "oropharyngeal candidiasis." The combined search terms used in the database were as follows: "denture stomatitis" and "etiology," "*candida*" and "denture," "oral candidiasis" and "denture," "*candida albicans*" and "denture," "*candida*" and "edentulism," "*candida*" and "denture stomatitis," "denture stomatitis" and "treatment," and "denture stomatitis" and "prognosis."

A total of four reviewers completed the review by reading full-text articles and collecting relevant information in a data extraction table. Categories included in this table were as follows: primary authors, study design, the number of included subjects, and the follow-up period. The remaining categories of the table included the treatment and outcome of treatment evaluated. One table was made for healthy subjects, and one was made for immunocompromised subjects. A comprehensive statistical meta-analysis was not performed.

RESULTS

The electronic search identified 2360 articles. Title and abstracts were screened by two authors independently for possible inclusion in the review. Following this review, 1766 were excluded, as they did not meet inclusion criteria. A total of 594 articles judged to be relevant by the title and abstract were read by a team of reviewers. Following article review, an additional 387 were excluded, as they did not meet inclusion criteria or were duplicates. Of the final 207 articles, 67 were relevant to complete denture stomatitis treatment methodology, and these were included in this review.

The included papers represented different levels of evidence. Among them, 64 prospective studies and 3 retrospective studies were reviewed. Among the prospective studies, 22 were cohort studies and 7 were cross-sectional studies. There were 33 randomized control trials (RCTs).

The included studies reflected outcomes of 5255 subjects. Patients were followed for a period of 1 day to 1 year. Among the studies, many did not differentiate between treatments for the maxillary versus the mandibular arch; however, most studies focused on the maxillary arch.

The included studies are summarized in Table 1 (for healthy patients) and Table 2 (for immunocompromised patients). A total of 62 articles evaluated healthy patients. A total of five articles evaluated immunocompromised patients. The studies range from prospective and retrospective cohort investigations, to cross-sectional observations to RCTs. The diagnostic criteria for oral candidiasis were not standardized among the studies.

The populations studied and the data collection methods are exceptionally varied. Treatments evaluated were grouped into eight main treatment categories. These include:

1. Antifungal therapy, including both systemic and topical application
2. Disinfectants and cleansers
3. Laser treatment of palatal tissue
4. Oral hygiene instructions
5. Fabrication of a new denture
6. Hard reline
7. Placement of a resilient liner or a tissue conditioner
8. Microwave disinfection

The treatments evaluated in healthy patients are summarized in Table 3. Thirty-six papers evaluated the effect of antifungal agents applied both locally and systemically. Of those, 34 papers revealed that treatment with an antifungal agent reduced DS in healthy patients. Two papers[15,35] showed no difference in outcome (Table 1). One article[37] compared single-agent anti-fungals to combination therapy. The results revealed that combination therapy of antifungal agents showed an increased benefit compared to single agent antifungals (Table 1).

Sixteen papers evaluated the use of disinfectants and/ or denture cleansers in DS treatment. Thirteen of 16 papers reported that treatment improved the condition (e.g., Table 1 [6,21]). Interestingly, nine papers included the use of alternative medicines (extracts, pollens) for the treatment of DS (Table 1[5,8,13–15,31,45,52]). Among these, the majority of studies demonstrated reduction of DS and equivalence with comparisons to antifungal agents. No negative control (sham treatment or simple cleansing) was included in these studies. Two papers[39,62] demonstrated that hard reline material placement successfully reduced DS (Table 1). Denture disinfection was also examined. Five articles evaluating microwave disinfection resulted in a positive outcome (Table 1[44,49]). Fabrication of a new complete denture was shown to be effective (Table 1[4]). Seven papers evaluated the use of resilient liners or tissue conditioners to treat DS. Of the seven evaluated, four showed an improvement in DS when a liner or tissue conditioner was placed. One article[28] (Table 1)

revealed an initial improvement, but an overall increase in DS when tissue conditioner was used. Two articles[11,15] showed no difference (Table 1). Targeting of the denture was a broadly successful, common therapeutic strategy, yet with reported limitations.[12]

Besides the direct treatment of the denture, laser treatment of tissues of DS patients was evaluated in three articles,[38,41,48] and all three revealed a decrease in DS (Table 2). In addition, control of biofilm through oral hygiene education and programming was discussed in five articles. Four showed an improvement in outcome, while one showed no difference (Table 2[24]). Of the 62 articles that evaluated healthy patients, a majority (42 studies) invoked some type of combined treatment strategy.

Far fewer studies have evaluated DS treatment in immunocompromised patients (Table 4). Four of these five papers evaluated the effect of antifungal agents applied both locally and systemically. Two[63,64] of the four studies involving antifungal agents showed a decrease in DS (Table 2), while two[66,67] showed no difference in DS (Table 2). No investigations examined the effects of disinfectants and cleansers on DS of immunocompromised patients. In addition, no studies evaluated the effect of a hard reline, laser treatment, microwave disinfection, new complete denture provision, or the use of tissue conditioners on the DS of immunocompromised individuals.

DISCUSSION

This systematic review identified the spectrum of treatments used for DS and summarized the treatment outcomes. Recently, a systematic review with meta-analysis reported on the comparison of antifungal therapies versus alternative methods for treatment of DS. That review concluded that both disinfection and antiseptic methods were as effective as antifungal therapy in treatment of DS.[13] The present findings (Table 1) from a broader assessment of the literature are consistent with this recent meta-analysis. Further, when considering immunocompromised individuals with DS separately, antifungal therapy was consistently reported to reduce or eliminate DS (Table 2).

While the intent of this review was to include a broad set of reports in an effort to gain more information, several limitations are imposed by the nature of these studies. Foremost among them is that the diagnostic criteria (Newman Classification) for DS were not fully represented and employed among the studies. Comparisons and resulting conclusions suffer from clinical heterogeneity due to unknown inclusion based on severity. The standardization of diagnostic criteria among inclusion criteria for these studies may influence or improve assessments. Future studies are needed to define the influence of diagnostic classification (severity) on treatment outcomes.

TABLE 1   Included studies evaluating the treatment of complete denture stomatitis in healthy patients

Authors, year	Prospective, retrospective	Number of subjects (N total)	Follow-up period	Treatment evaluated	Treatment outcome
Abaci, 2011[18]	Prospective	110		Amphotericin B, Fluconazole, 5-fluorocytosine, caspofungin terbinafine	Sensitivity of *C. albicans* to amphotericin B (61%), fluconazole (44%), 5-fluorocytosine (100%). *C. glabrata* (second most isolated species) susceptibility to caspofungin terbinafine (100%) and 5-fluorocytosine (100%). Caspofungin terbinafine and 5-fluorocytosine are suggested to be used in the treatment of fungal infections
Amanlou et al, 2006[19]	Prospective	24	0,7, 14,21, and 28 days	Miconazole 2% gel versus Zatana multiflora 0.1%	Miconazole reduced colony count more than Zatana multiflora. Zatana multiflora reduced erythema more than miconazole.
Andrucioli et al, 2004[20]	Prospective	24	60 days	Mechanical method with experimental denture paste and soft-bristle toothbrush for biofilm removal	Experimental product was efficient in the removal of denture plaque biofilm.
Arikan et al, 1995[21]	Prospective	60	14 days	Fluconazole, fluconazole plus, chlorhexidine, new fitting denture	For generalized simple DS fluconazole in conjunction with chlorhexidine resulted in greater improvement of palatal inflammation. Localized simple stomatitis patients improved with new fitting dentures.
Bakhshi et al, 2012[22]	Prospective	40	4 weeks	Compared nystatin to garlic extract	The changes in the length and width of erythema at different times (4-week treatment) according to the type of treatment were found to be significant, while an accelerated recovery was demonstrated for nystatin ($p < 0.001$). Both regimens resulted in significant recovery ($p < 0.0001$). Greater satisfaction with the use of garlic rather than nystatin was mentioned ($p < 0.0001$). Nystatin was more effective at earlier time points.
Banting et al, 1995[23]	Prospective	23	3 months	The effectiveness of an antifungal soaking solution (nystatin) as an adjunct to a nystatin lozenge compared to soaking dentures in tap water and using lozenges.	Compared to tap water, use of antifungal denture soaking solution showed no detectable difference in presence of *C. albicans* over a 3-month period, but the signs and symptoms of oral candidiasis resolved in all subjects after therapy. Nystatin denture soaking solution was not shown to provide any added benefit compared to nystatin lozenges alone.
Banting and Hill, 2001[24]	Prospective	34		(1) Scrub and microwave max denture for 1 minute at 850 W versus (2) soak denture in chlorhexidine overnight. All subjects received the same course of topical antifungal medication (nystatin 300,000 IU lozenges 3× daily for 14 days	After 3 months, one (8%) patient in the microwave group and 12 (63%) patients in the denture soak group demonstrated pseudohyphae on the cytological smears.

Study	Study type	N	Intervention	Duration	Findings
Barnabe et al, 2004[25]	Prospective	28	Coconut soap versus coconut soap with 0.05% sodium hyperchlorate	15days	$p < 0.05$ confidence level is (1) significantly reduced DS signs, (2) *C. albicans* count not reduced, (3) *S. mutans* reduced, (4) controlled biofilm.
Beyari, 2011[14]	Prospective	40	Three types of denture cleansers versus control (no cleanser)	6 months	Chemical cleansing of dentures decreased the total number of CFU of microorganisms and the number *S. mutans*. Condition of mucosa also improved with the decrease in microorganisms.
Blomgren et al, 1998[27]	Retrospective	60	Oral fluconazole and nystatin		No significant difference between the two groups treated with fluconazole and nystatin. Fluconazole showed considerable improvement in 87% of patients, nystatin showed improvement in 80% of patients. Fluconazole was reportedly easier to take. For immunocompromised patients, systematic treatment is recommended. Local antifungal is recommended in case of local predisposing factors (hyposalivation, local steroids, etc.).
Brosky et al, 2003[28]	Prospective	20	Molloplast B and MPDS-SL—experimental (resilient denture liners)		Candida growth on Molloplast B was not significantly different from growth on MPDS-SL. The rates of culture-positive testing (65% on Molloplast B samples and 45% on MPDS-SL samples) did not differ between the two resilient denture liners. Most common species were *C. albicans* and *C. glabrata*.
Budtz-Jorgensen etal, 2000[15]	Prospective	272	Preventative oral health program		Preventative program was effective in reducing the colonization of the oral mucosa and dentures by *Candida*. Reduction of number of patients with positive cultures.
Campelo et al, 2002[29]	Prospective	75	Essential oil Cymbopogom citratus (cream and spray), nystatin		CCR-2000 cream and spray are as effective as nystatin in reducing oral *Candida*. CCR-2000 cream and spray could be recommended to reduce oral yeasts, to prevent oral lesions related to *Candida*.
Capistrano et al, 2013[30]	Prospective	45	(1) 2% concentration miconazole gel, (2) 2.5% concentration propolis gel, (3) 24% concentration propolis mouthwash (propolis—a resinour MH collected by bees from various plants)	4 weeks	No difference among groups; all had a significant reduction or a complete remission of DS and a significant reduction of *C. albicans* colonies.
Catalan et al, 2008[31]	Prospective	27	Melaleveca alternifolia oil + CoeComfort treatment, Nystatin + Coe Comfort, and Coe Comfort	12 days	No difference
Cross et al, 2000[33]	Prospective	40	Cyclodextrin solution of itraconazole (compared) itraconazole capsules 100 mg twice daily for 15 days	6 months	Liquid and capsule preparations of itraconazole are equally effective adjuncts in the treatment of DS. The side effect profile reveals that itraconazole capsules are the preferred formulation.

(continued)

TABLE 1 (*Continued*)

Authors, year	Prospective, retrospective	Number of subjects (N total)	Follow-up period	Treatment evaluated	Treatment outcome
Cross et al, 1998[32]	Prospective	20		Fluconazole capsules (50 mg daily for 14 days)/itraconazole capsules (100 mg a day for 15 days)	Fluconazole and itraconazole were of comparable efficacy in the treatment of DS, on the basis of reduction in palatal erythema and mycological culture. Mycological cure was rare.
Cross et al, 2004[17]	Prospective	22	3 years	(1) capsular form of itraconazole (100 mg 2× a day) versus (2) 100 mg of itraconazole in the form of a mouthwash (10 mL 2× a day), swished and swallowed	A complete and consistent change of yeast species from baseline was observed in six patients after 6 months and at 3 years. The remaining five patients were yeast-free at the follow-up assessments. The recurrence of DS in patients who maintained a high standard of denture cleanliness was low. Although itraconazole was beneficial in reducing the fungal load, there may be strain persistence or subsequent recolonization of the oral cavity by a broader range of potentially less sensitive yeast species.
Czerminski et al, 2010[34]	Retrospective	14		Clotrimazole varnish (sustained release) compared to commercial varnish	Developed sustained (slow) release varnish can be applied in patients at lower frequency. Novel Clotrimazole sustained-release varnish can serve as the basis of a new treatment approach for Candidiasis.
Dar-Odeh and Shehabi, 2003[35]	Prospective	167		Amphoterecin B, Fluconazole	100% of Candida isolates were susceptible to amphotericin B, and only 25 (75%) were susceptible to fluconazole.
de Andrade et al, 2011[36]	Prospective	77	Baseline and 21 days	(1) Effervescent tablets, (2) ultrasound device, (3) effervescent tablets and ultrasound, (4) water on species of *Candida* and *S. mutans*.	Effervescent tablets decreased *S. mutans* count. Candida did not show a difference among the methods examined.
de Andrade et al, 2012[37]	Prospective	60	21 days	(1) Brushing and soak in water overnight, (2) brush with water and 12% chlorhexidine soak nightly, (3) brush with water and 2% chlorhexidine soak nightly at 21 days	Soaking nightly in 12% chlorhexidine and 2% chlorhexidine both had the same effect on biofilm detection at 21 days. The effect was greater than brushing with water and soaking in water alone.
de Resende et al, 2006[38]	Prospective	136		Fluconazole and 5-flucytosine, amphotericin B, and itraconazole	Fluconazole and 5-flucytosine showed increased efficacy over amphotericin B and Itraconazole.

Reference	Study type	N	Timepoints	Intervention	Findings
De Souza et al, 2009[39]	Prospective	11	21 days	(1) Oral and denture hygiene instructions and (2) instructions associated with the home use of a disclosing agent (1% neutral red)	Counts were low for all the tested species, and no significant difference was found between the tested interventions (Wilcoxon test, p values ranged from 0.157 to 1.000). The home use of a disclosing agent does not remarkably change the composition of denture biofilm.
Duyck et al, 2013[40]	Prospective	51	7 and 14 days	(1) H_2O storage, (2) dry storage, (3) H_2O and alkaline peroxide-based cleansing tablet storage	Water + alkaline peroxide-based cleansing tablet storage resulted in lowest bacterial level and lowest C. albicans level.
Egusa et al, 2000[41]	Prospective	12		PAFE (postantifungal effects) and CSH (cell surface hydrophobicity) to amphotericin and nystatin	PAFE nystatin = 5.99 (±0.49H) → decrease in CSH 17.32%, and 83% of isolates. PAFE Amphotericin B = 8.73 (±0.93) → decrease in CSH 14.26% and 66% of isolates.
Frenkel et al, 2001[16]	Prospective	412	Baseline, 1, 6 months	Oral health care education	DS reduced significantly over 6 months compared to the control group ($p < 0.0001$).
Geerts et al, 2008[12]	Prospective	40	14 days	(1) Tissue conditioner, (2) tissue conditioner and 500,000 nystatin	(1) Yeast goes down to day 4 then up higher than pretreatment level. (2) Decreased up to day 7, increased, but lower than pretreatment.
Glass et al, 2011[43]	Prospective	51		Denture cleanser: Polident at room temperature, Polident and microwave	Most effective methods for sanitization of contaminated dentures; Polident cleanser at 65 °C for 5 minutes or soaking the dentures in US or European Polident for 8 hours daily.
Grimoud et al, 2005[44]	Prospective	110	3 months	Oral hygiene protocol implemented and evaluated at 3 months	A reduction was observed in the number of patients showing the highest degree of C. albicans and C. glabrata colonization (>50 CFU) from 41.9% at T1 to 24.9% at T2 ($p < 0.05$), and from 56.4% at T1 to 13.0% at T2 ($p < 0.05$), respectively. The number of patients with candidiasis fell significantly from 43.2% at T1 to 10.2% at T2. The OH protocol led to an overall decrease in Candida spp. colonization, a significant reduction in the number of candidiasis.
Herrera et al, 2010[45]	Prospective	21		Six commercial propolis extracts	Propolis extracts are capable of inhibiting the development of Candida spp.
Jose et al, 2010[47]	Prospective	16		Four types of denture cleansers were evaluated	Denture cleansers tested exhibit effective anti-C. albicans biofilm activity both in terms of removal and disinfection. Residual biofilm retention was observed then can lead to regrowth and denture colonization. Still need mechanical disruptive methods. All cleansers reduced the metabolic activity by more than 80% following overnight immersion.
Kadir et al, 2007[48]	Prospective	55		Chlorhexidine gluconate (brief exposure of 30 min). Two subtherapeutic concentrations: 0.002% to 0.012%	Exposure of isolates to chlorhexidine reduced the phospholipase production significantly. No significant difference in the number of C. albicans isolates (isolates producing phospholipase). Subtherapeutic levels of chlorhexidine gluconate can modulate Candida phospholipase activity, thus suppressing the pathogenecity of C. albicans.

(continued)

TABLE 1 *(Continued)*

Authors, year	Prospective, retrospective	Number of subjects (N total)	Follow-up period	Treatment evaluated	Treatment outcome
Kisnisci et al, 1997[49]	Prospective	21		(1) Systemic antifungal therapy with fluconazole (14 days, 1 tablet of 50 mg a day), (2) topical nystatin mouthwashes (14 days, 4 times a day), (3) control	Systemic and topical antifungal therapies are both effective. Somewhat high success rates were obtained by only cleaning dentures. Topical treatment with nystatin is found more effective than fluconazole. The first choice for treatment would be topical therapy and cleaning of denture. Systematic therapy may be suggested as an alternative.
Koga-Ito et al, 2006[50]	Retrospective	60		Fluconazole, itraconazole, amphotericin B, flucytosine	Resistance to antifungal was not observed in isolates.
Koray M et al, 2005[51]	Prospective	61		Influence of Fluconazole capsules and of Hexitidine mouth rinses	*C. albicans* counts in saliva, lesions, and denture were significantly lower after treatment with all three protocols. No significant difference between results from each group. Group 2, Hexitidine mouthrinse only showed similar results with the least complications.
Lamfon et al, 2005[52]	Prospective	10	72 hours	Antifungals: (1) Miconazole, (2) Fluconazole, (3) Chlorhexidine, (4) Combinations.	Single agent miconazole, fluconazole, or chlorhexidine resulted in no inhibitory effects. The combination therapy did result in inhibition.
Marei et al, 1997[54]	Prospective	18		Denture removal versus relined dentures with TC, versus application of laser irradiation for lesions while continuing to wear dentures	The results revealed that lesions in the group treated with laser irradiation were clinically superior in healing when compared with the other groups. Histologic evidence of the therapeutic effect of lasers in healing denture-induced mucosal lesions was demonstrated. Densitometric evaluation showed an increase in the optical density of alveolar bone underneath the irradiated lesions compared with untreated lesions. These findings suggest the effect of therapeutic laser treatment on both soft tissue and bone with subsequent improvement of denture foundation after treatment of denture-induced mucosal lesions.
Marin Zuluaga et al, 2011[55]	Prospective	44		Tissue conditioner (changed weekly) versus acrylic hard reline material	Tissue conditioner had significantly ($p < 0.001$) greater resolution time, but both treatments were effective.
Martín-Mazuelos et al, 1997[53]	Prospective	335	Initial visit, 14 days, 15 days, and 1 month	(1) Fluconazole administered, then (2) Itraconazole administered to fluconazole-resistant subjects	(1) Clinical 97%, microbial 78% cure after fluconazole. (2) Itraconazole. Clinically cured: 100%. Microbially cured: 77%

Study	Type	N	Treatment	Duration	Results
Maver-Biscanin et al, 2004[56]	Prospective	70	(1) Irradiation 685-nm laser for 10 minutes (30 mW), (2) irradiation with 830-nm laser for 5 minutes (60 mW), (3) placebo (sham irradiation), (4) antimycotic antifungal oral gel	5 days	Had a fungicidal effect: Irradiation 685-nm laser for 10 minutes (30 mW) and irradiation with 830-nm laser for 5 minutes (60 mW). Placebo had no effect.
Mima et al, 2012[57]	Prospective	40	(1) Nystatin (100,000 IU) 4× daily for 15 days (clinical success rate 53%), (2) photodynamic therapy (PDT) 455 nm 3× daily for 15 days (clinical success rate 45%)	0, 15,30, 60, and 90 days	Both treatments reduced CFU/mL at end of treatment ($p < 0.05$). Photodynamic therapy was found to be as effective as topical treatment.
Mohammad et al, 2004[58]	Prospective	30	Dioxident 2× daily for 1 minute and soak overnight ClO_2 for 10 days		ClO_2 significantly improved clinical experience and microbial count ($p < 0.001$) after treatment.
Neppelenbroek et al, 2008[59]	Prospective	60	(1) Control, (2) microwave 650 W, 6 minutes 2× a day for 30 days, (3) microwave 650 W, 6 minutes 2× a day for 30 days+Miconazole 3x a day for 30 days, (4) Miconazole three times a day for 30 days	30 days	Microwave (650 W) and microwave + miconazole were effective. Microwaving dentures dramatically reduced *Candida* recurrence at follow-up.
Pinelli et al, 2013[62]	Prospective	30	*Ricinus communis* versus nystatin and miconazole	30 days (two examinations, one at 15 days and one at 30 days)	For MIC, *R. communis* significant differences showing clinical improvement were observed between the 15th and 30th days. No differences were seen in the nystatin group. *R. communis* is an effective treatment for reducing the clinical signs of DS. *R. communis* effectiveness was similar to that of miconazole and can be considered a viable treatment to conventional treatments in institutionalized elderly.
Pinto et al, 2008[63]	Prospective	140	Fluconazole		All *C. albicans* strains showed sensitivity to fluconazole.
Pinto et al, 2008[64]	Prospective	55	Night time immersion 10% vinegar overnight for 45 days	45 days, then 64 days and after	Significant decrease in *C. albicans* and significant decrease in DS 70.8% to 47.9%.

(continued)

TABLE 1 (*Continued*)

Authors, year	Prospective, retrospective	Number of subjects (N total)	Follow-up period	Treatment evaluated	Treatment outcome
Ribeiro et al, 2012[66]	Prospective	60		PDT procedures (P505, P1005, P50G, and P100G)	No microbial growth after PDT was observed in 60%, 53%, 47%, and 40% of dentures (no colony growth on all culture media after PDT). PDT was effective in disinfecting dentures (four treatments disinfected 90% of microorganisms on the dentures)
Ribeiro et al, 2009[65]	Prospective	30		Two exposure times of microwave irradiation (2 minutes and 3 minutes at 650 W)	Microwave irradiation for 3 minutes resulted in sterilization of dentures. 2-minute significant decrease in *Candida spp*. Microwave irradiation for 3 minutes may be a potential treatment to prevent cross contamination.
Salonen et al, 1996[67]	Prospective	49		(1) Miconazole 2% gel 3× to 4× daily on denture for 4 weeks, (2) Fluconazole 50 mg 1× a day for 2 weeks, (3) control group received new dentures. (Patients instructed not to wear dentures at night during study and for 6 months afterward)	(1) Group treated with miconazole showed healing in 58% of subjects. (2) Group treated with fluconazole showed healing in 77% of subjects. Overall 64% of patients receiving antifungal therapy showed healing. Control group showed positive healing in 20% of subjects. Method of medication (local or systemic) did not contribute significantly to the healing.
Sanita et al, 2012[68]	Prospective	40	90 days	Microwave denture disinfection versus nystatin treatment	40% of treated patients were cured by the end of treatment. There was no statistically significant difference in microbiologic and clinical outcomes between the two groups. Both treatments were considered successful in reducing the clinical signs of DS and significantly reducing the values of CFU's/MI from the palates and dentures.
Santos et al, 2008[69]	Prospective	33	Baseline and 1 week	Propolis versus miconazole gel (Daktarin)	Both Propolis gel and miconazole gave complete clinical remission.
Sefidgar et al, 2010[70]	Prospective	30		Artemisia Sieberi mouthwash (1%) versus nystatin mouthwash	No statistically significant difference in healing time between the 2 groups. Outcomes of treatments between groups were the same. Artemisia mouthwash (1%) could be as effective as nystatin in treatment of DS.
Sholapurkar et al, 2009[71]	Prospective	89	2 weeks	Fluconazole mouth rinse, clotrimazole mouth paste	Mycological eradication, 88.8%. Clotrimazole mouth paste 85.71%.
Silva et al, 2012[72]	Prospective	60		(1) Nystatin oral rinse, (2) Microwave disinfection, 3× daily for 14 days	Both nystatin oral rinse and microwave disinfection reduced clinical signs of DS. Species isolated in subsequent appointments were reduced in frequency from 98% to 53%, *C. glabrata* frequency reduced from 22% to 12% and *C. tropicalis* frequency was reduced from 25% to 7%.
Taillandier et al, 2000[73]	Prospective	305	2 weeks	Fluconazole oral suspension versus Amphotericin B oral suspension	122 (81%) fluconazole-treated and 135 (87%) amphotericin B-treated patients were clinically cured or improved. Mycological cure rates were 35% and 46% for fluconazole and amphotericin B, respectively. The symptoms of burning sensation and buccal pain resolved significantly sooner ($p < 0.05$) in fluconazole-treated patients.

Author, year	Study type	N	Intervention	Duration	Results
Uludamar et al, 2010[74]	Prospective	90	3 brands of alkaline peroxide tablets (Polident, Efferdent, Fittydent) and 2 mouthwashes (CloSYS II and Corsodyl)		No statistically significant difference among Polident, Efferdent, and control group in any treatment period. Fittydent showed a significantly greater decrease in *Candida* after the 60-minute time. CloSYS II and Corsodyl had a significant decrease in the number of CFU compared to control group at all time periods.
Uludamar et al, 2011[75]	Prospective	60	(1) Tissue conditioner only, (2) Dioxident mouthrinse (0.8% chlorine dioxide medication) and denture soak in the solution overnight, (3) Corsodyl mouthrinse (0.2% Chlorhexidine gluconate) and denture soak in the solution	15 days	Group 1: 65% responded to treatment, 40% cured, 25% showed improvement. *C. Albicans* colony count decreased slightly. Group 2: 85% of group responded to treatment, 60% cured, 25% showed improvement. Group 3: 90% responded to treatment, 70% cured, 20% showed improvement. Groups 1 and 2: Statistically significant decrease at end of treatment of *C. albicans* colonies. The treatment of DS with tissue conditioner alone is not sufficient to control *Candida* pathogenicity. The use of a tissue conditioner for the treatment of DS had no effect on eradicating the hyphal form of *C. albicans* identified in smears, and its effect on eradicating yeast cells was insignificant, but it did contribute to decreased palatal inflammation. Mouthrinses of both Dioxident and Corsodyl are more effective in eliminating palatal inflammation, candidal colonization, and hyphae.
Vasconcelos et al, 2003[76]	Prospective	60	*Punica granatum* (pomegranate) gel versus miconazole gel. Treatment prescribed: use gel 3× a day for 15 days		*P. granatum* showed a similar response rate to Miconazole, and *Candida* colonization was reduced as well. A similar performance compared to miconazole gel was observed for the negativity of *Candida*. The clinical and laboratory results show improvement with the use of *P. granatum*. No side effects were noted.
Vigild et al, 1998[77]	Prospective	264	Professional dental care and education	1 year	There was a significant decrease in the presence of DS. An improvement in denture hygiene was also observed.
Webb et al, 2005[78]	Prospective	60	(1) Sodium hypochlorite soak, (2) microwaving, (3) control	1 week	Results: Both hypochlorite and microwave irradiation significantly reduced the numbers of *Candida* and aerobic bacteria on both dentures, and both methods significantly reduced *Candida* on the palate; however, palatal aerobic bacteria were not significantly reduced by either method, and the controls showed insignificant changes at all three sites for both *Candida* and aerobes.
Zuluaga et al, 2011[79]	Prospective	44	Tissue conditioner (TC) replaced weekly versus acrylic hard reline material (AHRM)	4 weeks	Both TC and AHRM were effective in the management of DS. Significant differences were found in the DS resolution time ($p < 0.001$), taking longer for the TC. As such, AHRM required fewer appointments for the patient.

TABLE 2   Included studies evaluating the treatment of complete denture stomatitis in immunocompromised patients

Authors, year	Prospective or retrospective	Number of subjects (N total)	Follow-up period	Treatment evaluated	Treatment outcome
Blignaut et al, 2002[26]	Prospective	589		(1) Amphotericin B, (2) Nystatin, (3) 5-fluorocystosine, (4) Clotrimazole, (5) Miconazole, (6) Ketoconazole, (7) Itraconazole, (8) Fluconazole	100% susceptibility to fluconazole was observed. *Candida krusei* (the second most common isolate) only 2.6% of isolates were susceptible to fluconazole and itraconazole. Very little difference was observed between the antifungal profile of South African isolates compared to isolates from the United States, *Candida* and South America.
Finlay et al, 1996[42]	Prospective	73	20 weeks posttreatment	Amphotericin B, Fluconazole	Improvement seen in 72% of Amphotericin B patients and 92% of patients receiving fluconazole. Mycological cure at end of treatment: 31% amphotericin B and 46% fluconazole. Fluconazole is safe and well-tolerated antifungal agent. Antifungal prophylaxis useful for patients undergoing radiotherapy.
Hilton et al, 2004[46]	Prospective	35	6 months	Instructions by dentist on improving oral hygiene; minimize sugar intake, self-diagnosis of candidiasis	Candidiasis recurrence at 6 months: 78% among intervention and 88% among controls.
Nittayananta et al, 2008[60]	Prospective	75		Clotrimazole troche was prescribed until lesions eradicated; then, two groups: txt with 0.12% chlorhexidine or 0.9% normal saline	The time to recurrence of oral candidiasis between the chlorhexidine and the saline group was not statistically significant.
Nittayananta et al, 2013[61]	Prospective	38	2 weeks	Lawsone methyl ether mouthwash versus chlorhexidine mouthwash	Use of lawsone methyl ether mouthwash for 2 weeks neither led to antifungal drug resistance nor significant changes in genotype of oral *Candida*. Thus, lawsone methyl ether may be an alternative mouthwash in prophylaxis of oral candidiasis among those at risk for developing the disease.

Edentulism is a chronic condition influencing the individual for a lifetime. Yet, DS and its treatment were considered in terms of acute interventions by most of the included studies. This systematic review revealed few studies that evaluated therapy longer than 90 days. In a 6-month evaluation, the authors concluded that the use of denture cleansers reduced the number of microorganisms and diminished stomatitis.[14] In a 3-year follow-up study involving a small number of patients, Cross et al[17] stated that the recurrence of DS in patients who maintained a high standard of denture cleanliness was low. It is unknown if recurrent or repetitive infection and inflammation is prevalent among denture wearers.

Most studies included in this review represent small cohort studies or small prospective comparative trials. In an alternative epidemiological approach, Budtz-Jorgensen et al[4] evaluated the effectiveness of an oral health program on the prevalence of high risk, frail, or dependent adults. Of the 237 residents, 147 wore dentures. There were no significant differences in the numbers of mucosal yeast cultures for experimental and control groups or between individuals with slight, moderate, or severe stomatitis at baseline; however, 18 months following the institution of an oral health program, there was a highly significant reduction in the number of yeast colonies and a trend to reduced DS among the affected population (24% reduction in prevalence of moderate or

TABLE 3 **Treatment evaluated by strategies (healthy patients)**

Treatment categories	Number of papers in this category	Number of papers with a positive outcome (*decrease in denture stomatitis*)	Number of papers with a negative outcome (*increase in denture stomatitis*)	Number of papers showing no difference in outcome	Paper (listed by reference number)
Antifungal (pharmacotherapy): includes both local and systemic	36	34	0	2	1, 2, 4*. 5, 10**, 13, 14, 15*, 16, 17, 18, 20, 23, 26, 28*, 31,33, 34, 35, 36, 37+, 40, 41*, 42, 45, 46, 50, 51*, 52, 53**, 54, 55*, 56, 57*, 58*, 59
Disinfectant/cleansers	16	13	0	3	3, 6, 7*, 8, 9, 19, 21, 22, 25, 29*, 32, 43, 47, 57*, 58*, 61*
Hard reline	2	2	0	0	39*, 62*
Oral hygiene program	5	4	0	1	12, 24, 27, 30, 60
Laser treatment	3	3	0	0	38*, 41*, 48
Microwave disinfection	5	5	0	0	7*, 29*, 44, 49, 51*, 55*, 61*
New complete denture	1	1	0	0	4*
Resilient liners and/or tissue conditioners	7	4	1	2	11, 15*, 28*, 38*, 39*, 58*, 62*

*Paper combined treatment strategies (paper included in each treatment strategy group);
**no difference between tested interventions; +Single-agent antifungal showed no effect. Combination therapy showed positive effect

severe stomatitis). This study underscores the importance of managing oral hygiene for the edentulous patient.

In a single-blind randomized study that invoked an oral education program in nursing homes, Frenkel et al[16] enrolled 412 individuals of whom 294 wore complete dentures. Oral hygiene education was associated with a significant reduction ($p < 0.001$) in denture plaque scores at all visits during the 6-month investigation. Specifically regarding denture-induced stomatitis, significant reductions were observed at 6 months for Newton class II and III individuals who received oral

TABLE 4 **Treatment evaluated by strategies (immunocompromised patients)**

Treatment categories	Number of papers in this category	Number of papers with a positive outcome (*decreased denture stomatitis*)	Number of papers with a negative outcome (*increased denture stomatitis*)	Number of papers showing no difference in outcome	Paper (listed by reference number)
Antifungal (pharmacotherapy): includes both local and systemic	4	2	0	2	63, 64, 66, 67
Disinfectant/cleansers	0	0	0	0	n/a
Hard reline	0				
Oral hygiene program	1	1	0	0	65
Laser treatment	0	0	0	0	n/a
Microwave disinfection	0	0	0	0	n/a
New complete denture	0	0	0	0	n/a
Resilient denture liners and/or tissue conditioners	0	0	0	0	n/a

hygiene education. The authors concluded that the simple education program resulted in sustained improvement in denture hygiene and denture-induced stomatitis.

There is variability in the management of patients within studies. For example, Cross et al,[17] who evaluated the impact of itraconazole on *Candida* species counts, indicated that patients who removed their dentures for sleeping increased from base- line (25%) to 70% at the 6-month follow up. Managing this and other variables (denture quality, denture hygiene, etc.) may be needed in further investigation. Among the management strategies represented by the included publications, many involved antifungal agents applied to the tissues locally or systemically. In a recent investigation by Altarwaneh et al,[7] measurement of denture, mucosal, and salivary fungal counts revealed that the denture may be the prevalent site of infection and that saliva may be a reservoir of biofilm-derived pathogens. The importance of treating the denture of the affected patient should be emphasized.

The treatment of DS in healthy versus immuno-compromised individuals suggested an approach to intervention that favored pharmacological treatment of the patient rather than other methods that targeted the prosthesis. While studies of healthy edentulous individuals suggest that targeted treatment of the prosthesis by direct mechanical or indirect hygiene measures is effective, the importance of managing immunocompromised individuals using a prosthesis-targeted approach with or without pharmacological antifungal agents requires investigation. The observations made regarding immunocompromised individuals with DS indicate that the host response to infection is a key feature of DS. The individual susceptibility to biofilm-mediated stomatitis remains largely unexplored among otherwise healthy individuals.

CONCLUSION

This review revealed many strategies for treatment of denture stomatitis patients. The investigated treatments did reduce DS. The scope of treatment is broad and included strategies that targeted biofilm formation on the prosthesis as well as targeted approaches focused on treatment of a fungal infection of tissues. Clinical strategies commonly involved multiple approaches with a combined goal of eliminating pathogenic microorganisms and preventing reestablishment of a pathogenic biofilm through preventive hygiene measures. The common limitation of these studies was the duration of study. The period of time necessary to develop a DS-evoking pathogenic biofilm remains to be determined.

REFERENCES

1. Gendreau L, Loewy ZG: Epidemiology and etiology of denture stomatitis. *J Prosthodont* 2011;20:251–260.

2. Girard B Jr, Landry RG, Giasson L: Denture stomatitis: etiology and clinical considerations. *J Can Dent Assoc* 1996;62:808–812.

3. Allison RT, Douglas WH: Micro-colonization of the denture-fitting surface by *Candida albicans. J Dent* 1973;1:198–201.

4. Budtz-Jorgensen E, Stenderup A, Grabowski M: An epidemiologic study of yeasts in elderly denture wearers. *Community Dent Oral Epidemiol* 1975;3:115–119.

5. Thein, Z, Samaranayake Y, Samaranayake, L: Characteristics of dual species *Candida* biofilms on denture acrylic surfaces. *Arch Oral Biol* 2007;52:1200–1208.

6. Martori E, Ayuso-Montero R, Martinez-Gomis J, et al: Risk factors for denture-related oral mucosal lesions in a geriatric population. *J Prosthet Dent* 2014;111:273–279.

7. Altarawneh S, Bencharit S, Mendoza L, et al: Clinical and histological findings of denture stomatitis as related to intraoral colonization patterns of Candida albicans, salivary flow, and dry mouth. *J Prosthodont* 2013;22:13–22.

8. Martori E, Ayuso-Montero R, Martinez-Gomis J, et al: Risk factors for denture-related oral mucosal lesions in a geriatric population. *J Prosthet Dent* 2014;111:273–279.

9. Newton AV: Denture sore mouth. A possible etiology. *Br Dent J* 1962;112:357–360.

10. Shepherd MG: The pathogenesis and host defence mechanisms of oral candidosis. *NZ Dent J* 1986;82:78–81.

11. Greenspan D, Greenspan JS: Management of the oral lesions of HIV infection. *J Am Dent Assoc* 1991;122:26–32.

12. Geerts, GAVM, Stuhlinger ME, Basson NJ: Effect of an antifungal denture liner on the saliva yeast count in patients with denture stomatitis: a pilot study. *J Oral Rehabil* 2008;35:664–669.

13. Emami E, Kabawat M, Rompre PH, et al: Linking evidence to treatment for denture stomatitis: a meta-analysis of randomized controlled trials. *J Dent* 2014;42:99–106.

14. Beyari M: Tissue inflammatory response and salivary *Streptococcus mutans* count with three different denture cleansers. *Afr J Microbiol Res* 2011;5:965–974.

15. Budtz-Jørgensen E, Mojon P, Rentsch A, et al: Effects of an oral health program on the occurrence of oral candidosis in a long-term care facility. *Commun Dent Oral Epidemiol* 2000;28:141–149.

16. Frenkel H, Harvey I, Newcombe RG: Improving oral health in institutionalized elderly people by educating caregivers: a randomized controlled trial. *Community Dent Oral Epidemiol* 2001;29:289–297.

17. Cross L, Williams D, Sweeney C, et al: Evaluation of the recurrence of denture stomatitis and Candida colonization in a small group of patients who received itraconazole. *Oral Surg Oral Med Oral Pathol* 2004;97:351–358.

18. Abaci O, Haliki-Uztan A: Investigation of the susceptibility of *Candida* species isolated from denture wearers to different antifungal antibiotics. *Afr J Microbiol Res* 2011;5:1398–1403.

19. Amanlou M, Beitollahi JM, Abdollahzadeh S, et al: Miconazole Gel compared with *Zataria multifora* Boiss. gel in the treatment of denture stomatitis. *Phytother Res* 2006;20:966–969.

20. Andrucioli MC, de Macedo LD, Panzeri H, et al: Comparison of two cleansing pastes for the removal of biofilm from dentures and palatal lesions in patients with atrophic chronic candidiasis. *Braz Dent J* 2004;15:220–224.

21. Arikan A, Kulak Y, Kadir T: Comparison of different treatment methods for localized and generalized simple denture stomatitis. *J Oral Rehabil* 1995;22:365–369.

22. Bakhshi M, Taheri JB, Shabestaii SB, et al: Comparison of therapeutic effect of aqueous extract of garlic and nystatin mouthwash in denture stomatitis. *Gerodontology* 2012;29:e680–e684.

23. Banting DW, Greenhorn PA, McMinn JG: Effectiveness of a topical antifungal regimen for the treatment of oral Candidiasis in older, chronically ill, institutionalized, adults. *J Can Dent Assoc* 1995:61:199–200.

24. Banting DW, Hill SA: Microwave disinfection of dentures for the treatment of oral candidiasis. *Spec Care Dent* 2001;21:4–8.

25. Barnabe W, Neto TD, Pimenta FC, et al: Efficacy of sodium hypochlorite and coconut soap used as disinfecting agents in the reduction of denture stomatitis, *Streptococcus mutans* and *Candida albicans*. *J Oral Rehabil* 2004;31:453–459.

26. Blignaut E, Messer S, Hollis RJ, et al: Antifungal susceptibility of South African oral yeast isolates from HIV/AIDS patients and healthy individuals. *Diagn Microbiol Infect Dis* 2002;44:169–174.

27. Blomgren J, Berggren U, Jontell M: Fluconazole versus nystatin in the treatment of oral candidosis. *Acta Odontol Scand* 1998;56:202–205.

28. Brosky ME, Pesun I, Morrison B, et al: Clinical evaluation of resilient denture liners. Part 2: *Candida* count and speciation. *J Prosthodont* 2003;12:162–167.

29. Campelo RS, Queiroz, MV, Lima EO, et al: C. Identification of Candida species in palatal mucosa and denture surface and antifungal therapy Cymbopogom citratus [abstract]. *J Dent Res* 2002;81:B135.

30. Capistrano H, de Assis EM, Leal R, et al. Brazilian green propolis compared to miconazole gel in the treatment of *Candida*-associated denture stomatitis. *Evid Based Complement Alternat Med* 2013;2013:947980. doi: 10.1155/2013/947980. Epub 2013 May 2

31. Catalan A, Pacheco JG, Martinez A, et al: In vitro and in vivo activity of melaleuca alternifolia mixed with tissue conditioner on *Candida albicans*. *Surg Oral Med Oral Pathol Oral Radiol Endod* 2008;105:327–332.

32. Cross LJ, Bagg J, Wray D, et al: A comparison of fluconazole and itraconazole in the management of denture stomatitis: a pilot study. *J Dent* 1998;26:657–664.

33. Cross LJ, Bagg J, Wray D, et al: Efficacy of the cyclodextrin liquid preparation of itraconazole in treatment of denture stomatitis: comparison with itraconazole capsules. *Antimicrob Agents Chemother* 2000;44:425–427.

34. Czerninski R, Sivan S, Steinberg D, et al: A novel sustained-release clotrimazole varnish for local treatment of oral candidiasis. *Clin Oral Investig* 2010;14:71–78.

35. Dar-Odeh NS, Shehabi AA: Oral Candidosis in patients with removable dentures. *Mycoses* 2003;46:187–191.

36. de Andrade IM, Cruz P, da Silva CH, et al: Effervescent tablets and ultrasonic devices against *Candida* and mutans streptococci in denture biofilm. *Gerodontology* 2011;28:264–270.

37. de Andrade IM, Cruz P, da Silva CH, et al: Effect of chlorhexidine on denture biofilm accumulation. *J Prosthodont* 2012;21:2–6.

38. de Resende MA, de Sousa L, Oliveira R, et al: Prevalence and antifungal susceptibility of yeasts obtained from the oral cavity of elderly individuals. *Mycopathologia* 2006;162:39–44.

39. de Souza RF, Nascimenta C, Regis RR, et al: Effects of the domestic use of a disclosing solution on the denture biofilm: a preliminary study. *J Oral Rehabil* 2009;36:491–497.

40. Duyck J, Vandamme K, Muller P, et al: Overnight storage of removable dentures in alkaline peroxide-based tablets affects biofilm mass and composition. *J Dent* 2013;41:1281–1289.

41. Egusa H, Ellepola ANB, Nikawa H, et al: Sub-therapeutic exposure to polyene antimycotics elicits a post-antifungal effect (PAFE) and depresses the cell surface hydrophobicity of oral *Candida albicans* isolates. *J Oral Pathol Med* 2000;29:206–213.

42. Finlay PM, Richardson MD, Robertson AG: A comparative study of the efficacy of fluconazole and amphotericin B in the treatment of oropharyngeal candidosis in patients undergoing radiotherapy for head and neck tumors. *Br J Oral Maxillofac Surg* 1996;34:23–25.

43. Glass RT, Conrad R, Bullard J, et al: Evaluation of cleansing methods for previously worn prostheses. *Compendium* 2011;32:68–73.

44. Grimoud AM, Lodter JP, Marty N, et al: Improved oral hygiene and *Candida* species colonization level in geriatric patients. *Oral Dis* 2005;11:163–169.

45. Herrera C, Alvear M, Barrientos L, et al: The antifungal effect of six commercial extracts of Chilean propolis on *Candida* spp. *Cien Inv Agr* 2010;37:75–84.

46. Hilton JF, MacPhail LA, Pascasio L, et al: Self-care intervention to reduce oral candidiasis recurrences in HIV-seropositive persons: a pilot study. *Commun Dent Oral Epidemiol* 2004;32:190–200.

47. Jose A, Coco B, Milligan S: Reducing the incidence of denture stomatitis: are denture cleansers sufficient? *J Prosthodont* 2010;19:252–257.

48. Kadir T, Gumru B, Uygun-Can B: phospholipase activity of *Candida albicans* isolates from patients with denture stomatitis: the influence of chlorhexidine gluconate on phospholipase production. *Arch Oral Biol* 2007;52:691–696.

49. Kisnisci R, Akal U, Ozden N: Comparison of treatment modalities in chronic atrophic candidosis: a clinical and microbiologic study. *Turk J Med Sci* 1997;27:337–340.

50. Koga-Ito CY, Lyon JP, Vidotto V, et al: Virulence factors and antifungal susceptibility of *Candida albicans* isolates from oral candidosis patients and control individuals. *Mycopathologia* 2006;161:219–223.

51. Koray M, Ak G, Kurklu E: Fluconazole and/or hexetidine for management of oral candidiasis associated with denture-induced stomatitis. *Oral Dis* 2005;11:309–313.

52. Lamfon H, Al-Karaawi Z, McCullough M, et al: Composition of in vitro denture plaque biofilms and susceptibility to antifungals. *FEMS Microbiol Lett* 2005;242:345–351.

53. Martin-Mazuelos E, Aller AI, Romero MJ, et al: Response to fluconazole and itraconazole of *Candida* spp. in denture stomatitis. *Mycoses* 1997;40:283–289.

54. Marei MK, Abdel-Meguid SH, Mokhtar S, et al: Effect of low-energy laser application in the treatment of denture-induced mucosal lesions. *J Prosthet Dent* 1997;77:256–264.

55. Marin Zuluaga D, Gomez Velandia OC, Ruedo Clauijo DM: Denture-related stomatitis managed with tissue conditioner and hard autopolymerising reline material. *Gerodontology* 2011;28:258–263.

56. Maver-Biscanin M, Mravak-Stipetic M, Jerolimov V, et al: Fungicidal effect of diode laser irradiation in patients with denture stomatitis. *Lasers Surg Med* 2004;35:259–262.

57. Mima EG, Vergani CE, Machado AL, et al: Comparison of photodynamic therapy versus conventional antifungal therapy for the treatment of denture stomatitis: a randomized clinical trial. *Clin Microbiol Infect* 2012;18:E380–E388.

58. Mohammad AR, Giannini PJ, Preshaw P, et al: Clinical and microbiological efficacy of chlorine dioxide in the management of chronic atrophic candidiasis: an open study. *Int Dent J* 2004;54:154–158.

59. Neppelenbroek KH, Pavarina AC, Palomari DM, et al: Effectiveness of microwave disinfection of complete dentures on the treatment of *Candida*-related denture stomatitis. *J Oral Rehabil* 2008;35:836–846.

60. Nittayananta W, DeRouen TA, Arirachakaran P: A randomized clinical trial of chlorhexidine in the maintenance of oral candidiasis-free period in HIV infection. *Oral Dis* 2008;14:665–670.

61. Nittayananta W, Pangsomboon K, Panichayupakaranant P, et al: Effects of lawsone methyl ether mouthwash on oral *Candida* in HIV-infected subjects and subjects in denture stomatitis. *J Oral Path Med* 2013;42:698–704.

62. Pinelli LA, Montandon AB, Corbi SC, et al: *Ricinus communis* treatment of denture stomatitis in institutionalized elderly. *J Oral Rehabil* 2013;40:375–380.

63. Pinto E, Ribeiro IC, Ferreira NJ, et al: Correlation between enzyme production, germ tube formation and susceptibility to fluconazole in *Candida* species isolated from patients with denture-related stomatitis and control individuals. *J Oral Pathol Med* 2008;37:587–592.

64. Pinto T, Neves A, Pereira M, et al: Vinegar as an antimicrobial agent for control of *Candida* spp in complete denture wearers. *J Appl Oral Sci* 2008;16:385–390.

65. Ribeiro DG, Pavarina AC, Dovigo LN, et al: Denture disinfection by microwave irradiation: a randomized clinical study. *J Dent* 2009;37:666–672.

66. Ribeiro DG, Pavarina AC, Dovigo LV, et al: Photodynamic inactivation of microorganisms present on complete dentures. A clinical investigation. *Lasers Med Sci* 2012;27:161–168.

67. Salonen MA, Raustia AM, Oikarinen KS: Effect of treatment of palatal inflammatory papillary hyperplasia with local and systemic antifungal agents accompanied by renewal of complete dentures. *Acta Odontol Scand* 1996;54:87–91.

68. Sanita PV, Machado A, Pavarina AC, et al: Microwave denture disinfection versus nystatin in treating patients with well-controlled type 2 diabetes and denture stomatitis: a randomized clinical trial. *Int J Prosthodont* 2012;25:232–244.

69. Santos VR, Gomes RT, de Mesquita RA, et al: Efficacy of Brazilian Propolis gel for the management of denture stomatitis: a pilot study. *Phytother Res* 2008;22:1544–1547.

70. Sefidgar SA, Moghadamnia A, Tafti A, et al: Evaluation of the effect of Artemisia Sieberi mouthwash 1% on denture stomatitis (A preliminary study). *Casp J Intern Med* 2010;1:47–49.

71. Sholapurkar AA, Pai KM, Rao S: Comparison of efficacy of fluconazole mouthrinse and clotrimazole mouthpaint in the treatment of oral candidiasis. *Aust Dent J* 2009;54:341–346.

72. Silva M, Mima E, Colombo A, et al: Comparison of denture microwave disinfection and conventional antifungal therapy in the treatment of denture stomatitis: a randomized clinical study. *Oral Surg Oral Med Oral Pathol Oral Radiol* 2012;114:469–479.

73. Taillandier J, Esnault Y, Alemanni M, et al: A comparison of fluconazole oral suspension and amphotericin B oral suspension in older patients with oropharyngeal candidosis. *Age Ageing* 2000;29:117–123.

74. Uludamar A, Ozkan Y, Kadir T, et al: *In vivo* efficacy of alkaline peroxide tablets and mouthwashes on *Candida albicans* in patients with denture stomatitis. *J Appl Oral Sci* 2010: 18:291–296.

75. Uludamar A, Ozyesil AG, Oskan Y: Clinical and microbiological efficacy of three different treatment methods in the management of denture stomatitis. *Gerodontology* 2011;28:104–110.

76. Vasoncelos A, Sampaio M, Sampaio F, et al: Use of *Punica granatum* as an antifungal agent against candidosis associated with denture stomatitis. *Mycoses* 2003;46:192–196.

77. Vigild M, Brinck J, Hede B: A one-year follow-up of an oral health care programme for residents with severe behavioral disorders at special nursing homes in Denmark. *Comm Dent Health* 1998;15:88–92.

78. Webb B, Thomas C, Whittle T: A 2-year study of *Candida*-associated denture stomatitis treatment in aged care subjects. *Gerodontology* 2005;22:168–176.

79. Zuluaga, D, Velandia O, Claujo R: Denture-related stomatis managed with tissue conditioner and hard autopolymerising reline material. *Gerodontology* 2011;28:258–263.

PART III

TREATMENT INNOVATIONS

15

FABRICATING COMPLETE DENTURES WITH CAD/CAM AND RP TECHNOLOGIES

Mehmet Selim Bilgin, dds, phd,[1] Ali Erdem, dds, phd,[1] Osman Sami Aglarci, dds, phd,[2] and Erhan Dilber, dds, phd[1]

[1]Department of Prosthodontics, Faculty of Dentistry, Sifa University, Izmir, Turkey
[2]Department of Oral and Maxillofacial Radiology, Faculty of Dentistry, Sifa University, Izmir, Turkey

Keywords
Rapid prototyping; 3D printing; complete denture; digital; CAD/CAM; tooth alignment

Correspondence
Mehmet Selim Bilgin, Sifa University, Faculty of Dentistry, Department of Prosthodontics Mansuroglu Mah. 293/1 No:14, 35100, Bayrakli, Izmir, Turkey.
E-mail: mselimbilgin@gmail.com

Conflict of interest: None declared

Accepted January 4, 2015

Published in *Journal of Prosthodontics* 2015; Vol. 24, pp. 576–79

doi: 10.1111/jopr.12302

ABSTRACT

Two techological approaches for fabricating dentures; computer-aided design and computer-aided manufacturing (CAD/CAM) and rapid prototyping (RP), are combined with the conventional techniques of impression and jaw relation recording to determine their feasibility and applicability. Maxillary and mandibular edentulous jaw models were produced using silicone molds. After obtaining a gypsum working model, acrylic bases were crafted, and occlusal rims for each model were fabricated with previously determined standard vertical and centric relationships. The maxillary and mandibular relationships were recorded with guides. The occlusal rims were then scanned with a digital scanner. The alignment of the maxillary and mandibular teeth was verified. The teeth in each arch were fabricated in one piece, or set, either by CAM or RP. Conventional waxing and flasking was then performed for both methods. These techniques obviate a practitioner's need for technicians during design and provide the patient with an opportunity to participate in esthetic design with the dentist. In addition, CAD/CAM and RP reduce chair time; however, the materials and techniques need further improvements. Both CAD/CAM and RP techniques seem promising for reducing chair time and allowing the patient to participate in esthetics design. Furthermore, the one-set aligned artificial tooth design may increase the acrylic's durability.

Seventy-seven years ago, a new age for complete dentures was ushered in with the clinical evaluation of methyl methacrylate (MMA). Within a decade, MMA was the preferred material for 95% of the dentures manufactured because it fulfilled the requirements for an ideal base material.[1] Furthermore, MMA is used as a major component in artificial tooth sets, which consist of several materials such as poly (methyl methacrylate) (PMMA) and various ceramics and composites. Since 1940, acrylic teeth have been used in the fabrication of complete dentures. Acrylic teeth are preferred for their price and esthetics and because they chemically bond to an acrylic denture base.[2] In contrast, ceramics do not bond chemically to acrylic; however, they are resistant to surface wear, and porcelain teeth are believed to transmit forces to bone directly.[3]

For these reasons, manufacturers were motivated to develop alternative denture materials by factoring in esthetics, bonding, biocompatibility, and stress distribution.[4] With the development of new technologies, patients are required to spend less time in clinics and make fewer visits. Consequently, even chairside and other laboratory personnel work fewer hours.[5,6]

Computer-aided design (CAD) and computer-aided manufacturing (CAM) technologies have been used for single-visit restorative treatments. Previous studies have shown how accurate results can be obtained through digital impression techniques.[7,8] According to the findings of more recent studies, mistakes that previously occurred during the clinical and laboratory phases can now be prevented, owing to the extreme accuracy afforded by digital impression devices,[9,10] and the repetitions required for conventional impression techniques can now be avoided. Furthermore, obtaining direct digital impressions from edentulous patients is a topic of much discussion because of the displaceability of soft tissues.[11] An advantage of virtual design is that any shape can be digitally prototyped. Rapid prototyping (RP) is an innovative technique currently employed in dentistry. With the appropriate design software and hardware, it is possible to arrange the dentition, occlusion, shape, angulations, and even the flange itself with different colors.[12] Therefore, in the near future, complete dentures are expected to be commercially produced by medical informatics institutions rather than laboratory technicians.

EXPERIMENTAL TECHNIQUE

In our experimental laboratory procedure, a combination of conventional techniques with two approaches, CAD/CAM and RP, was used to fabricate complete dentures. Maxillary and mandibular edentulous jaw models were made using silicone molds (B-3 NHG; Frasaco GmbH, Tettnang, Germany). After fabricating a gypsum (Sherapremium; Shera Werkstoff Technologie GmbH, Lemförde, Germany)

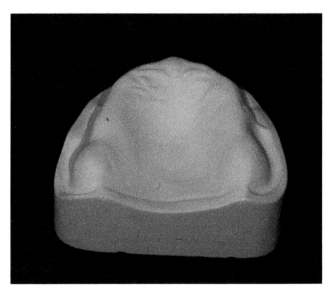

FIGURE 1   Maxillary working model.

working model (Fig 1), acrylic (Sherapress, Shera Werkstoff Technologie GmbH) bases were crafted, and wax rims (Fig 2) for each model were fabricated. A bite registration block with edentulous maxillary and mandibular models was used for mounting the working models on the articulator to provide standardized vertical and centric relationships. With the guidance of the plaster model's anatomic landmark (labial frenulum, corners of the arch), midline and canine zones were marked on the occlusal and labial surfaces of the wax rims. The smiling zone was adjusted according to the height of the bite registration blocks of the

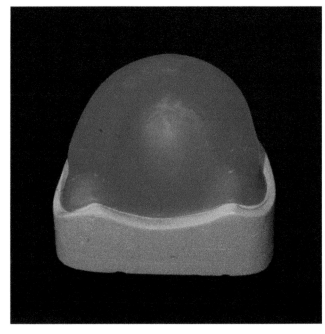

FIGURE 2   Maxillary working model with acrylic base and wax rim.

upper rim. A one-set aligned artificial tooth (1SA) system was designed and manufactured as one piece for the maxillary and mandibular arch using CAD/CAM and RP, respectively.

CAD/CAM

The occlusal rims were scanned with a digital scanner (D810; 3Shape, Copenhagen, Denmark) to obtain 3D images of the rims and base (Fig 3) together with the guides as the midline, maxillary canine locations, and smiling zone. The scanned images of the rims are important for the curve of the arches as well as the height and width of the artificial teeth. In addition to these guides, the locations of the rims in the artificial design are required to ensure that the rims are a support for soft tissues such as lips and cheeks. According to the fabricated guides and occlusal rim shape, the design of the 1SA of the maxillary and mandibular arches (Fig 4) and occlusion was digitally completed using a computer (Precision T5400 workstation; Dell, Round Rock, TX) using dwos software (Dental Wings Inc., Montreal, Canada). The monochromatic PMMA block (Tempo Cad; On-Dent Ltd, Izmir, Turkey) used for the temporary fixed restoration was milled (Fig 5). The 1SA artificial teeth were embedded in wax rims, and waxing and flasking procedures were fabricated using the conventional methods with metal flasks to obtain the definitive prosthesis (Figs 6, 7).

RAPID PROTOTYPE (RP)

The 1SA digital design was sent to EnvisionTEC Laboratories for manufacturing with an RP machine (P4 DDP Mini;

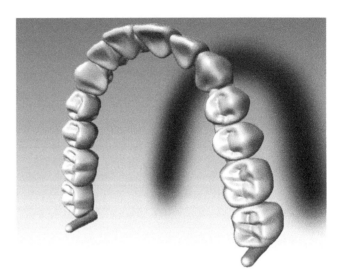

FIGURE 4   Designed maxillary teeth.

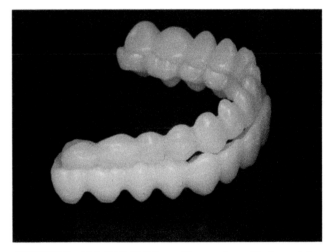

FIGURE 5   1SA CAD/CAM maxillary and mandibularmodels.

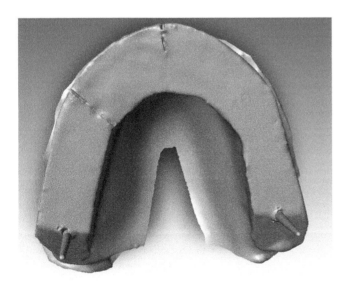

FIGURE 3   Digitally scannedmaxillary wax rim and acrylic base.

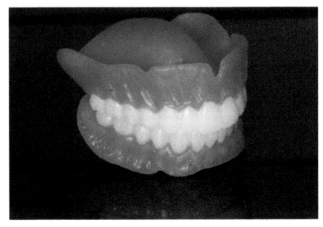

FIGURE 6   1SA CAD/CAM with wax modelling.

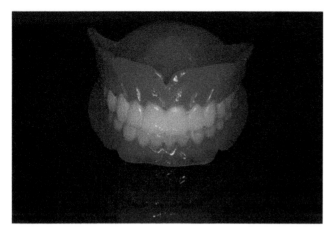

FIGURE 7   Definitive prostehesis with 1SA CAD/CAM.

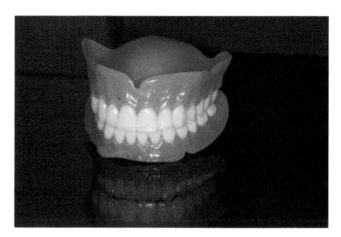

FIGURE 10   Definitive prosthesis with 1SA RP.

EnvisionTEC GmbH, Gladbeck, Germany) using an A2 shade light-cured, micro-hybrid, nano-filled resin (E-Dent 100; EnvisionTEC GmbH). Then the resins were photo-polymerized on a voxel-by-voxel basis (volumetric pixel) of the liquid resin. It took 76 minutes to build the design with a 50-^m-thick layer. The light power was 180 mW/dm^2, and

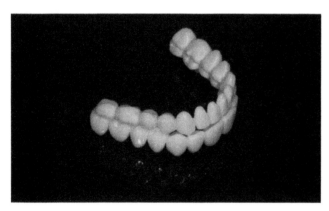

FIGURE 8   1SA RP maxillary and mandibularmodels.

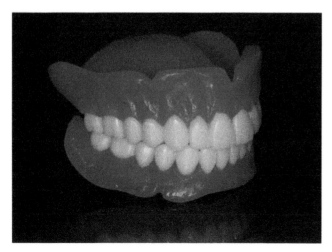

FIGURE 9   1SA RP with wax modeling.

the number of flashes was 6×1000. After achieving the maxillary and mandibular1SA design (Fig 8), wax (Cavex Set Up Wax, Cavex, Haarlem, The Netherlands) modeling was performed. Flasking procedures were fabricated according to the conventional methods with metal flasks, and the definitive prosthesis was obtained similar to the CAD/CAM technique (Figs 9, 10).

DISCUSSION

Since 3D scanners were introduced to dentistry, the accuracy of the obtained images has been a subject of much discussion and research. Several studies have been conducted to measure the accuracy of these devices, and the measurement of working models with calipers is assumed to be the standard. These measurements have been compared with digital measurements.[7–10,13]

Inokoshi et al[12] fabricated trial dentures with RP. According to the results of a deviation analysis, RP offers high processing accuracy compared to conventional wax dentures. The mucosa has a displaceability of approximately 0.14 to 0.34 mm. Compensation for these deviations can be performed clinically. A trial insertion appointment can still be included to advance the quality of denture fabrication with RP. Even though the devices and techniques are promising, it is necessary to acquire impressions in the same manner as in the conventional method, that is, taken in impression compound with custom trays.

In the near future, cone-beam computed tomography (CBCT) or magnetic resonance imaging (MRI) could be used instead of taking impressions or scanning for complete dentures with some apparatus; however, the depth of the sulcus and the displaceability of removable soft tissues are problems that remain unsolved. Infante et al[6] studied a maxillary and mandibular anatomic measuring device (Avadent) used for recording the vertical and centric relationships of the upper and lower jaws, and they found it challenging to record the jaw relationships because the system does not provide all occlusion schemes.

RP and CAD/CAM systems will reduce chair time for patients. Although some systems build the entire structure, failures will require remanufacturing of the prosthesis at a high cost. In our study, 1SA has the advantage of avoiding occlusal vertical relationship and centric relation errors due to the technician's potential manipulation errors while transferring models to the articulator and arranging teeth manually. Therefore the design and manipulation phases are extracted from the technician's process in the RP and the CAD/CAM methods. In addition, it is possible to consider the personal choices of patients, and dentists can directly relate their knowledge of occlusion and esthetics to the design without the assistance of a laboratory technician.[12] As is widely known, the three essential variables in the selection of complete dentures are composition, color, and shape. The denture tooth selection process may be eliminated chairside and provided by the 1SA system digitally.

It is also possible that 1SA may provide extra strength to the denture due to the one-piece construction when compared to individually placed denture teeth. A limitation for complete dentures fabricated with RP is the manufacturing expense, which is still high for clinics. The high price is consequently passed on to the patients. Furthermore, the safety of these RP acrylic materials is still being tested, and these materials are being assessed for long-term use.

CONCLUSION

The proposed and tested CAD/CAM and RP techniques obviate a practitioner's need for technicians during design and provide the patient with an opportunity to participate in esthetic de sign with the dentist. In addition, CAD/CAM and RP reduce chair time. Although further improvements in techniques and materials are needed regarding the production, toxicity, and machinery, the final product demonstrates that denture fabrication can be accomplished with self-designed esthetics, occlusion, and potentially increased durability using 1SA, especially with single complete dentures opposing natural dentition when the dentures are fabricated using RP or CAD/CAM.

REFERENCES

1. Murray MD, Darvell BW: The evolution of the complete denture base. Theories of complete denture retention-a review. Part 1. *Aust Dent J* 1993;38: 216–219.

2. Thean HP, Chew CL, Goh KI: Shear bond strength of denture teeth to base: a comparative study. *Dent Dig* 1996;27: 425–428.

3. Sipahi C, Ozcan M, Piskin B: Effect of physicochemical surface treatments on the bond strength and adhesion of porcelain denture teeth to heat-polymerized acrylic resin denture base material. *J Adhes* 2012;88: 200–212.

4. Rickman LJ, Padipatvuthikul P, Satterthwaite JD: Contemporary denture base resins: Part 2. *Dent Update* 2012;39: 176–178, 80–82, 84 passim.

5. Kanazawa M, Inokoshi M, Minakuchi S, et al: Trial of a CAD/CAM system for fabricating complete dentures. *Dent Mater J* 2011;30: 93–96.

6. Infante L, Yilmaz B, McGlumphy E, et al: Fabricating complete dentures with CAD/CAM technology. *J Prosthet Dent* 2014;111: 351–355.

7. Sousa MV, Vasconcelos EC, Janson G, et al: Accuracy and reproducibility of 3-dimensional digital model measurements. *Am J Orthod Dentofacial Orthop* 2012;142: 269–273.

8. Alcan T, Ceylanoğlu C, Baysal B: The relationship between digital model accuracy and time dependent deformation of alginate impressions. *Angle Orthod* 2009;79: 30–36.

9. Dincel M, Gumus HO, Buyuk SK, et al: The evaluation of the accuracy of the 3 dimensional digital model measurements. *J Dent Fac Atatürk Uni* 2013;21: 366–370.

10. Yuan FS, Sun YC, Wang Y, et al: Accuracy evaluation of a new three-dimensional reproduction method of edentulous dental casts, and wax occlusion rims with jaw relation. *Int J Oral Sci* 2013;5: 155–161.

11. Hobrink J, Zarb GA, Bolender CL, et al: *Prosthodontic Treatment for Edentulous Patients: Complete Dentures and Implant-Supported Prostheses (ed 12)*. St. Louis, Mosby, 2004, pp. 298–328.

12. Inokoshi M, Kanazawa M, Minakuchi S: Evaluation of a complete denture trial method applying rapid prototyping. *Dent Mater J* 2012;31: 40–46.

13. Gümüş HÖ, Dinçel M, Büyük SK, et al: The effect of pouring time on the dimensional stability of casts made from conventional and extended-pour irreversible hydrocolloids by 3D modelling. *J Dent Sci* 2014 DOI: 10.1016/j.jds.2014.05.003.

16

PART-DIGITIZING SYSTEM OF IMPRESSION AND INTEROCCLUSAL RECORD FOR COMPLETE DENTURE FABRICATION

TAKASHI MATSUDA, DDS, TAKAHARU GOTO, DDS, PHD, KAZUTOMO YAGI, DDS, PHD, TOSHIYA KASHIWABARA, DDS, PHD, AND TETSUO ICHIKAWA, DDS, PHD
Department of Oral & Maxillofacial Prosthodontics, Tokushima University Graduate School, Institute of Biomedical Sciences, Tokushima, Japan

Keywords
CAD/CAM; digital; complete denture; impression; interocclusal record

Correspondence
Tetsuo Ichikawa, DDS, PhD, Department of Oral & Maxillofacial Prosthodontics, Tokushima University Graduate School, Institute of Biomedical Sciences, 3-18-15 Kuramoto, Tokushima 770-8504, Japan.
E-mail: ichi@tokushima-u.ac.jp

The authors deny any conflicts of interest.

Accepted March 3, 2015

Published in *Journal of Prosthodontics* 2016; Vol. 25, Issue 6, pp. 503–9

doi: 10.1111/jopr.12375

ABSTRACT

Few studies have reported the application of digital technology to removable dentures, particularly for the process of impression and interocclusal recording for complete denture fabrication. This article describes a part-digitizing system of impression and interocclusal records for complete denture fabrication. The denture foundation area in an edentulous mouth, including the border areas and residual ridge, is outlined by tracing the surfaces with a 3-D pen-type digitizer. Specialized trays for final impressions and interocclusal records were generated using computer-aided design and manufactured using the digital data. Final impression and interocclusal records were carried out using these specialized trays. The computer-aided method using preliminary digital impressions and specialized trays would be feasible for clinical use for complete denture fabrication.

Prosthodontic treatments and laboratory techniques have been conducted by indirect methods using various impression materials for more than 400 years, because the wax impression technique was first developed in the 1600s.[1,2] The lost-wax process involves the extraoral fabrication of prostheses; however, the associated chairside and laboratory procedures are complex, and the amount of dental waste generated has also increased. Standard prosthodontic procedures also require many visits to fabricate a set of complete dentures, even if attempts have been made to reduce the number of visits needed.

Digital technology has advanced rapidly, and various digital systems for prosthetic dentistry have been developed in recent years. Computer-aided design (CAD) and computer-aided manufacturing (CAM) technology have been commercialized for the fabrication of inlays, crowns, fixed partial dentures (FPDs), and implant superstructure frames.[3,4] Few studies, however, have reported the application of digital technology to removable dentures, particularly for the process of impressions and interocclusal recording for complete denture fabrication.

We developed a part-digitizing system for complete denture fabrication, specifically for the process of acquiring preliminary impressions and manufacturing a novel custom tray that could be employed for both the final impression and interocclusal record using digital impression data. The purposes of this article are to describe the processes involved in our part-digitizing system, explain its potential for clinical use, and discuss the current status and future perspectives regarding digital technology for complete denture fabrication.

PART-DIGITIZING SYSTEM USING THE BITE-IMPRESSION TECHNIQUE

Figures 1 to 4 show the part-digitizing system for complete denture fabrication using the "bite-impression" technique. The system consists of three steps, described below.

Step 1: Digital Preliminary Impression

The denture foundation area in an edentulous mouth, including the border areas and residual ridge, is outlined by tracing the surfaces with a 3-D pen-type digitizer (MicroScribe G2X; Solution Technology Inc., Omaha, NE). This type of contact scanner provides coordinates using a stylus pen top (Fig 1). The foundation area is scanned, while the stylus pen top touches the mucosa gently. After cubic spline interpolation and smoothing are applied to the raw digital data, each foundation area is reconstructed using CAD software (Rhinoceros 3.0; AppliCraft, Tokyo, Japan). In addition, the intra- and extraoral anatomical landmarks, such as labial frenum, hamular notch, and ala-tragus line, are inserted into the digital data for the fabrication of specialized custom trays.

Step 2: CAD and Manufacturing of the Bite-Impression Tray

Specialized trays for the final impressions and interocclusal record are generated using CAD, based on the digital data (Figs 2, 3). The trays have a specialized cross-arch occlusal rim for the interocclusal record. The lower tray has three posterior hemispherical projections and an anterior occlusion rim to determine arch form. The upper tray has a concave box rim, resulting in the application of paraffin wax into each molar region and the anterior occlusion rim. Each of the occlusion rims is positioned with reference to anatomical landmarks recorded digitally at the time of the preliminary impression so that the treatment time for the interocclusal record is reduced as much as possible. The CAD data are used to generate specialized plastic trays using a 3-D printer.

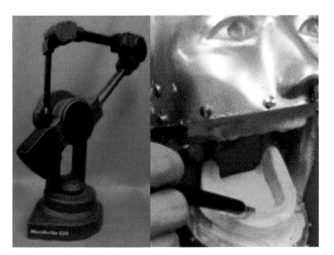
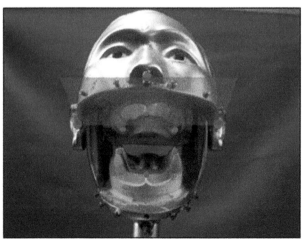

FIGURE 1 Description of part-digitizing system, part 1. Digital preliminary impression. Three-dimensional coordinate input of denture foundation area (left), 3-D coordinate input of anatomical landmarks (right).

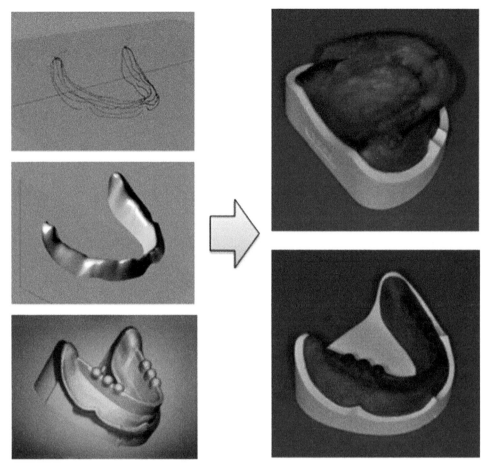

FIGURE 2   Description of part-digitizing system, part 2. CAD and manufacturing of bite-impression trays. CAD image of mandible by raw data (top left), CAD image of mandible after cubic spline interpolation and smoothing (middle left), CAD final design of lower tray (bottom left). CAM fabrication of specialized trays (right).

The design of these specialized trays could also be used for conventional handmade fabrication.

Step 3: Final Impression and Interocclusal Record Using Specialized Trays

The final impression and interocclusal record are made using specialized trays (Fig 4). The final upper impression is obtained using the upper tray according to a conventional procedure, which involves border modeling and distribution of the final impression material. After lower modeling is performed using the lower tray, the upper and lower trays are placed in the mouth. Standard gentle tapping movements result in the three hemispherical projections of the lower tray being plotted onto the wax rim of the upper tray, and the interocclusal relationship is thus determined. The final lower impression is performed under bite pressure.

Accuracy of Digital Impression

In this study, the accuracy of the digital impressions was confirmed in the following manner. The participants were five young dentists (mean age, 30.4 ± 5.1 years), each with less than 5 years' experience at Tokushima University Hospital. They were asked to trace upper and lower plaster edentulous models (G-2 402; Nissin, Kyoto, Japan) using the procedure described above. Figure 5 shows four types of tracing instructions that were followed:

1. Trace the alveolar ridge freehand for 30 seconds.
2. Trace the alveolar ridge with a tracing interval of 10 mm, including the top and reflection.
3. Trace the alveolar ridge with a tracing interval of 5 mm, including the top and reflection.
4. Trace the alveolar ridge with a tracing interval of 3 mm, including the top and reflection.

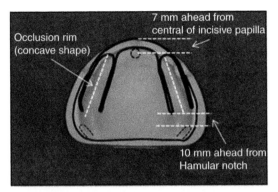

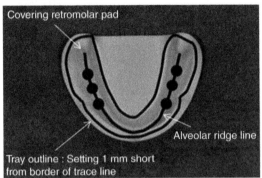

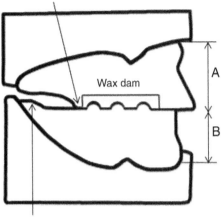

FIGURE 3   Design of bite-impression trays. (A) Twenty-two millimeters under the deepest part of the upper gingivobuccal fold or the same height as the inferior border of the upper lip. (B) Eighteen millimeters over the deepest part of the lower gingivobuccal fold or the same height as the superior border of the lower lip.

The master edentulous models were also scanned at a resolution of 15 μm using a dental scanner (Dental Wings 7 Series; Dental Wings, Montreal, Canada), and the resulting digital images were constructed as reference images. Experimental and reference digital images were automatically superimposed using specialized software (Gom Inspect; GOM, Braunschweig, Germany) so the least mean square error between each of the two images was lowest. The error distributions were qualitatively inspected, and the mean errors were calculated.

In each of the upper and lower jaws, the mean errors were less than 1.0 mm, irrespective of the tracing conditions, when the master edentulous model dimension was referenced (Fig 6). The mean error tended to decrease with decreasing tracing intervals (30-second freehand tracing, 0.60 ± 0.11 mm; 10-mm tracing interval, 0.67 ± 0.04 mm; 5-mm tracing interval, 0.48 ± 0.04 mm; 3-mm tracing interval, 0.43 ± 0.03 mm; analysis of variance, $p < 0.05$). In both jaws, there were significant differences in the measurement error between the four tracing conditions, but there were no significant differences between the maxilla and mandible. No significant interaction was found between the jaws and the tracing intervals.

DISCUSSION

There are very few published reports regarding the digitalization of complete denture fabrication. In the context of impression data acquisition, two indirect procedures have been reported. In one, existing dentures are digitized all together using cone-beam computed tomography, the dentures are polished, and occlusal and foundation surfaces are reconstructed on a computer.[5,6] In the other, the impression surface and interocclusal record are digitized separately by optical metrology using equipment such as a laser scanner and charge-coupled device (CCD) camera, and the images are then integrated on a computer.[7] A study in which intraoral scanners were used to directly digitize edentulous jaws has recently been published. In this in vitro trial, the mean errors were 0.05 to 0.59 mm in the maxilla and in 0.04 to 0.56 mm in the mandible.[8] The accuracy of our procedure was greater than or comparable to that in the report; however, our procedure required approximately 1 minute of scanning time, whereas intraoral scanners require about 10 minutes.[9] In our procedure, reducing the interval would increase the tracing time and result in error caused by head and jaw movements. The accuracy of our procedure is acceptable for

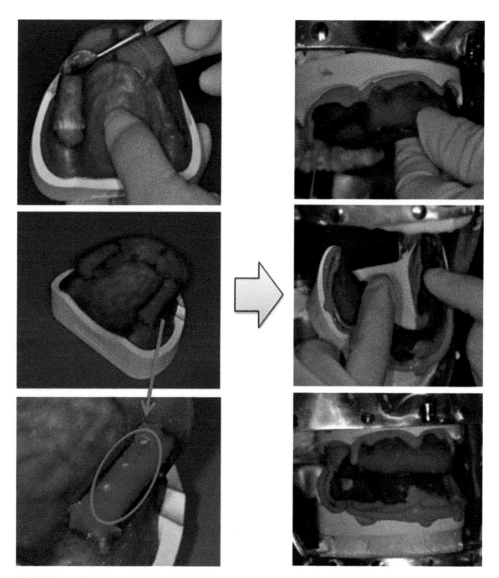

FIGURE 4   Description of part-digitizing system, part 3. Final impression and interocclusal record using bite-impression trays. Preparation of wax rim of upper tray (top left), indentation of three projections on wax rim produced by tapping movements (middle and bottom left), final impression of maxilla (top right), placement of lower tray for final impression (middle right), and final lower impression under bite pressure (bottom right).

preliminary impressions, considering the above results regarding accuracy and tracing time. A conventional final impression using silicone material is necessary to successfully produce a complete denture, using the engineering methods now available.

For manufacturing, 3-D printing has been used for rapid prototyping, and computed numerical control milling machines have been used.[6,10–15] The artificial teeth and denture base can each be manufactured separately using specialized material, and the two parts can then be integrated using cementation.[6] Alternatively, ready-made artificial teeth are prepared, and the denture base is manufactured so that the artificial teeth can be cemented to particular sites of the denture base. Two commercially available CAD/CAM systems, AvaDent (Global Dental Science LLC, Scottsdale, AZ) and Dentca (Dentca Inc., Los Angeles, CA), can be used to manufacture complete dentures using this technology.[16]

Previous studies have compared the accuracy of fabrication yielded by conventional procedures with that yielded by CAD/CAM procedures and have reported satisfactory

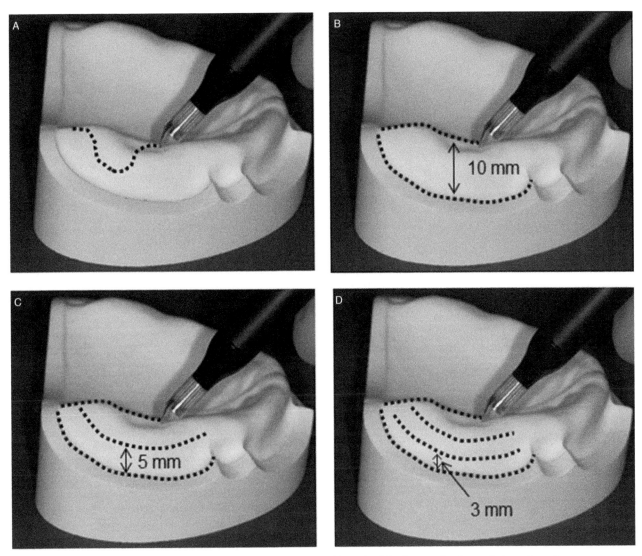

FIGURE 5   Instructions used to prompt tracing with each of the four tracing intervals investigated with regard to digital preliminary impressions. (A) Freehand tracing for 30 seconds; (B–D) 10-, 5-, and 3-mm tracing intervals, respectively.

results.[6,10] The accuracy required for the fabrication of complete dentures is generally lower than that required for crowns and FPDs; therefore, it is not difficult to digitize the denture surfaces and manufacture dentures with satisfactory accuracy using CAD/CAM.

When using a digitization system for complete denture fabrication, it is important to design the overall outline of the denture and arrangement of artificial teeth and then to develop specialized software for them. It is also important to directly obtain the digital information to design the overall outline of the dentures, as was done in this study. It has been suggested that the acquisition of impressions for complete dentures is not a process of taking, but rather one of making, particularly with regard to determining the denture border.

A stylus pen-type digitizer is more accurate than an optical scanner for determining the denture outline and anatomical landmarks.

Compromised and elderly patients are at a relatively high risk of accidental ingestion and aspiration during impression-taking. This system could reduce this risk by shortening the impression time. It is also minimally invasive. In a trial calculation, the cost of treatment using this system from the time of preliminary impression acquisition to interocclusal record was estimated to be 30% higher than that of conventional procedures. The higher cost of this system is due to depreciation of the 3-D printer; therefore, this type of apparatus will become less expensive with more widespread use.

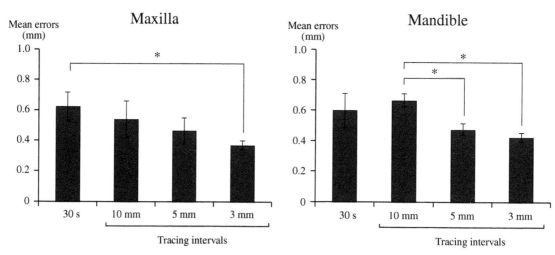

FIGURE 6   Accuracy of digital preliminary impressions.

CONCLUSION

The investigation of this part-digitizing system for acquiring preliminary digital impressions and specialized trays suggests that it has potential for clinical use in complete denture fabrication, although further improvement of the system is required.

REFERENCES

1. Hofmann-Axthelm W: *History of Dentistry*. Chicago, Quintessence, 1981, pp. 16–286.

2. Mutlu G, Harrison A, Huggett R: A history of denture base materials. *Quintessence Dent Tech* 1989;13:145–150.

3. Bidra AS, Taylor TD, Agar JR: Computer-aided technology for fabricating complete dentures: systematic review of historical background, current status, and future perspectives. *J Prosthet Dent* 2013;109:361–366.

4. Lima JM, Anami LC, Araujo RM, et al: Removable partial dentures: use of rapid prototyping. *J Prosthodont* 2014;23:588–591.

5. Inokoshi M, Kanazawa M, Minakuchi S: Evaluation of a complete denture trial method applying rapid prototyping. *Dent Mater J* 2012;31:40–46.

6. Kanazawa M, Inokoshi M, Minakuchi S, et al: Trial of a CAD/CAM system for fabricating complete dentures. *Dent Mater J* 2011;30:93–96.

7. Maeda Y, Minoura M, Tsutsumi S, et al: A CAD/CAM system for removable denture. Part I: Fabrication of complete dentures. *Int J Prosthodont* 1994;7:17–21.

8. Patzelt SB, Vonau S, Stampf S, et al: Assessing the feasibility and accuracy of digitizing edentulous jaws. *J Am Dent Assoc* 2013;144:914–920.

9. Grünheid T, McCarthy SD, Larson BE: Clinical use of a direct chairside oral scanner: an assessment of accuracy, time, and patient acceptance. *Am J Orthod Dentofacial Orthop* 2014;146:673–682.

10. Wu J, Gao B, Tan H, et al: A feasibility study on laser rapid forming of a complete titanium denture base plate. *Lasers Med Sci* 2010;25:309–315.

11. Goodacre CJ, Garbacea A, Naylor WP, et al: CAD/CAM fabricated complete dentures: concepts and clinical methods of obtaining required morphological data. *J Prosthet Dent* 2012;107:34–46.

12. Zhang YD, Jiang JG, Liang T, et al: Kinematics modeling and experimentation of the multi-manipulator tooth-arrangement robot for full denture manufacturing. *J Med Syst* 2011;35:1421–1429.

13. Sun Y, Lü P, Wang Y: Study on CAD&RP for removable complete denture. *Comput Methods Programs Biomed* 2009;93:266–272.

14. Kawahata N, Ono H, Nishi Y, et al: Trial of a duplication procedure for complete dentures by CAD/CAM. *J Oral Rehabil* 1997;24:540–548.

15. Busch M, Kordass B: Concept and development of a computerized positioning of prosthetic teeth for complete dentures. *Int J Comput Dent* 2006;9:113–120.

16. Kattadiyil MT, Goodacre CJ, Baba NZ: CAD/CAM complete dentures: a review of two commercial fabrication systems. *J Calif Dent Assoc.* 2013;41:407–416.

17

ENHANCING FRACTURE AND WEAR RESISTANCE OF DENTURES/OVERDENTURES UTILIZING DIGITAL TECHNOLOGY: A CASE SERIES REPORT

Ahmed Afify, DMD and Stephan Haney, DDS, FACP

Department of Comprehensive Dentistry, Graduate Prosthodontics, UT Health Science Center, San Antonio, TX

Keywords

Fracture; wear; denture; overdenture; CAD/CAM; zirconia; framework; SLM; milled

Correspondence

Ahmed Reda Afify, Department of Comprehensive Dentistry, Graduate Prosthodontics, UT Health Science Center, 8210 Floyd Curl Dr., San Antonio, TX 78229. E-mail: afify@uthscsa.edu

The authors deny any conflicts of interest.

Accepted December 12, 2015

Published in *Journal of Prosthodontics* 2016; Vol. 25, pp. 489–94

doi: 10.1111/jopr.12462

ABSTRACT

Since it was first introduced into the dental world, computer-aided design/computer-aided manufacturing (CAD/CAM) technology has improved dramatically in regards to both data acquisition and fabrication abilities. CAD/CAM is capable of providing well-fitting intra- and extraoral prostheses when sound guidelines are followed. As CAD/CAM technology encompasses both surgical and prosthetic dental applications as well as fixed and removable aspects, it could improve the average quality of dental prostheses compared with the results obtained by conventional manufacturing methods. The purpose of this article is to provide an introduction into the methods in which this technology may be used to enhance the wear and fracture resistance of dentures and overdentures. This article will also showcase two clinical reports in which CAD/CAM technology has been implemented.

Within the last decade, computer-aided design and computer-aided manufacturing technology, collectively referred to as CAD/CAM, has been solidly established as a viable technology in dentistry. CAD/CAM has a proven record of success and is now an efficient and cost-effective alternative to traditional methods for the design and fabrication of dental restorations. This technology is used in prosthodontics to create a wide range of products from fixed (full contour crowns, copings, implant abutments, etc.) to removable prostheses (tissue- and implantassisted dentures).

Computer-aided technology can either involve additive manufacturing (such as rapid prototyping) or subtractive manufacturing (such as computerized numerical control machining). Additive manufacturing, or 3D printing, converts a virtual image from a digital file to a 3D object by laying down successive layers of a chosen material. Subtractive manufacturing uses images from a digital file to create an object by machining (cutting/milling) to physically remove material from a blank, leaving the desired geometry.[1]

The purpose of this manuscript is to showcase the different innovative methods for the treatment of the edentulous prosthodontic patient to improve wear and fracture resistance of their dental prostheses.

WEAR RESISTANCE

Wear of occluding denture tooth surfaces is an inevitable sequela of successful treatment with removable prostheses. Although the severity of this wear process relies on several factors, major determinants include the length of service, the physical nature of opposing dentition, and presence of parafunctional habits. When the extent of wear becomes more significant, the patient's occlusal vertical dimension, chewing efficiency, and esthetics are increasingly compromised.[2,3]

Various solutions have been discussed in the literature to address the issue of wear, including highly cross-linked acrylic resin teeth,[9] amalgam or metal inserts on occlusal surfaces, and the use of composites.[10] Of the assorted solutions, however, gold occlusal surfaces have been the most frequently referenced option.

Since the concept was first introduced to dental literature in 1964,[2] a number of methods to construct gold occlusal surfaces have been described. Some authors have advocated construction after the prosthesis has been processed, inserted, and adjusted,[2–5] while others described techniques to incorporate gold occlusal surfaces prior to processing.[6–8] Whether gold occlusal surfaces are created before or after the denture processing, extra steps such as waxing, investing, casting, and polishing are required, which are time consuming and expensive, and require considerable technical expertise. After creating gold occlusal surfaces, a variety of cementing and bonding agents have been recommended to attach the gold occlusal surfaces to the prepared prosthetic teeth, including composite resin, adhesive resin cement, and chemically activated acrylic resin.

As the cost of gold has risen, and as patient acceptance of metal display has declined, alternative materials for durable yet esthetic occlusal surfaces have come to the market. The fabrication of a maxillary denture with posterior occlusal onlays in one of those alternative materials, zirconia, is now possible with CAD/CAM subtractive (milling) technology.

FRACTURE RESISTANCE

Similarly, CAD/CAM technology can be used to enhance the fracture resistance of conventional and implant-supported prostheses. Fracture of an acrylic resin denture base can be an inconvenient and vexing complication to treatment. The etiology of denture fractures has been extensively investigated and reported in the literature.[11–13] Causes of these fractures include occlusal disharmony, excessive occlusal forces, flexure and fatigue of the denture base as a result of alveolar resorption, thin spots in the denture base, impact damage as a result of dropping the denture,[11] as well as fractures by neuropsychiatric patients.[14]

Denture base fractures are more commonly seen with implant-supported removable complete dentures than tissue-supported prostheses. This is an inherent complication in the anterior portion of bar-retained mandibular overdentures when an inadequate thickness of acrylic resin exists to house the dimensions of the bar and clips.[15,16] This tendency also holds true in cases of limited interarch space for Locator or ball attachment retained implant overdentures.

The use of a metal base or metal framework for a removable prosthesis is not a new concept. A "suspended" internal framework in a denture prosthesis was described by Morrow et al in 1968.[17] A number of authors have since formulated additional techniques to incorporate reinforcing metal frameworks within a denture base before processing.[16,18–20]

Dental laboratory fabrication of a framework and the subsequent prosthesis remains a labor-intensive, technique-sensitive task typically performed by an experienced dental laboratory technician. With the introduction of the additive selective laser melting (SLM) technology to fabricate partial removable dental prosthesis (RDP) frameworks,[21] a more cost-effective method to manufacture metal frameworks is now available.

This article documents and examines the use of both additive and subtractive methods to create conventional dentures and implant-assisted overdentures with enhanced wear and fracture resistance.

PATIENT 1: MAXILLARY COMPLETE DENTURE WITH MILLED POSTERIOR ZIRCONIA ONLAYS

A 55-year-old male was referred to the graduate prosthodontics clinic for fabrication of a maxillary complete RDP. Four years

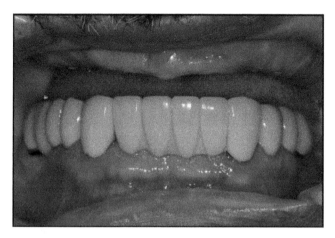

FIGURE 1   Pretreatment photo.

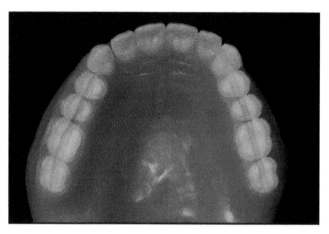

FIGURE 3   Zirconia onlay preparations on premolars/molars.

ago, his mandibular dentition had been successfully restored in an outside practice with metal ceramic crowns and a fixed dental prosthesis (Fig 1). In the interval following his mandibular rehabilitation, he reported replacement of his maxillary denture five times due to the severe wear of the denture teeth opposing his porcelain restorations. His last maxillary complete denture also fractured, and he had no maxillary prosthesis for 1 year. A treatment option to remake the maxillary denture with milled gold occlusal onlays was presented to the patient, but was rejected due to esthetic concerns. An alternative milled zirconia onlay approach was selected.

Technique

1. A new maxillary complete denture was fabricated, optimizing patient esthetics and phonetics (Fig 2). Masticatory efficiency and comfort were maximized with clinical remount and occlusal refinement of the clinically fitted prosthesis. After a period of comfortable denture wear, the final denture occlusal anatomy

was digitally scanned (3Shape; 3Shape A/S, Copenhagen, Denmark). An interocclusal record made in centric relation (CR) was scanned as well.

2. All posterior acrylic resin teeth were prepared for zirconia onlays with 1 mm of occlusal reduction and a 2-mm central isthmus. The preparations included the palatal cusps but ended on the lingual inclines of the buccal cusps (Figs 3 and 4). An additional scan was performed of the prepared teeth and merged with the original scan.

3. In the design phase, preparation finish lines were outlined and proximal margins connected to virtually create a single splinted framework covering all premolars and molars. The milling parameters for zirconia were entered according to the manufacturer's recommendations.

4. Using the merging function of the 3Shape software, a zirconia framework design was selected to reproduce the original tooth shape and form. Occlusal contacts

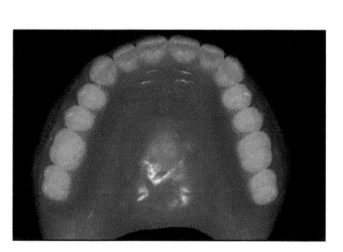

FIGURE 2   Complete maxillary denture.

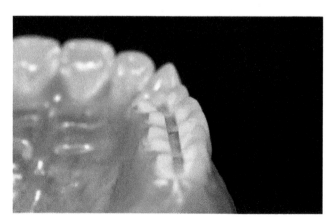

FIGURE 4   Onlay preparations on posterior acrylic resin teeth.

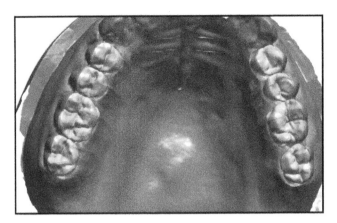

FIGURE 5 Designed splinted zirconia onlays.

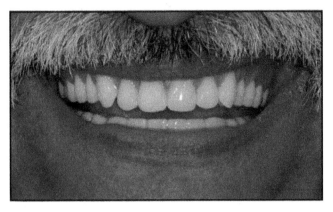

FIGURE 7 Definitive prosthesis delivered.

were refined and brought to idealized positions via the scanned interocclusal CR registration (Fig 5).

5. After approval, the virtual splinted zirconia onlay designs were transmitted to the milling center for fabrication (Whip Mix Corporation, Louisville, KY). Upon receipt from the milling center, the external onlay surfaces were polished and tried in. After fit and occlusal accuracy were verified, onlay intaglio surfaces were treated with Z-prime (Bisco, Shaumburg, IL) prior to final cementation to enhance the bond to the resin cement. Retentive undercuts were made in the onlay preparations to create both chemical and mechanical retention of the resin cement to the acrylic teeth.

6. Bonding was completed using translucent dual cure resin cement (Rely X Unicem; 3M ESPE, St. Paul, MN). Excess cement flash was removed, and occlusal refinement was accomplished on the articulator via the previously fabricated remount cast (Fig 6). Minimal adjustments were required intraorally before definitive prosthesis delivery (Fig 7).

PATIENT 2: MAXILLARY COMPLETE DENTURE WITH METAL PALATE OPPOSING A MANDIBULAR IMPLANT OVERDENTURE WITH INTERNAL METAL FRAMEWORK

A 72-year-old female patient presented to the graduate prosthodontics clinic for complete denture care. She reported dissatisfaction with her previous prosthesis due to the thickness of the palatal area and the repeated fracture of her mandibular implant-assisted overdenture.

Technique

1. After a wax try-in appointment, the dentures were flasked using the split stone flasking technique (SSFT), and all wax boiled out. This innovative technique was devised by Dr. Russell Johnson and presented in the poster competition at the 2013 Annual Session of the American College of Prosthodontists. The SSFT permits rigid indexing of denture tooth positions for space analysis (Fig 8).

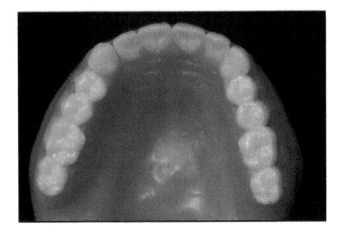

FIGURE 6 Zirconia onlays bonded to maxillary denture resin teeth.

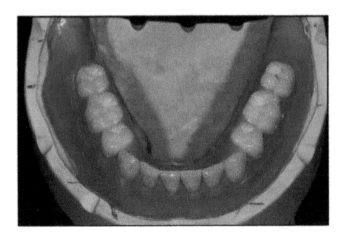

FIGURE 8 Final tooth setup for mandibular implant-assisted overdenture.

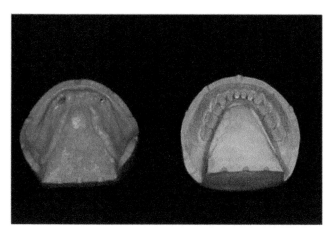

FIGURE 9   Split stone flask index for space analysis.

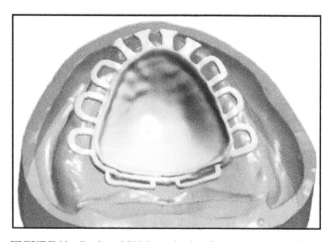

FIGURE 11   Designed SLM metal palate framework for maxillary denture.

2. The space between the teeth and the edentulous ridge was filled with lab condensation silicone putty (Sil-Tech; Ivoclar Vivadent, Amherst, NY; Fig 9) and digitally scanned (3Shape). The scanned silicone mold provided a 3D representation of the space available for the metal framework.

3. Using the removable partial denture design software for the 3Shape, a metal framework with tripodal cast stops and metal struts over the Locator housings was created virtually within the restorative space and transmitted to the manufacturer for sintering (Argen Dental Laboratory, San Diego, CA; Fig 10). The maxillary metal palate framework was designed in a similar fashion (Fig 11).

4. Upon receipt from the manufacturer, fit and reproduction fidelity were verified (Figs 12 and 13). Both frameworks were opaqued in areas of planned acrylic resin retention with a light-cured pink opaquer (Ropak UV; XPDent, Miami, FL) and allowed to cure for 15 minutes in a curing oven. The SSF was used to verify sufficient space between the opaqued frame and overlying denture resin teeth before processing (Fig 14).

5. Framework tissue stops were luted to the casts with chemically cured acrylic resin (Lang Dental Manufacturing Co., Wheeling, IL). The SSF for both prostheses were incorporated in the conventional brass flasks, as

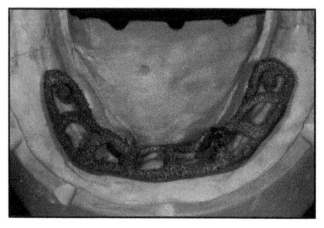

FIGURE 12   SLM metal framework tried on mandibular cast.

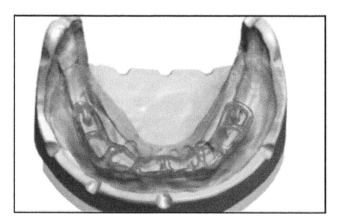

FIGURE 10   Completed metal framework design.

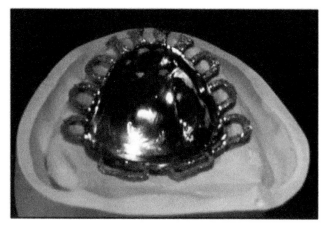

FIGURE 13   SLM framework fitted to final cast.

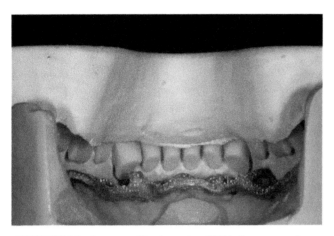

FIGURE 14 Space verification using SSF before processing.

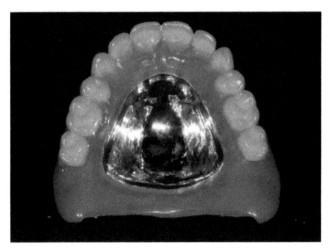

FIGURE 15 Final maxillary prosthesis, occlusal view.

described by Johnson, and heat processed per the manufacturer's recommendations. Locator attachments were picked up intraorally in the mandibular prosthesis.

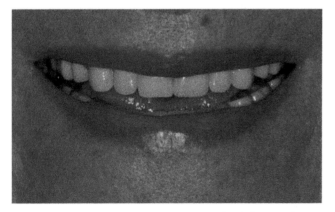

FIGURE 16 Post-insertion with prosthesis delivered, frontal view.

6. The definitive prosthesis was inserted and the patient reevaluated in 1 week to verify phonetic competency, occlusal accuracy, and patient satisfaction with the comfort and esthetics (Figs 15 and 16).

DISCUSSION

This report has examined two examples of care that highlight the potential of CAD/CAM technology to enhance wear and fracture resistance for bothconventional and implant overdentures. Theuse of milled zirconiarestorations for complete dentures has been reported in the literature: examples used full occlusal coverage with zirconia mechanically connected tothe underlyingacrylic resin teeth by diatorics.[22] However, inone of the presented patients, only the palatal cusps were onlaid with preparations ending on lingual inclines of the buccal cusps for esthetic purposes. The shade matching between resin acrylic teeth and polished zirconia is a challenge and represents a point of concern for some patients, especially those with high esthetic expectations or with a high smile line. The fear of weakening the buccal cusp by not incorporating it in the onlay design was addressed by employing a lingualized occlusal scheme for the tooth setup.

The use of porcelain denture teeth has also been suggested as a remedy for excessive wear when opposing porcelain restorations; however, porcelain teeth require considerable restorative space to be considered as a viable option. The main form of connection between porcelain teeth and the acrylic resin denture base is purely mechanical. In circumstances of limited restorative space, grinding the intaglio of porcelain teeth may compromise the retentive diatorics and result in the eventual separation of the porcelain tooth from the acrylic resin denture base. The use of zirconia over prepared acrylic teeth takes advantage of the chemical bond strength of acrylic teeth in relation to the denture base, while simultaneously providing a good bonding substrate for the milled zirconia. Other materials have been described in the literature for onlays, including milled lithium disilicate.[23] The reported design requires individually milled crowns at a cost considerably more significant than that of zirconia milled in quadrants. The use of splinted zirconia may also enhance the retentive properties compared to individual crowns. Additionally, lithium disilicate requires greater thickness than zirconia for adequate fracture resistance and is less appropriate in circumstances of limited restorative spaces. Finally, polished zirconia has been shown to have superior wear characteristics when opposing unrestored natural teeth.[24–26]

For SLM framework fabrication, the physical properties of base metal alloys make them the material of choice for this purpose. Allergies to such materials have been reported in the literature, with an estimated frequency of 10% in females and 1% in males.[27] Careful medical history and allergy testing should be considered to make an appropriate material choice for each patient. Metal palate designs create limitations for relining and rebasing such dentures. Garfield has described an acid etch technique that can be used to mitigate this concern somewhat.[28] The rough surface texture created by SLM framework production is ideal for mechanical retention between the framework and the denture resin. Conversely, polishing such highly irregular exposed portions of these SLM frames is time consuming and requires considerable technical expertise.

CONCLUSION

These clinical reports demonstrated the following:

1. The total estimated time from initial scanning through design, milling, shipping, and receipt of CAD/CAM frames is 3 to 4 days.
2. The cost of CAD/CAM products represents a considerable savings from that of conventionally fabricated frames.
3. SLM products are particularly suited for fabrication of frames that will be totally incorporated within a prosthesis, negating the finish and polish issues with raw SLM surfaces.
4. After 2 years of service, a stable occlusion was confirmed for both patients presented, with no clinical signs of occlusal wear or prosthesis fracture.
5. Digital technology is being used to efficiently create clinically successful and reliable dental restorations. In the near future, CAD/CAM may well become the preferred fabrication method for most dental prostheses.

ACKNOWLEDGMENTS

The authors thank Dr. Ryan Sheridan of Lackland Air Force Base, Graduate Prosthodontics; and Dr. Russell Johnson of the UT Health Science Center, San Antonio, Graduate Prosthodontics.

REFERENCES

1. Dankwort CW, Weidlich R, Guenther B, et al: Engineers' CAx education—it's not only CAD. *Comput-Aided Design* 2004;36:1439–1450.
2. Wallace DH: The use of gold occlusal surfaces in complete and partial dentures. *J Prosthet Dent* 1964;14:326–333.
3. Nicholas WT, Flamme J: Gold occlusal surfaces for acrylic denture teeth with vertical parallel pin castings. *Quintessence Dent Tech* 1987;11:119–122.
4. Imbery TA, Evans DB, Koeppen RG: A new method of attaching cast gold occlusal surfaces to acrylic resin denture teeth. *Quintessence Int* 1993;24:29–33.
5. Woodward JD, Gattozzi JG: Simplified gold occlusal technique for removable restorations. *J Prosthet Dent* 1972;27:447–450.
6. Koehne CL, Morrow RM: Construction of denture teeth with gold occlusal surfaces. *J Prosthet Dent* 1970;23:449–455.
7. Engelmeier RL: Fabricating denture teeth with custom anatomic and nonanatomic metal surfaces. *J Prosthet Dent* 1980;43:352–356.
8. Lloyd PM: Laboratory fabrication of gold occlusal surfaces for removable and implant-supported prostheses. *J Prosthodont* 2003;85:8–12.
9. Kamonwanon P, Yodmongkol S, Chantarachindawong R, et al: Wear resistance of a modified polymethyl methacrylate artificial tooth compared to five commercially available artificial tooth materials. *J Prosthet Dent* 2015;114:286–292.
10. Suzuki S: In vitro wear of nano-composite denture teeth. *J Prosthodont* 2004;13:238–243.
11. Jagger DC: The fractured denture-solving the problem. *J Prim Dent Care* 1998;5:159–162.
12. Darbar UR, Huggett R, Harrison A: Denture fracture—a survey. *Br Dent J* 1994;176:342–345.
13. Chaffee NR, Felton DA, Cooper LF, et al: Prosthetic complications in an implant-retained mandibular overdenture population: initial analysis of a prospective study. *J Prosthet Dent* 2002;87:40–44.
14. Vallittu PK: A review of methods used to reinforce polymethyl methacrylate resin. *J Prosthodont* 1995;4:183–187.
15. Polyzois GL, Andreopoulos AG, Lagouvardos PE: Acrylic resin denture repair with adhesive resin and metal wires: effects on strength parameters. *J Prosthet Dent* 1996;75:381–387.
16. Rodrigues AH: Metal reinforcement for implant-supported mandibular overdentures. *J Prosthet Dent* 2000;83:511–513.
17. Morrow RM, Reiner PR, Feldmann EE, et al: Metal reinforced silicone-lined dentures. *J Prosthet Dent* 1968;19:219–229.
18. Massad JJ: A metal-based denture with soft liner to accommodate the severely resorbed mandibular alveolar ridge. *J Prosthet Dent* 1989;57:707–711.
19. Jameson WS: Fabrication and use of a metal reinforcing frame in a fracture-prone mandibular complete denture. *J Prosthet Dent* 2000;83:476–479.
20. Balch JH, Smith PD, Marin MA, et al: Reinforcement of a mandibular complete denture with internal metal framework. *J Prosthet Dent* 2013;109:202–205.
21. Williams RJ, Bibb R, Eggbeer D, et al: Use of CAD/CAM technology to fabricate a removable partial denture framework. *J Prosthet Dent* 2006;96:96–99.
22. Livaditis JM, Livaditis GJ: The use of custom-milled zirconia teeth to address tooth abrasion in complete dentures: a clinical report. *J Prosthodont* 2013;22:208–213.
23. Yoon TH, Madden JC, Chang WG: A technique to restore worn denture teeth on a partial removable dental prosthesis by using ceramic onlays with CAD/CAM technology. *J Prosthet Dent* 2013;110:331–332.

24. Lawson NC, Janyavula S, Syklawer S, et al: Wear of enamel opposing zirconia and lithium disilicate after adjustment, polishing and glazing. *J Dent* 2014;42:1586–1591.

25. Stober T, Bermejo JL, Rammelsberg P, et al: Enamel wear caused by monolithic zirconia crowns after 6 months of clinical use. *J Oral Rehabil* 2014;41:314–322.

26. Mundhe K, Jain V, Pruthi G, et al: Clinical study to evaluate the wear of natural enamel antagonist to zirconia and metal ceramic crowns. *J Prosthet Dent* 2015;114:358–363.

27. Workshop: Biocompatibility of metals in dentistry. National Institute of Dental Research. *J Am Dent Assoc* 1984;109:469–471.

28. Garfield RE: An effective method for relining metal-based prostheses with acid-etch techniques. *J Prosthet Dent* 1984;51:719–721.

18

DESIGN OF COMPLETE DENTURES BY ADOPTING CAD DEVELOPED FOR FIXED PROSTHESES

Yanfeng Li, md,[1] Weili Han, mm,[2] Jing Cao, md,[1] Yuan Iv, mm,[1] Yue Zhang, mm,[1] Yishi Han, mm,[1] Yi Shen, mm,[3] Zheng Ma, bm,[1] and Huanyue Liu, bm[1]

[1]Department of Stomatology, First Affiliated Hospital of Chinese PLA General Hospital, Beijing, China
[2]Department of Stomatology, Fengtai Community Health Service Center, Beijing, China
[3]Department of Stomatology, Beijing Shen Yi Denture Processing Center, Beijing, China

Keywords
CAD; complete dentures; baseplates; occlusal rims; three-dimensional (3D) digital edentulous models

Correspondence
Yanfeng Li, Department of Stomatology, First Affiliated Hospital of Chinese PLA General Hospital, No. 51, Fucheng Road, Haidian District, Beijing 100048, China.
E-mail: m.god@yeah.net

Authors Yanfeng Li and Weili Han contributed equally to this work.

All authors declare that they have no conflict of interest.

Accepted August 13, 2016

Published in *Journal of Prosthodontics* 2016; Vol. 00, pp. 1–8

doi: 10.1111/jopr.12554

ABSTRACT

The demand for complete dentures is expected to increase worldwide, but complete dentures are mainly designed and fabricated manually involving a broad series of clinical and laboratory procedures. Therefore, the quality of complete dentures largely depends on the skills of the dentist and technician, leading to difficulty in quality control. Computer-aided design and manufacturing (CAD/CAM) has been used to design and fabricate various dental restorations including dental inlays, veneers, crowns, partial crowns, and fixed partial dentures (FPDs). It has been envisioned that the application of CAD/CAM technology could reduce intensive clinical/laboratory work for the fabrication of complete dentures; however, CAD/CAM is seldom used to fabricate complete dentures due to the lack of suitable CAD software to design virtual complete dentures although the CAM techniques are in a much advanced stage. Here we report the successful design of virtual complete dentures using CAD software of 3Shape Dental System 2012, which was developed for designing fixed prostheses instead of complete dentures. Our results demonstrated that complete dentures could be successfully designed by the combination of two modeling processes, single coping and full anatomical FPD, available in the 3Shape Dental System 2012.

Edentulism remains a big public health problem in both developed countries due to population aging and developing countries due to poor oral care.[1] It has been estimated that the prevalence of edentulism is 26% in the United States, 15% to 78% in Europe, 24% in Indonesia, 11% in China, and 23% in Brazil among seniors.[2] Complete dentures are among the main dental prosthetic restorations for edentulous patients.[3,4] It is expected that the demand for complete dentures will continuously increase, despite an anticipated decrease in the age-specific rates of edentulism.[5–7]

Conventional design and fabrication of complete dentures involve a series of clinical and laboratory procedures.[8] Traditionally, five appointments are needed to make complete dentures, including preliminary impressions, final impressions, recording jaw relations, trial placement of wax denture, and placement/insertion of complete dentures. The design and fabrication of complete dentures are mainly performed manually involving a broad series of clinical and laboratory procedures. Therefore, the quality of the fabricated dentures is highly dependent on the skills of the dentist and technician, leading to difficulty in quality control.

Computer-aided design (CAD) has been extensively used to define the geometry of an object, while computer-aided manufacturing (CAM) has gained popularity in the fabrication process to transform raw materials into the specified object.[9,10] CAD/CAM has been extensively used to design and fabricate various dental restorations including dental inlays, veneers, crowns, partial crowns, and fixed partial dentures (FPDs).[10–12] CAD/CAM technology has apparent advantages over conventional methods in the design and fabrication of dental restorations, since fewer appointments are needed, and the procedures are simplified for better quality control.[13] It has been envisioned that the application of CAD/CAM technology could reduce intensive clinical/laboratory work for the fabrication of complete dentures; however, CAD/CAM is not widely used to fabricate complete dentures due to the lack of suitable CAD software. Only recently several commercial CAD software systems have become available for designing complete dentures, including AvaDent digital dentures (Global Dental Science, LLC, Scottsdale, AZ).[14–17] By using CAD/CAM technology, impressions, jaw relations, occlusal plane orientation, tooth mold and shade selection, and maxillary anterior tooth positioning could be finished in one patient visit for the fabrication of complete dentures.[18]

Here we report our attempts to design complete dentures using modeling processes available in 3Shape Dental System 2012 (3Shape A/S, Copenhagen, Denmark). The modeling processes in this CAD software were developed for the design of fixed prostheses, not complete dentures; however, we found that virtual complete dentures could be designed by combining the single coping and full anatomical FPD modeling processes based on 3D digital edentulous models by scanning the physical master cast, wax occlusal rims and baseplates (i.e., record bases) followed by alignment using point-to-point matching. To our best knowledge, this is the first study on the design of complete dentures by adopting CAD software developed for the design of fixed prostheses.

MATERIALS AND METHODS

Material and Equipment

The equipment included 3Shape D810 scanner with 15 μm accuracy (3Shape A/S) and Dell Optiplex 780 (Core 2 Duo E8400, cache 8G; Dell Inc., Round Rock, TX) with Windows 7 operating system and 3Shape Dental System 2012 CAD software. Dental alginate impression material and die-stone were purchased from Heraeus Kulzer (Hanau, Germany).

Generation of Physical Edentulous Master Cast, Wax Occlusal Rims, and Baseplates

A female edentulous patient with missing teeth for 30 years and order II alveolar ridge resorption (according to the classification proposed by Atwood[19] and Cawood and Howell[20]) was selected to obtain customized physical wax occlusal rims, baseplates, and master cast. Before the impression, the patient gave informed consent approved by the institutional review board. Alginate impression material was used to obtain the impression, after which the physical master cast, wax occlusal rims, and baseplates were produced as described previously.[9,13] The following information was recorded during the patient's visit: the vertical distance and horizontal jaw relations between the maxillary and mandibular jaws, occlusal plane position, fullness of anterior teeth, facial midline, cuspid line, high lip line, and lower lip line. To get an accurate occlusal plane and stable occlusal record, the occlusal plane of wax occlusal rims was lowered by 1 mm except for positions 17, 24, 27, 37, 34, and 47. Moreover, a 3-mm wax layer was evenly removed from the labial and buccal faces of physical wax occlusal rims to better observe the fullness of the arranged teeth.

Design of Virtual Complete Denture

We attempted to design virtual complete dentures by combining a single coping and full anatomical FPD, which were developed for designing a fixed prosthesis (Fig 1). In the first part of this approach, we initially generated the 3D digital edentulous models by scanning the physical master cast, wax occlusal rims, and baseplates followed by trimming and alignment. Then we treated each edentulous jaw as one single abutment tooth, and designed one single inner crown for each using the modeling process of single coping in the software, followed by presetting six abutment teeth on the alveolar ridge crest. In the second part of this approach, we designed the 7-7 full anatomical bridge using the modeling

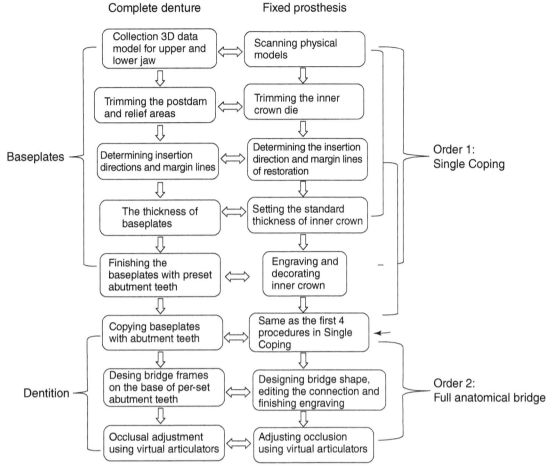

Complete denture   Fixed prosthesis

FIGURE 1   The procedure flowchart for designing fixed prosthesis using CAD and the corresponding procedures in the design of complete denture.

process of full anatomical bridge. By this approach, we successfully designed the virtual complete dentures from the 3D digital edentulous models (Fig 2).

Design Virtual Baseplates by Using the Modeling Process of Single Coping in Order 1

Trimming Maxillary and Mandibular 3D Digital Edentulous Models   Edentulous 3D digital models (data format STL) were obtained by scanning the maxillary and mandibular master cast, and spraying occlusal rims and baseplates using 3ShapeD810 scanner according to the manufacturer's instruction, followed by alignments using the point-to-point matching method (Fig 2). The modeling process of single coping included smoothening, removing, and adding. Small protrusions on the models were removed to make the model smooth. The maxillary zygomatic process, maxillary tuberosity, incisive papilla, maxillary hard palate, mandible external oblique ridge, and mandible mylohyoid ridge were then relieved according to the requirements for designing complete dentures. A line was drawn along the pterygomaxillary

notches and the points at 2 mm behind the fovea palatinae to reduce the thickness of the model. A bow shape was formed by gradually shallowing the area from this line to 5 mm before this line, in parallel to the mucosal surface of the palate.

Design Denture Base and Abutment Teeth   Each single edentulous jaw in the 3D digital models was treated as a single abutment tooth at position 16 for the maxilla or position 46 for the mandible to design an inner crown with a thickness of 2 mm (data format STL). The crown margin lines were designed to meet the requirement for complete dentures and form the base for complete dentures. In particular, the labial and buccal ended at the mucobuccal fold between the alveolar mucosa and the labial and buccal mucosa, and avoided the labial/buccal frenulum. The mandible ended at the lingual frenulum, thus avoiding the lingual frenulum, while the rear margin ends at 1/3 to 1/2 of retromolar pad. The rear margin of the maxilla ended at the line of pterygomaxillary notches and points at 2 mm behind the fovea palatinae. Abutment teeth were preset at six

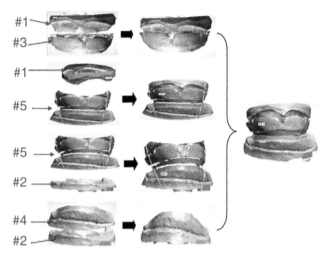

FIGURE 2 The process to generate 3D digital edentulous models for CAD, including separated 3D digital models of maxillary master cast (#1), mandibular master cast (#2), maxillary occlusal rim with maxillary baseplate (#3), mandibular occlusal rim with mandibular baseplate (#4), and maxillary occlusal rim with maxillary baseplate and mandibular occlusal rim with mandibular baseplate (#5).

points (16, 24, 26, 34, 36, and 46) on the alveolar ridge crest. The height at these positions was increased on the baseplates, and inner crowns were created at these positions via engraving (Fig 3).

Design Virtual Dentitions Using Full Anatomical Bridge in Order 2

The denture bases with preset abutment teeth designed in order 1 (Figs 3C and F) were copied into order 2 using the modeling process of full anatomical bridge. An FPD of 17 to 27 was created based on the abutment teeth at 16, 24, and 26;

an FPD of 37 to 47 was created based on abutment teeth at 34, 36, and 46. Quantitative movements of artificial teeth could be easily achieved in all directions by using 3Shape Dental System 2012. The arrangement of teeth was in the order of maxillary anterior teeth, mandibular anterior teeth, maxillary posterior teeth, and finally mandibular posterior teeth. The high points of labial surfaces for the anterior teeth were arranged to be on the labial surfaces of the customized occlusal rims.

In particular, the teeth were arranged in the order of $1_\perp 1$ (maxillary central incisor), $2_\perp 2$ (maxillary lateral incisor), $3_\perp 3$ (maxillary canine), $1^\top 1$ (maxillary central incisor), $2^\top 2$ (mandibular lateral incisor), $3^\top 3$ (mandibular canine), $4_\perp 4$ (mandibular first premolar), $5_\perp 5$ (maxillary second premolar), $6_\perp 6$ (maxillary first molar), and $7_\perp 7$ (maxillary second molar) according the standard protocols, except for the specification listed in Table 1. Finally, $4\text{-}7^\top 4\text{-}7$ teeth were arranged to establish the most extensive occlusal relationship with the maxillary posterior teeth.

Occlusal Adjustment The designed virtual complete dentures with master cast models were placed in the virtual articulators provided in 3Shape Dental System 2012 for adjusting the occlusal relationship via the movements of occlusion, laterotrusion, pro-/retrusion, and side shift. The articulator parameters were adjusted for Bennett L, Bennett R, Cond. incl. L, Cond. incl. R values. The interfering points were removed from the maxillary and mandibular dentitions using the function available in the software.

RESULTS

CAD software could facilitate fast and easy modeling of complex dental restorations and enable automatic

TABLE 1 **The position of teeth arranged in relation to the occlusal plane**

Teeth	Position in relation to the occlusal plane
$1_\perp 1$	Incisal edges are 1 mm below the occlusal plane of the customized occlusal rims.
$2_\perp 2$	Incisal edges are on the occlusal plane.
$3_\perp 3$	Cusp tips are 1 mm above the occlusal plane.
$1^\top 1$	Incisal edges are 2 mm above the occlusal plane.
$2^\top 2$	Incisal edges are 2 mm above the occlusal plane.
$3^\top 3$	Cusp tips are 2 mm above the occlusal plane.
$4_\perp 4$	Mesial fossa is in line with the alveolar ridge crest of mandibular posterior teeth, being 1 mm away from the occlusal plane; buccal cusps of 24 are 1 mm above the occlusal plane.
$5_\perp 5$	Lingual cusps are in line with the alveolar ridge crest of mandibular posterior teeth; lingual cusps and buccal cusps are 1 mm above the occlusal plane.
$6_\perp 6$	Lingual cusps are in line with the alveolar ridge crest of mandibular posterior teeth; mesiolingual (26) is 1 mm above the occlusal plane, distal cusps and mesiobuccal cusps are on the occlusal plane, and distobuccal cusps are 0.5 mm above the occlusal plane.
$7_\perp 7$	Lingual cusps are 1 mm above the occlusal plane, their mesiobuccal cusps are 2 mm above the occlusal plane, distobuccal cusps are 2.5 mm above the occlusal plane.

Note: Unless otherwise noted, the occlusal plane used later is the occlusal plane of the customized occlusal rims.

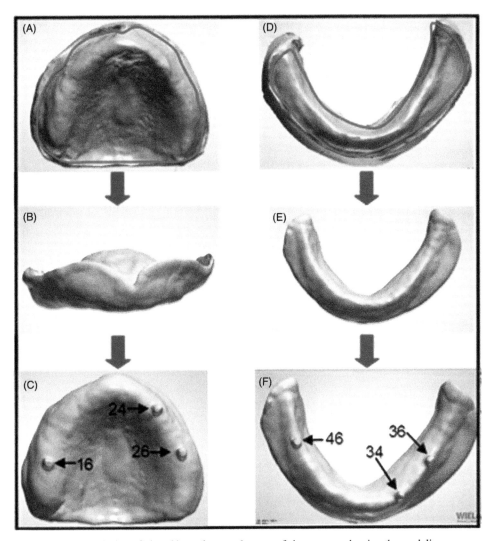

FIGURE 3 The design of virtual baseplates and preset of abutment teeth using the modeling process of single coping. (A) determining the margin line of maxillary baseplate; (B) designed maxillary baseplate; (C) abutment teeth preset on the maxillary baseplate; (D) determining the margin line of mandibular baseplate; (E) designed mandibular baseplate; (F) abutment teeth (16, 24, 26, 34, 36, and 46) preset on the mandibular baseplate.

manufacturing of a designed restoration model on computer-aided production equipment; however, we found no report on the methodology to design complete dentures using CAD systems developed for designing fixed prostheses. In this study, we utilized the single coping and full anatomical bridge available in the CAD software of 3Shape Dental System 2012 to design complete dentures. Figures 4 to 6 show the designed maxillary dentition on the maxillary baseplate, mandibular dentition on the mandibular baseplate, and the relationship of the virtual maxillary dentition and mandibular wax rim or virtual mandibular dentition and maxillary wax rim. Figure 7 shows the results from the adjustment procedures, with different colors indicating the contact regions for different movements. Finally, virtual

complete dentures (Figs 7C and F) were successfully designed according to the scheme shown in Figure 1; however, we failed to generate virtual complete dentures using any single modeling process available in the CAD software of 3Shape Dental System 2012, including full anatomical bridge, full anatomical crown, single coping, and bridge framework.

DISCUSSION

More than ten CAD/CAM systems have been made available for the design of fixed prostheses,[4] including FrameWork 3D (Siemens, Erfurt, Germany), Procera Software 2.0 (Nobel

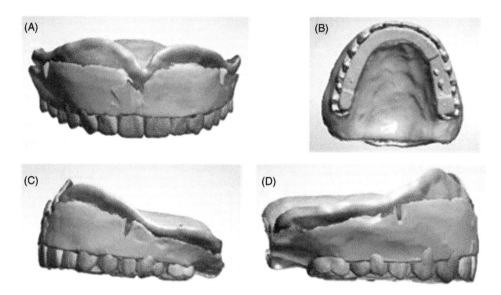

FIGURE 4 The front view (A), view from the occlusal plane (B), view from the left (C), and view from the right (D) for designed virtual maxillary dentition and wax rim.

Biocare, Kloten, Switzerland), Cercon Art CAD (Dentsply, York, PA), Cercon System, Lava Design 5.0 (3M ESPE, St. Paul, MN), Energy CAD (Kavo, Biberach, Germany), and some "self-assembled" open-end CAD/CAM systems. For those open-end systems, the data collection system, CAD system, and CAM system can be created by different companies and assembled into one whole system later. Currently, the two relatively mature open-end systems available on the market are: (1) 3Shape Dental special scanner + 3Shape CAD software + German mills, which can process all brands of zirconia and plastics; (2) 3Shape Dental special scanner

+ 3Shape CAD software + US 3D system wax machine, which can be used to embed cast metal and produce all-ceramic crowns after finishing wax-up. The open-end systems have advantages that extensive materials can be processed, and manufacturing cost is lower. 3Shape Dental System 2012 has been proven to be suitable for the repair and implanting of various fixed prostheses, and the design of removable partial dentures. In this study we aimed to investigate the feasibility of using the modeling processes in 3Shape Dental System 2012 developed for designing fixed prostheses to design virtual complete dentures.

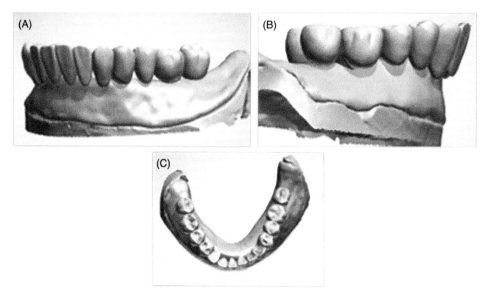

FIGURE 5 The view from the left (A), view from the right (B) and view from the occlusal plane (C) for designed virtual mandibular dentition and wax rim.

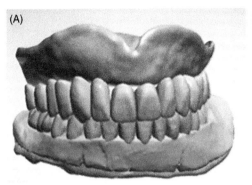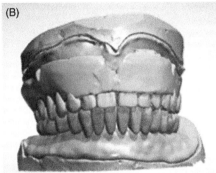

FIGURE 6 The virtual maxillary dentition and mandibular wax rim (A), and virtual mandibular dentition and maxillary wax rim (B).

We initially tried to generate virtual edentulous 3D digital models by direct scanning the patient's mouth, but it was time consuming, and it was difficult to reconstruct the 3D digital edentulous models. Therefore, 3D digital edentulous models used for CAD were obtained via indirect method. The modeling processes for fixed prostheses do not directly support the determination of relative positions of complete maxillary/mandibular edentulous jaws. Three-dimensional noncontact laser scanner 3Shape D810 was used to scan the physical master cast and wax occlusal rims with baseplates to obtain five separate 3D digital models of the maxillary master cast (#1), mandibular master cast (#2), maxillary occlusal rim with maxillary baseplate (#3), mandibular occlusal rim with mandibular baseplate (#4), and maxillary occlusal rim with maxillary baseplate and mandibular occlusal rim with mandibular baseplate (#5) (Fig 2). A point-by-point matching approach was used to match model #1 and model #3, model #1 and model #5, model #2 and model #5, and model #2 and model #4. After the matching, complete 3D digital models were obtained for use in CAD with the relative position relationship of the maxillary and mandibular jaws (Fig 3).

The CAD system of 3Shape Dental System 2012 contains 19 scanning and modeling processes for scanning physical models and designing dental restorations, including single coping, bridge framework, full anatomical crown, and full anatomical bridge. We investigated the feasibility of using a single modeling process such as single coping, bridge framework, full anatomical crown, or full anatomical bridge, and one combination of two single modeling processes of single coping and full anatomical bridge for complete denture design. Our results showed that only the approach of combining two single modeling processes is feasible for designing a virtual complete denture (Fig 7). In this approach, we used single coping to design the baseplates, meeting the requirement for complete denture design. Six abutment teeth were then preset on the baseplates at positions 16, 24, 26, 34, 36, and 46 to enhance the bonding of dentition to the baseplate (Fig 3). Based on the models designed using single

coping, we further used full anatomical bridge to design a 17 to 27 FPD for the maxillary dentition based on the abutment teeth of 16, 24, and 26, and a 37 to 47 FPD for the mandibular dentition based on the abutment teeth of 34, 36, and 46. Virtual teeth were arranged for the maxillary and mandibular dentitions. Denture bases and abutment teeth would be made of red resin, while the FPDs would be made of white resin. Thus, locating abutment teeth at the area of posterior teeth is suitable for better esthetics. Moreover, in this way the abutment teeth could be engraved slightly smaller, with smaller margins for the inner crown than for the full anatomical outer crown, thus compensating some position inaccuracies caused by abutment teeth.

CAD software of 3Shape Dental System 2012 contains some well-known articulators including 3Shape Generic, Sam2p, KaVo PROTAR evo, Denar Mark 330, ACR (Artex compatible), supporting occlusion, laterotrusion, pro-/retrusion, and side shift with adjustment parameters. Different colors could be used to indicate the contact regions for different movements (Figs 7A and D). The virtual articulation provides a complete articulation both automatically and precisely, thus saving time by reducing manual work.

The CAD of virtual complete dentures was completed after the occlusal adjustment to obtain the final virtual complete dentures (Figs 7C and F). In this study, our major goal was to demonstrate the feasibility of designing virtual complete dentures for patients using CAD developed for fixed prostheses, 3Shape Dental System 2012, and thus did not actually fabricate the physical complete dentures from the designed virtual complete dentures; however, the designed virtual complete dentures could be exported from 3Shape Dental System 2012 to a CAM software, and then used to guide the fabrication of physical complete dentures through computerized numerical control.[21] Either additive manufacturing such 3D printing or subtractive manufacturing such as milling and cutting could be used to fabricate the physical complete dentures, depending on the materials used for the denture.[22,23]

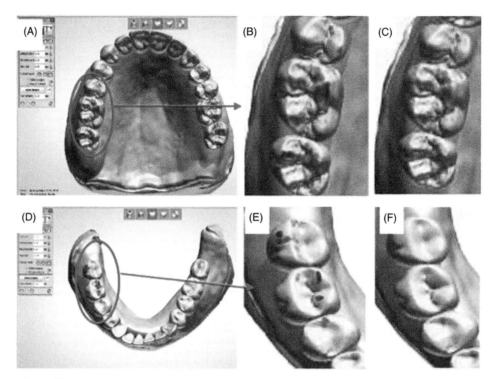

FIGURE 7   The detection of interfering points and subsequent removal of interfering points. (A) detected interfering points in maxillary jaw; (B) the enlarged image of the red cycle in A; (C) interference points removed from B; (D) detected interfering points in maxillary jaw; (E) the enlarged image of the red cycle in D; (F) interference points removed from B.

CONCLUSIONS

Our study demonstrated that virtual complete dentures could be successfully designed using a combination of two single modeling processes: single coping and full anatomical bridge, available in 3Shape Dental System 2012. To our best knowledge, this is the first report that complete dentures could be designed by selecting the modeling processes in CAD software developed for the complete denture design.

REFERENCES

1. Polzer I, Schimmel M, Muller F, et al: Edentulism as part of the general health problems of elderly adults. *Int Dent J* 2010;60: 143–155.

2. Paulino MR, Alves LR, Gurgel BC, et al: Simplified versus traditional techniques for complete denture fabrication: a systematic review. *J Prosthet Dent* 2015;113:12–16.

3. Bidra AS, Taylor TD, Agar JR: Computer-aided technology for fabricating complete dentures: systematic review of historical background, current status, and future perspectives. *J Prosthet Dent* 2013;109:361–366.

4. Sun Y, Lu P, Wang Y: Study on CAD&RP for removable complete denture. *Comput Methods Programs Biomed* 2009;93:266–272.

5. Carlsson GE, Omar R: The future of complete dentures in oral rehabilitation. A critical review. *J Oral Rehabil* 2010;37:143–156.

6. Douglass CW, Shih A, Ostry L: Will there be a need for complete dentures in the United States in 2020? *J Prosthet Dent* 2002;87:5–8.

7. Alfadda SA: The relationship between various parameters of complete denture quality and patients' satisfaction. *J Am Dent Assoc* 2014;145:941–948.

8. Cunha TR, Della Vecchia MP, Regis RR, et al: A randomised trial on simplified and conventional methods for complete denture fabrication: masticatory performance and ability. *J Dent* 2013;41:133–142.

9. Goodacre CJ, Garbacea A, Naylor WP, et al: CAD/CAM fabricated complete dentures: concepts and clinical methods of obtaining required morphological data. *J Prosthet Dent* 2012;107:34–46.

10. Davidowitz G, Kotick PG: The use of CAD/CAM in dentistry. *Dent Clin North Am* 2011;55:559–570.

11. van Noort R: The future of dental devices is digital. *Dent Mater* 2012;28:3–12.

12. Pascu N-E, Dobrescu T, Opran C, et al: Realistic scenes in CAD application. *Proc Eng* 2014;69:304–309.

13. Infante L, Yilmaz B, McGlumphy E, et al: Fabricating complete dentures with CAD/CAM technology. *J Prosthet Dent* 2014; 111:351–355.

14. Maeda Y, Minoura M, Tsutsumi S, et al: A CAD/CAM system for removable denture. Part I: fabrication of complete dentures. *Int J Prosthodont* 1994;7:17–21.

15. Li Y, Lv Y, Lu Y, et al: Design and finite element analysis of a novel sliding rod microscrew implantation device for mandibular prognathism. *Int J Clin Exp Med* 2015;8:10687–10695.

16. Bi Y, Wu S, Zhao Y, et al: A new method for fabricating orbital prosthesis with a CAD/CAM negative mold. *J Prosthet Dent* 2013;110:424–428.

17. Yamamoto S, Kanazawa M, Iwaki M, et al: Effects of offset values for artificial teeth positions in CAD/CAM complete denture. *Comput Biol Med* 2014;52:1–7.

18. McLaughlin JB, Ramos, Jr. V: Complete denture fabrication with CAD/CAM record bases. *J Prosthet Dent* 2015;114:493–497.

19. Atwood DA: Postextraction changes in the adult mandible as illustrated by microradiographs of midsagittal sections and serial cephalometric roentgenograms. *J Prosthet Dent* 1963;13:810–824.

20. Cawood JI, Howell RA: A classification of the edentulous jaws. *Int J Oral Maxillofac Surg* 1988;17:232–236.

21. Bidra AS, Taylor TD, Agar JR: Computer-aided technology for fabricating complete dentures: Systematic review of historical background, current status, and future perspectives. *J Prosthet Dent* 2013;109:361–366.

22. Abduo J, Lyons K, Bennamoun M: Trends in computer-aided manufacturing in prosthodontics: a review of the available streams. *Int J Dent* 2014;2014:783948.

23. Choi JW, Kim N: Clinical application of three-dimensional printing technology in craniofacial plastic surgery. *Arch Plast Surg* 2015;42:267–277.

19

TREATMENT OF EDENTULISM: OPTIMIZING OUTCOMES WITH TISSUE MANAGEMENT AND IMPRESSION TECHNIQUES

THOMAS J. SALINAS, DDS, FACP
Associate Professor, Department of Dental Specialties, Mayo Clinic, Rochester, MN

Keywords
Edentulism; tissue conditioning; impression; selective pressure; functional impression; base adaptation; patient outcome; denture adhesive

Correspondence
Thomas J. Salinas, Mayo Clinic, Department of Dental Specialties, 200 1st St. SW, Rochester, MN 55905.
E-mail: Salinas.thomas@mayo.edu

Presented as part of the FDI 2008 World Dental Congress: "Facing the Future of Edentulism: 21st Century Management of Edentulism—A World of Challenges in a Universe of Helpful Technologies." September 26, 2008, Stockholm, Sweden.

Accepted August 29, 2008

Published in *Journal of Prosthodontics* 2009; Vol. 18, pp. 97–105

doi: 10.1111/j.1532-849X.2009.00438.x

ABSTRACT

Significant numbers of patients throughout the world seek treatment for edentulism. The trend toward tissue-integrated prostheses has been a monumental step in restoring edentulous patients to function; however, this treatment can be out of reach for those who fail to qualify or those who do not have sufficient resources to afford it. In these cases, conventional dentures remain an important primary course of treatment. Attention to detail when diagnosing, treatment planning, and performing treatment for these patients is still a prime consideration for the best possible outcome. In particular, many experienced denture wearers are afflicted with chronically inflamed denture-bearing mucosa. Clinicians must recognize the need for tissue conditioning, choices of impression materials, and accepted fabrication techniques that can have favorable outcomes when matched with patients who are philosophical and realistic in their expectations. The purpose of this article is to review impression philosophies, associated materials, and methods of tissue conditioning. Retention and stability of the denture bases can be augmented by the routine use of denture adhesive, and indications for use of denture adhesive will be discussed.

Edentulous patients often seek treatment for replacement of their missing teeth for improvements in esthetics, function, and speech. According to recent studies, the incidence of edentulism worldwide has shown a decline, and the demand for treatment may be different than what it was several decades ago.[1–5] Despite this decline, however, there will be an increase in those adults in the United States who will need at least one or two complete dentures by the year 2020.[6] Further, there will be significant need for these patients to maintain their complete dentures due to residual ridge resorption phenomenon and material wear.

Successful outcomes of complete denture therapy have been associated with three variables: pretreatment expectations, satisfaction with the dental care received, and mental health.[7] Many patients who seek treatment for edentulism may fall into one of several personality classifications as described by House[8] and more recently by Gamer et al.[9] As a result of these classifications, patients and practitioners alike can be placed into one of several divisions based on their expectations from past treatment with complete dentures. Many patients who seek treatment for edentulism have realistic expectations in their ability to eat foods they desire, the esthetics they desire to achieve, and their overall psychologic improvement.[10] The ACP classification of edentulism is based primarily on anatomic factors and other modifiers to arrive at a diagnostic index.[11] With questionnaires and evaluations, it is important for clinicians to quantify the patient's level of satisfaction with his/her current prostheses as a predictor of the treatment outcome.[12] This can facilitate arriving at a diagnosis that aids in developing a prognosis when considering differential treatment. In fact, just the ability to masticate comfortably with newly fabricated dentures often leads to a more favorable result based on a patient's own perceptions.[13] From a predictive standpoint, this has been validated with a screening questionnaire that identifies which type of patient may benefit from such intervention;[14] however, some patients are maladaptive in their ability to tolerate conventional removable prosthodontic treatment and may require more advanced treatments.[15] The advent of osseointegration has vastly improved the outcome related to treating edentulous patients;[16] however, the treatment requirements involved with using an osseointegration protocol may preclude some patients from participating. Additionally, the resources needed to provide even simplistic implant treatment may be out of reach financially for many patients. In some circumstances, osseointegrated implants in augmented jaws when compared to the results with newly fabricated conventional complete dentures do not always lead to a superior patient-perceived improvement over complete denture wear.[17] Therefore, the use of conventional denture treatment is the mainstay of treatment for many of these patients.

Human life expectancy has significantly increased over the last several decades,[18,19] resulting in many elderly patients medically managed with a myriad of pharmacologic regimens.[20,21] As such, many of these patients have drug interactions and drug side effects, which may predispose their oral environments to xerostomia. Dry mouth coupled with compromised denture-bearing tissues may render complete dentures intolerable. Even the most carefully selected patient and meticulous attention to technique may be insufficient to surpass the difficulties encountered with salivary dysfunction. Assuming proper adaptation of the denture base is obtained, the routine use of denture adhesives in xerostomic patients can help augment denture base contact with oral mucosa.[22]

HISTORICAL APPROACH TO DENTURE FABRICATION-DEFINITIVE IMPRESSIONS

Approaches to treating edentulous patients have been outlined over the last century and formed the foundation of philosophies for occlusion,[23,24] esthetics,[25–27] mandibular movement,[28] maxillofacial prosthodontics,[29,30] and other subdisciplines of prosthodontics.[31] These focus areas are all fundamental to complete denture fabrication, contributing their unique importance to the entire treatment. The impression technique has been a large area of focus due to its special consideration specific to each case.[32–34] It may be agreed upon that materials influenced impression techniques in the past, despite the criticism that this is an empiric approach.[35,36] Many impression materials have specific applications based on their unique properties. Conversely, as impression philosophy has changed and developed, concurrent development and application of newer materials have also taken place. The treatment of edentulous patients has historically undertaken a standard technique whereby the type of impression subscribes to one of several impression philosophies.[37]

The selective pressure technique has a long history of development, with impressions being made with vegetable or inorganic-based materials as far back as in the 1700s.[38] Frequently, a wash of wax, gutta-percha, or plaster was made inside a primary impression made with modeling plastic compound.[39,40] Some of these concepts were advocated by the Green Brothers in 1907 and were considered a significant advance in impression making.[41] Distinctions were made for maxillary and mandibular impressions, as it was recognized that there were significant differences between the two.[42,43] It was realized early on that excessive pressure applied to the edentulous maxilla could create significant tissue distortion. Therefore, a portion of the primary impression was removed to create space for secondary impression material that alleviated pressure created during the first phase of the impression. A variant of this technique was to create a vacuum on the tissue side using low-fusing material such as Adaptol (Kaye Research

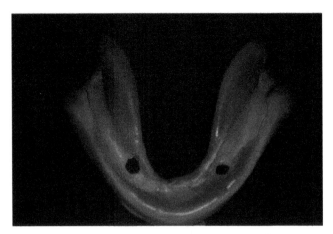

FIGURE 1   Border-molded custom tray with Adaptol® material to achieve peripheral seal.

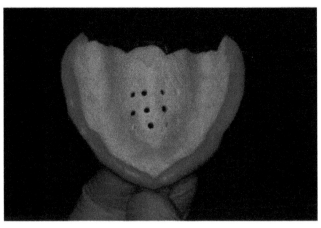

FIGURE 3   Border-molded custom tray using Iso Functional® material to capture peripheral tissues.

Laboratories, Ashaway, RI) to border-mold and create an effective seal (Figs 1, 2).[44] These techniques all used an open-mouth approach for creating a border seal with selectively directed pressure areas. More recent descriptions of border-molding techniques advocate the use of either polyether material or heavy body vinylpolysiloxane.[45,46] Border molding with heavy consistency polyether material has been suggested as an easier technique than impression modeling compound as its flow and temperature requirements are better achieved without overextending the base or potentially damaging tissue with superheated material. Additionally, polyether can be easily shaped or added to for modification after it has been formed. Other materials such as Iso Functional (GC Corporation, Tokyo, Japan) (Figs 3, 4) can provide this functional molding of the denture borders without trauma or undue tissue distortion. A properly extended custom tray is needed that is 2 to 4 mm short of full extension to accommodate space for border-molding materials. With the use of

carefully constructed and bordermolded custom trays, these steps are also achievable and result in a predictable outcome. Most of these techniques are applied in some fashion for obtaining impressions of edentulous arches today[47,48] (Figs 5, 6).

The mucostatic technique was discussed some years ago by Page[49] and was largely controversial due to its nonuniformity of application.[50] Mucostatic impressions were based on the use of recording materials that duplicated the tissues in a passive state. The borders of the dentures were also confined to only the stress-bearing mucosal areas, and were not refined to make a border seal.[44] The choices of impression material in these cases were thin zinc oxide eugenol pastes that accurately recorded the denture-bearing areas.

Although somewhat similar in principle to the mucostatic technique, the pressure-less or minimal pressure technique was different in tray design and choice of impression material. Light to heavy body elastomeric materials caused tissue displacement phenomena and could be anticipated to cause

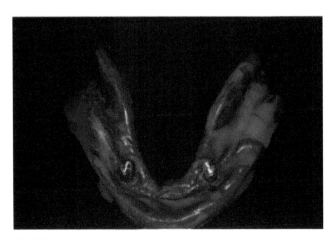

FIGURE 2   Secondary wash impression with polyether impression material. Implant analogs are in place.

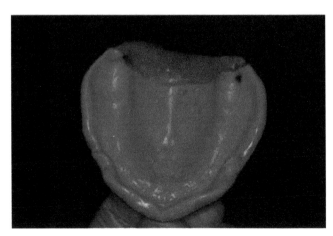

FIGURE 4   Secondary impression with vinylpolysiloxane material.

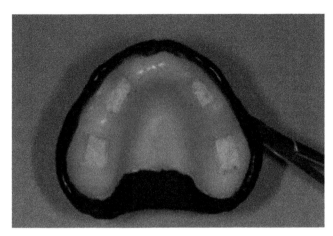

FIGURE 5 Border-molded impression tray with plastic modeling compound.

some distortion with their use.[37] The use of alternative materials such as thin mixes of alginate or zinc oxide eugenol pastes generated less pressure based on their flow properties.[51] Custom tray design has been suggested to include relief and escape holes to aid in reducing the pressures generated during the impression.[52] These combined features can reduce the pressures by almost half what is encountered without these features;[51] however, other studies do not support this finding and depict more of the choice of material used as a correlation of pressure generation.[53]

FUNCTIONAL IMPRESSIONS

Impressions can also be made with a closed-mouth technique, including a functional impression protocol that uses patients' musculature in stabilizing a record base or occlusion rim. This philosophy was introduced in the early 1900s[54] and often used wax,[55] modeling plastic compound, or more

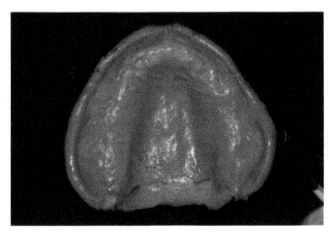

FIGURE 6 Rubber base secondary impression with functional use of mouth temperature wax to create a functional posterior palatal seal.

recently, tissueconditioning material. As described later, many experienced denture wearers have some degree of alveolar resorption with some associated abused tissue. In these cases, the use of tissue conditioning material may compensate for these changes, occlusally stabilize the denture base, and obtain an impression simultaneously. This has been an adjunct in achieving healthy tissues, while obtaining a functionally accurate impression. To properly use the closed-mouth technique, well-fitting record bases, accurately occluding rims, and an acceptable vertical dimension is needed.[56] This technique may also be used for reline impressions of existing complete dentures and may be used with a linear or a branched denture construction technique. A linear technique is well understood and commences with recording of the tissues with impressions, recording centric position and eccentric pathways, trial tooth arrangements, and insertion procedures. A branched technique includes the use of a diagnostic prosthesis to accommodate for tongue thrusting habits, maxillomandibular discrepancies and other scenarios that create difficulties in obtaining comfort and function with complete dentures.[57] This diagnostic prosthesis aids in making the functional impression and gives indication if the patient can comfortably function. The functional impression is inclusive within the branched technique and is effective in achieving an accurate recording in relation to stable occlusal relationships.

The use of functional impression material, such as a tissue conditioner, in its flowable state, accurately records the tissues in a functional state. These soft acrylic resins do not set hard. They have properties that allow them to flow when forces are placed upon them, optimizing the shape and distribution of the material dependent upon the functional displacement of the tissue beneath the denture base. Some tissue conditioners have extended periods of flow, conforming to tissues during several hours of eating, speaking, and swallowing. After a suitable evaluation period of several days, the patient returns, the denture base is inspected for retention and stability, and, if satisfactory, it is invested and cast in newly polymerized acrylic resin[57,58] (Fig 7).

Other products have been introduced recently, including anatomically correct impression trays, which can be modified by the use of heat molding, adaptation, and refinement with elastomeric materials. With repeated practice, the use of these trays can allow for a definitive impression to be accomplished in a single visit.[59]

These impression philosophies may also be considered for edentulous patients treated with dental implants. Dependent upon the number of implants, these patients should be treated differently in that the majority of the load may be supported by dental implants. In implant-retained or -supported prostheses, high pressure areas can be adjusted, or the attachment mechanisms modified without significant loss of retention. This is not the case for conventional complete denture impressions where extended coverage and intimate

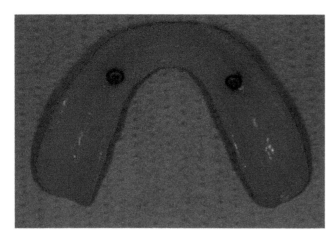

FIGURE 7   Tissue surface of functional impression/tissue conditioning with modified soft acrylic resin. Note matrix portion of stud attachment without intervening material.

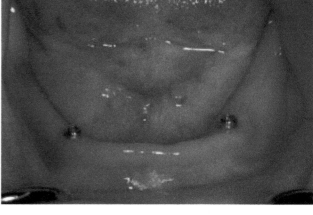

FIGURE 8   Patient treated for excessive pressure mucositis at day 1. Note erythema and edematous tissue surrounding and between the abutments.

base adaptation are essential to stability and retention. Complete but judicious extension of the impression into all possible supportive and retentive areas is the goal for conventional complete denture impression techniques.

TISSUE CONDITIONING

Understanding complete denture prostheses mandates an understanding of residual ridge resorption. It is also imperative that patients understand that residual ridge resorption is inevitable, and prostheses need to be modified appropriately to compensate for these changes on a timely, recurring basis. Residual ridge resorption has been reported and discussed by Tallgren,[60] Atwood,[61,62] and others.[63,64]

In light of changes inherent in edentulous jaws, continued use of complete dentures without prosthetic compensation (i.e., relining or rebase procedures) can result in significantly abused tissues. One of the key physical findings identifying abused tissues is the recognition of surface texture and color. Mobile tissues are especially susceptible to injury and are often found in anterior areas where combination syndrome has been identified.[65] Other commonly damaged areas are tissues in a chronic excessive state of positive or negative pressure (Figs 8–10). This diseased soft tissue state can be associated with overdentures where implants or natural teeth have been used as abutments. Some circumstances can precipitate formation of abused tissues in edentulous jaws:

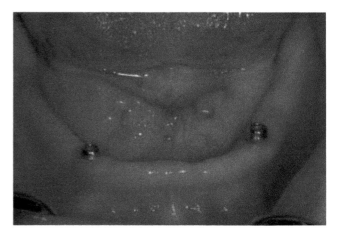

FIGURE 9   This image demonstrates partial resolution of erythema after tissue conditioner was applied 48 hours previously.

1. Tissues recorded with a nonactive impression protocol
2. Denture wear has traumatized the supporting tissues
3. Chronic infection
4. Poor denture base adaptation.

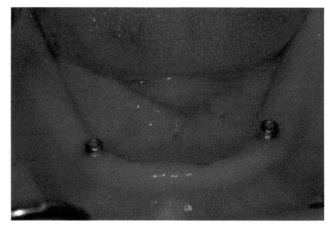

FIGURE 10   This image shows progress at 5 days. Note decreased tissue height around the abutments.

To reverse inflamed tissues to a state of health, the tissues will often benefit from conditioning techniques. From the work of Lytle[66] and others,[67,68] it is important to understand that conditioning may favorably change the edentulous tissues in a way so that complete dentures may be successfully worn. Impressions of healthy tissues will be beneficial to maintaining health.

To accomplish tissue conditioning, it is preferable to use soft acrylic resin polymers, although zinc oxide eugenol pastes and silicone impression materials have also been suggested.[69,70] Uniform reduction of the intaglio denture surface (1 to 2 mm) should create sufficient space for the material. This can be done with a marking pen and depth cutting bur to insure uniformity. Modified acrylic resin materials are composed of conventional poly-methyl methacrylate (PMMA) beads and a liquid preparation of ester and ethyl alcohol. When mixed, these substances gel and become resilient. In time, the alcohol evaporates, and the material becomes progressively harder. To maintain the softness and conditioning effect of the material, it is important to change all the material every 3 to 4 days.[71,72] One way to minimize this hardening phenomenon is to preserve resiliency by sealing it with a surface coating agent such as J-305 monopoly syrup (Factor II, Inc., Lakeside AZ) or Microseal (Kay See dental, Kansas City, MO).[73] These materials are light cured after application to slow the evaporation of alcohols and keep the material resilient, thereby conditioning the underlying tissues longer. Although objectionable to many patients, a more expedient tissue response is seen when the dentures are completely removed from use. A slower response is seen when the soft tissue conditioning technique described above is used over 10 to 14 days.[74]

IMPROVING FIT TO UNDERLYING TISSUES

Due to the polymerization shrinkage associated with PMMA resin, adaptation of the intaglio surface of complete dentures may have uneven pressure distribution. To ensure uniform pressure distribution, using a processed acrylic resin denture base has been advocated.[75,76] Also, the use of this technique in incrementalizing contraction of acrylic resin leads to greater occlusal accuracy upon processing. Jacob and Yen[77] and others[78–80] have popularized this technique in conventional and maxillofacial prosthetic cases and have produced fewer occlusal processing errors and improved the level of fit. The use of clear acrylic resin bases allows a better assessment on the fit of these bases covering tissues or implant substructures. The use of light-cured urethane dimethacrylate bases has recently become available (Eclipse™, Dentsply, York, PA) and can expedite the processing time and result in more intimate adaptation between the denture base and the underlying supporting tissues.[81] Additionally, this material shows a higher

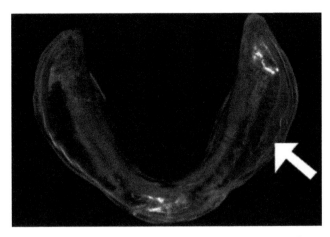

FIGURE 11   Occlusal view of a clear denture base to be used as a definitive denture base. Note the finish line for secondary addition of acrylic resin.

transverse strength than conventional heat-processed acrylic resins[82] (Fig 11).

Processing techniques are another consideration for improvement of fit and material quality of complete dentures. The biggest discrepancy in denture construction appears to be that of the acrylic resin processing. The classic use of compression molding acrylic resin has been well accepted for the last 70 years.[83,84] In recent years, it has been shown that injection molding techniques can improve the level of fit and adaptation of processed acrylic resin to the underlying stone cast.[85] Such injection molding techniques allow less dimensional change upon processing, thereby improving adaptation of the denture base to the underlying tissues. Craig has cited that linear dimensional change of acrylic resin approximates 6%.[86] Comparisons of the accuracy of compression and injection molding have been disputed over the years;[87,88] however, the most recent data indicate that injection molding is better than compression molding.[89–91] Although residual monomer content in injection molding is said to be similar to that of compression molding techniques, this may be more related to the length of processing rather than the technique itself.[92] Injection molding techniques, however, do not lend themselves to use in reline procedures, which are best accomplished by compression molding.

IMPROVING PATIENT ACCEPTANCE

The use of denture adhesives has been met with mixed reception from practitioners, but most agree that denture adhesives can be used as a helpful adjunct to conventional complete denture treatment.[93] Assuming proper denture construction and optimal fit to healthy tissues, denture adhesives have several indications.

Denture adhesives:

1. can be used for stabilization of trial denture bases and immediate dentures
2. may assist xerostomic patients with complete denture wear[94]
3. may help mentally handicapped or elderly patients with adapting to and using new complete dentures
4. can stabilize dentures against newly rehabilitated jaws with osseointegrated implants, and tissue-supported removable partial dentures.[22,95,96]

Contraindications for using denture adhesives are primarily ill-fitting prostheses.[22] Concern for masking underlying pathology may be an important contraindication for using denture adhesives as changes in denture base adaptation to the edentulous tissues should be suspect. As with other modes of therapy, regular care and discretionary follow-up are suggested.

The appropriate application of denture adhesive has been suggested to be in small pea-sized increments distributed throughout the denture base, as needed based on retention or lack thereof (Fig 12). This helps establish guidelines that may prevent overuse and excessive intake of material.[97] Zinc additions to denture adhesives were introduced in the 1980s to increase adhesive properties.[22] The effect of zinc copper depletion has been potentially implicated with neurological disease, where significant overuse and ingestion of the material is suspected.[98] Patients treated for this problem benefited from copper supplementation and cessation of denture adhesive use.

The use of patient-based outcomes can be further enhanced with custom tinting acrylic resin denture bases. Custom-tinted denture bases tend to yield a more realistic representation of soft tissue color and potentially better acceptance of the dentures. Incremental additions of tinted acrylic resin with the use of custom characterization kits (Candulor, USA, Inc., Los Angeles, CA) and the present-day

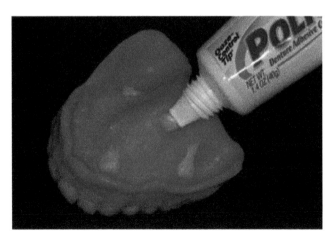

FIGURE 12 Suggested application of denture adhesive to the intaglio surface of a maxillary denture that minimizes excessive use.

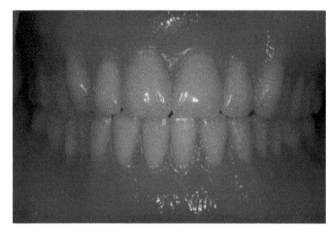

FIGURE 13 Clinical images of complete dentures in centric occlusion. These dentures have been fabricated with the traditional processing technique to produce color and surface texture.

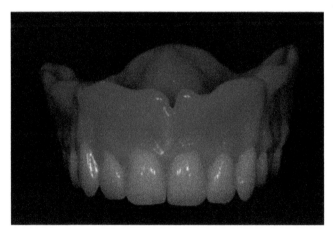

FIGURE 14 Maxillary complete denture fabricated with a characterized tinted denture to simulate soft tissues. (Courtesy Robert E. Kreyer, CDT).

selection of esthetic denture teeth have transcended the traditional denture acrylic resin red fiber appearance and provides patients with more natural esthetics (Figs 13, 14).[99]

CONCLUSIONS

Treatment of edentulous patients with specific impression techniques is often a topic of discussion when considering complete dentures for treating edentulous patients. To increase the prognosis for favorable outcomes, it is important that the appropriate patient personality be identified to understand realistic outcomes and limitations of treatment. Second, it is also critical to assess tissue health and determine if a conventional linear sequence of denture construction will be appropriate. Impression techniques can be selected based on the present state of basal tissue support; for instance, firm tissues may be well recorded with a spaced custom tray using elastomeric material. The use of processed denture bases where there is compromised support, significant maxillomandibular discrepancy, and neuromuscular deficits may enhance the recording of centric relation and minimize occlusal processing errors. Contemporary materials and processing techniques also optimize the chances of providing patients with well-constructed, well-fitting prostheses. Additionally, attention to esthetics with custom base tinting and realistic tooth selection can help optimize patient acceptance of treatment. The routine use of denture adhesives with specific indications has also been advocated to have an augmentative role in optimizing retention and stability of the complete denture prostheses.

TIPS FOR THE PRACTICING DENTIST

1. For patients who are wearing complete dentures requiring refabrication, ensure soft tissue health by serially relining with a 10- to 14-day period of conditioning with soft acrylic resin every 3 to 4 days. Alternatively, patients should leave their dentures out of the mouth for 48 hours prior to impressioning.

2. Use border-molded custom trays with relief for non-load-bearing tissues to record tissues in a state of displacement for selective pressure distribution. The choice of an elastomeric material should be based on flow properties and relative surface area to be recorded. For example, high flow materials should be used for the edentulous maxilla, and higher viscosity materials should be used for the mandible.

3. Where sufficient interarch distance exists, it is suggested to use injection-molded processed bases to aid in obtaining accurate interocclusal registration, decreased occlusal errors, and improved base adaptation. Insertion steps for complete dentures should follow laboratory and clinical remount verification procedures to minimize clinical impact of processing errors along with standard adaptation assessment with pressure indicating mediums.

REFERENCES

1. Osterberg T, Carlsson GE, Sundh V, et al: Number of teeth-a predictor of mortality in 70-year-old subjects. *Community Dent Oral Epidemiol* 2008;36:258–268.
2. Dye BA, Tan S, Smith V, et al: Trends in oral health status: United States, 1988–1994 and 1999–2004. *Vital Health Stat* 2007;248:1–92.
3. Chattopadhyay A, Arevalo O, Cecil JC, 3rd: Kentucky's oral health indicators and progress towards healthy people 2010 objectives. *J Ky Med Assoc* 2008;106:165–174.
4. Armour BS, Swanson M, Waldman HB, et al: A profile of state-level differences in the oral health of people with and without disabilities, in the U.S., in 2004. *Public Health Rep* 2008;123:67–75.
5. Zitzmann NU, Hagmann E, Weiger R: What is the prevalence of various types of prosthetic dental restorations in Europe? *Clin Oral Implants Res* 2007;18(Suppl 3):20–33.
6. Douglass CW, Shih A, Ostry L: Will there be a need for complete dentures in the United States in 2020? *J Prosthet Dent* 2002;87:5–8.
7. Diehl RL, Foerster U, Sposetti VJ, et al: Factors associated with successful denture therapy. *J Prosthodont* 1996;5:84–90.
8. House M: Full denture technique. In Conley FJ, Dunn AL, Quesnell AJ, et al (eds): *Classic Prosthodontic Articles: A Collector's Item*. Chicago, IL, American College of Prosthodontists, 1978.
9. Gamer S, Tuch R, Garcia LT: M. M. House mental classification revisited: intersection of particular patient types and particular dentist's needs. *J Prosthet Dent* 2003;89:297–302.
10. Lechner SK, Roessler D: Strategies for complete denture success: beyond technical excellence. *Compend Contin Educ Dent* 2001;22:553–559; quiz 60.
11. McGarry TJ, Nimmo A, Skiba JF, et al: Classification system for complete edentulism. *J Prosthodont* 1999;8:27–39.
12. Awad MA, Shapiro SH, Lund JP, et al: Determinants of patients' treatment preferences in a clinical trial. *Community Dent Oral Epidemiol* 2000;28:119–125.
13. Garrett NR, Kapur KK, Perez P: Effects of improvements of poorly fitting dentures and new dentures on patient satisfaction. *J Prosthet Dent* 1996;76:403–413.
14. Allen PF, McMillan AS, Walshaw D: A patient-based assessment of implant-stabilized and conventional complete dentures. *J Prosthet Dent* 2001;85:141–147.
15. Zarb GA, Schmitt A: The longitudinal clinical effectiveness of osseointegrated dental implants: the Toronto Study. Part II: the prosthetic results. *J Prosthet Dent* 1990;64:53–61.
16. Adell R, Lekholm U, Rockler B, et al: A 15-year study of osseointegrated implants in the treatment of the edentulous jaw. *Int J Oral Surg* 1981;10:387–416.
17. Kimoto K, Garrett NR: Effect of mandibular ridge height on patients' perceptions with mandibular conventional and implant-assisted overdentures. *Int J Oral Maxillofac Implants* 2005;20:762–768.

18. Minino AM, Heron MP, Smith BL: Deaths: preliminary data for 2004. *Natl Vital Stat Rep* 2006;54:1–49.

19. Hoyert DL, Heron MP, Murphy SL, et al: Deaths: final data for 2003. *Natl Vital Stat Rep* 2006;54:1–120.

20. Carter LM, McHenry ID, Godlington FL, et al: Prescribed medication taken by patients attending general dental practice: changes over 20 years. *Br Dent J* 2007;203:E8; discussion 200–201.

21. Jainkittivong A, Aneksuk V, Langlais RP: Medical health and medication use in elderly dental patients. *J Contemp Dent Pract* 2004;5:31–41.

22. Grasso JE: Denture adhesives. *Dent Clin North Am* 2004;48: 721–733.

23. Monson GS: Applied mechanics to the theory of mandibular movements. *Dental Cosmos* 1932;74:1039–1053.

24. Payne SH: A comparative study of posterior occlusion. *J Prosthet Dent* 1952;2:661–666.

25. Vig RG, Brundo GC: The kinetics of anterior tooth display. *J Prosthet Dent* 1978;39:502–504.

26. Frush JP: The dynesthetic interpretation on the dentogenic concept. *J Prosthet Dent* 1958;8:558–551.

27. Frush JP: Introduction to dentinogenic restorations. *J Prosthet Dent* 1955;5:586–595.

28. Gysi A: Simplifying the correct articulation of artificial teeth. *Dent Digest* 1913;19:1–8.

29. Curtis TA, Griffith MR, Firtell DN: Complete denture prosthodontics for the radiation patient. *J Prosthet Dent* 1976;36: 66–76.

30. Kelly EK: Retentive dentures for patients with mutilated jaws. *J Am Dent Assoc* 1965;71:1419–1425.

31. Pound E: Utilizing speech to simplify a personalized denture service. *J Prosthet Dent* 1970;24:586–600.

32. Zinner I, Sherman H: An analysis of the development of complete denture impression techniques. *J Prosthet Dent* 1981;46:242–249.

33. Drago CJ: A retrospective comparison of two definitive impression techniques and their associated postinsertion adjustments in complete denture prosthodontics. *J Prosthodont* 2003;12: 192–197.

34. Devan M: Basic principles of impression making. *J Prosthet Dent* 1952;2:26.

35. Petrie CS, Walker MP, Williams K: A survey of U.S. prosthodontists and dental schools on the current materials and methods for final impressions for complete denture prosthodontics. *J Prosthodont* 2005;14:253–262.

36. Firtell DN, Koumjian JH: Mandibular complete denture impressions with fluid wax or polysulfide rubber: a comparative study. *J Prosthet Dent* 1992;67:801–804.

37. Koran A: Impression materials for denture bearing mucosa. *Dent Clin North Am* 1980;24:97–111.

38. Lindsay L: *A Short History of Dentistry*. London, John Bale and Sons and Danielsson, 1933.

39. Turner C, Anthony L: *American Textbook of Prosthetic Dentistry (ed 1)* Philadelphia, PA, Lea and Febiger, 1928.

40. Tench R: Impressions for dentures. *J Am Dent Assoc* 1934;21: 1005–1018.

41. Greene J: *"Greene Brothers" Clinical Course in Dental Prostheses*, Revised Edition. Detroit, MI, Detroit Dental Manufacturing Company, 1913.

42. Neil E: *The Master Impression: An Important Feature of Standardized Full Denture Practice* (ed 4) Nashville, TN, Marshall Bruce Co., 1932.

43. Schlosser R: *Complete Denture Prosthesis*. Philadelphia, PA, Saunders, 1939.

44. Heartwell CM: *Syllabus of Complete Dentures* (ed 2). Philadelphia, PA, Lea and Febiger, 1974.

45. Smith DE, Toolson LB, Bolender CL, et al: One-step border molding of complete denture impressions using a polyether impression material. *J Prosthet Dent* 1979;41:347–351.

46. Chaffee NR, Cooper LF, Felton DA: A technique for border molding edentulous impressions using vinyl polysiloxane material. *J Prosthodont* 1999;8:129–134.

47. Massad JJ, Cagna DR: Immediate complete denture impressions: case report and modern clinical technique. *Dent Today* 2008;27:58, 60, 62–65.

48. Cagna DR, Massad JJ: Vinyl polysiloxane impression material in removable prosthodontics. Part 2: immediate denture and reline impressions. *Compend Contin Educ Dent* 2007;28: 519–526; quiz 27–28.

49. Page H: *Mucostatics-A Principle Not A Technique*. Chiacgo, IL, published by author, 1946.

50. Tuckfeld W: Review of impression techniques in full denture prosthesis. *Int Dent J* 1950;1:112–130.

51. Frank RP: Analysis of pressures produced during maxillary edentulous impression procedures. *J Prosthet Dent* 1969;22: 400–413.

52. Campbell D: *Full Denture Prosthesis*. St. Louis, MO, Mosby, 1924.

53. Masri R, Driscoll CF, Burkhardt J, et al: Pressure generated on a simulated oral analog by impression materials in custom trays of different designs. *J Prosthodont* 2002;11:155–160.

54. Lieberthal R: *Advanced Impression Taking*. New York, NY, Professional Publishing Company, 1919.

55. Schlosser R, Gehl D: *Complete Denture Prosthesis* (ed 3). Philadelphia, PA, Saunders, 1953.

56. Winkler S: *Essentials of Complete Denture Prosthodontics*. Philadelphia, PA, Saunders, 1979.

57. Pound E: *Personalized Denture Procedures Dentist's Manual*. Anaheim, CA, Denar Corporation, 1973.

58. Grant A HJ, McCord JF: *Complete Prosthodontics* (ed 1). London: Mosby-Wolfe, 1994.

59. Massad JJ, Cagna DR: Vinyl polysiloxane impression material in removable prosthodontics part 3: implant and external impressions. *Compend Contin Educ Dent* 2007;28:554–560; quiz 61.

60. Tallgren A: The continuing reduction of the residual alveolar ridges in complete denture wearers: a mixed-longitudinal study covering 25 years. *J Prosthet Dent* 1972;27:120–132.

61. Atwood DA: Reduction of residual ridges: a major oral disease entity. *J Prosthet Dent* 1971;26:266–279.

62. Atwood DA: Bone loss of edentulous alveolar ridges. *J Periodontol* 1979;50:11–21.

63. Lkeman PR, Watt DM: Morphological changes in the maxillary denture bearing area. A follow up 14 to 17 years after tooth extraction. *Br Dent J* 1974;136:500–503.

64. Wical KE, Swoope CC: Studies of residual ridge resorption. I. Use of panoramic radiographs for evaluation and classification of mandibular resorption. *J Prosthet Dent* 1974;32:7–12.

65. Kelly E: Changes caused by a mandibular removable partial denture opposing a maxillary complete denture. *J Prosthet Dent* 1972;27:140–150.

66. Lytle R: Management of abused tissues in complete denture construction. *J Prosthet Dent* 1957;7:27–42.

67. Chase W: Tissue conditioning utilizing Dynamic Adaptive Stress. *J Prosthet Dent* 1961;11:804–15.

68. Dukes BS: An evaluation of soft tissue responses following removal of ill-fitting dentures. *J Prosthet Dent* 1980;43:251–253.

69. Pound E. Preparatory dentures: A protective philosophy. *J Prosthet Dent* 1965;15:5–18.

70. Lytle R: Compolete denture construction based on a study of the deformation of the underlying soft tissues. *J Prosthet Dent* 1959;9:539–551.

71. Murata H, Iwanaga H, Shigeto N, et al: Initial flow of tissue conditioners–influence of composition and structure on gelation. *J Oral Rehabil* 1993;20:177–187.

72. Graham BS, Jones DW, Sutow EJ: Clinical implications of resilient denture lining material research. Part II: Gelation and flow properties of tissue conditioners. *J Prosthet Dent* 1991;65:413–418.

73. Malmstrom HS, Mehta N, Sanchez R, et al: The effect of two different coatings on the surface integrity and softness of a tissue conditioner. *J Prosthet Dent* 2002;87:153–157.

74. Laney WR: *Diagnosis and Treatment in Prosthodontics*. Philadelphia, PA, Lea and Febiger, 1983.

75. Brewer AA: Prosthodontic research in progress at the School of Aerospace Medicine. *J Prosthet Dent* 1963;13:49–69.

76. Langer A: The validity of maxillomandibular records made with trial and processed acxrylic resin bases. *J Prosthet Dent* 1981;45:253–258.

77. Jacob RF, Yen TW: Processed record bases for the edentulous maxillofacial patient. *J Prosthet Dent* 1991;65:680–685.

78. Crane K: Processed bases for complete dentures. *Trends Tech Contemp Dent Lab* 1992;9:21–24.

79. Thomas-Weintraub A, Weintraub GS: Processed permanent record bases in complete denture therapy: rationale and technique. *Compend Contin Educ Dent* 1985;6:660–665, 668.

80. Jackson AD, Lang BR, Wang RF: The influence of teeth on denture base processing accuracy. *Int J Prosthodont* 1993;6:333–340.

81. Gunji K: A basic study on newly developed light-curing resins-Fitness, flexural properties and bond strength to self-curing resins. *Kokubyo Gakkai Zasshi* 2005;72:7–12.

82. Machado C, Sanchez E, Azer SS, et al: Comparative study of the transverse strength of three denture base materials. *J Dent* 2007;35:930–933.

83. Souder W, Paffenbarger G: Physical properties of dental materials. In Office GP (ed): *Circular C433 of the National Bureau of Standards*. Washington, DC, National Bureau of Standards, 1942.

84. Academy of DP: Final report of the workshop on clinical requirements of ideal denture base materials. *J Prosthet Dent* 1968;20:101–105.

85. Ganzarolli SM, de Mello JA, Shinkai RS, et al: Internal adaptation and some physical properties of methacrylate-based denture base resins polymerized by different techniques. *J Biomed Mater Res B Appl Biomater* 2007;82:169–173.

86. Craig R: *Craig's Restorative Dental Materials* (ed 12) St. Louis, MO, Elsevier, 2006.

87. Jackson AD, Grisius RJ, Fenster RK, et al: Dimensional accuracy of two denture base processing methods. *Int J Prosthodont* 1989;2:421–428.

88. Haug SP, Duke P, Dixon SE, et al: A pilot clinical evaluation of a new injection denture base system. *Compend Contin Educ Dent* 2001;22:847–852, 54; quiz 56.

89. Campos MS, Cavalcanti BN, Cunha VP: Occlusal changes in complete dentures processed by pack-and-press and injection-pressing techniques. *Eur J Prosthodont Restor Dent* 2005;13:78–80.

90. Keenan PL, Radford DR, Clark RK: Dimensional change in complete dentures fabricated by injection molding and microwave processing. *J Prosthet Dent* 2003;89:37–44.

91. Nogueira SS, Ogle RE, Davis EL: Comparison of accuracy between compression- and injection-molded complete dentures. *J Prosthet Dent* 1999;82:291–300.

92. Lung CY, Darvell BW: Minimization of the inevitable residual monomer in denture base acrylic. *Dent Mater* 2005;21:1119–1128.

93. Slaughter A, Katz RV, Grasso JE: Professional attitudes toward denture adhesives: A Delphi technique survey of academic prosthodontists. *J Prosthet Dent* 1999;82:80–89.

94. Stafford GD: Denture adhesives-a review of their uses and compositions. *Dent Pract Dent Rec* 1970;21:17–19.

95. Adisman IK: The use of denture adhesives as an aid to denture treatment. *J Prosthet Dent* 1989;62:711–715.

96. Folse GJ: Denture adhesives: when, why, and how. *Dent Today* 2004;23:70–71.

97. Grasso JE: Denture adhesives: changing attitudes. *J Am Dent Assoc* 1996;127:90–96.

98. Nations SP, Boyer PJ, Love LA, et al: Denture cream. An unusual source of excess zinc, leading to hypocupremia and neurologic disease. *Neurology* 2008;71:639–643.

99. Donovan TE, Derbabian K, Kaneko L, et al: Esthetic considerations in removable prosthodontics. *J Esthet Restor Dent* 2001;13:241–253.

PART IV

FUNCTIONAL PARAMETERS AND ASSESSMENT

20

THE POSITION OF THE OCCLUSAL PLANE IN NATURAL AND ARTIFICIAL DENTITIONS AS RELATED TO OTHER CRANIOFACIAL PLANES

Firas A.M. Al Quran, phd, msc med, bds,[1] Abdalla Hazza'a, phd, msc med, bds,[2] and Nabeel Al nahass, msc dent, dds[3]

[1]Associate Professor in Prosthetic Dentistry, Faculty of Dentistry, Jordan University of Science and Technology (JUST), Irbid, Jordan
[2]Associate Professor in Oral and Maxillofacial Radiology, Faculty of Dentistry, Jordan University of Science and Technology (JUST), Irbid, Jordan
[3]Private Practice, Dubai, United Arab Emirates

Keywords
Occlusion; cephalometric; plane; orientation

Correspondence
Firas A.M. AL Quran, PO Box 3030, Irbid 22110, Jordan.
E-mail: firasalquran@yahoo.com, firasq@just.edu.jo

Accepted December 10, 2009

Published in *Journal of Prosthodontics* 2010; Vol. 19, Issue 8, pp. 601–5

doi: 10.1111/j.1532-849X.2010.00643.x

ABSTRACT

Purpose: This study aimed at determining the most reliable ala-tragus line as a guide for the orientation of the occlusal plane in complete denture patients by use of cephalometric landmarks on dentate volunteers.
Materials and Methods: Analysis was made for prosthodontically related craniofacial reference lines and angles of lateral cephalometric radiographs taken for 47 dentate adults. Variables were determined and data were analyzed using SPSS (SPSS, Inc., Chicago, IL).
Results: Occlusal plane angle formed between the occlusal plane and Camper's plane had the lowest mean value in the angle formed with Camper's I, which represents the measure taken from the superior border of the tragus of the ear with a score of 2.1°. The highest was measured in the angle formed with Camper's III with a score of 6.1°, while the angle formed with Camper's II was 3.2°. The differences between the three planes in relation to the occlusal plane was significant ($p < 0.001$).
Conclusion: The superior border of the tragus with the inferior border of the ala of the nose was most accurate in orienting the occlusal plane.

Occlusal plane orientation is one of the most important clinical procedures in removable prosthodontic treatment for edentulous patients. It is the most important plane to be determined in complete denture work, as it is a vital and important basis for tooth arrangement. The occlusal plane position is considered to be the primary link between function and esthetics. The orientation of the occlusal plane is lost in patients rendered edentulous and should be relocated if complete dentures are to be esthetic and to function satisfactorily. For example, if the occlusal plane is placed too high, the tongue cannot rest on the lingual cusps of the mandibular denture and prevents the denture's displacement. There is also a tendency for accumulation of food in the buccal and lingual sulci. On the other hand, if the occlusal plane is placed too low, it could lead to tongue and cheek biting.[1]

Complete dentures are constructed to function in the mouth as an integral part of the masticatory system; therefore, they should be designed to conform to the patient's physiologic jaw relations. The plane of occlusion forms one essential physiologic concept of jaw relation and occlusion. The plane of occlusion in complete dentures has often been oriented anteriorly to fulfill esthetic requirements and posteriorly parallel to Camper's line, which is a horizontal line drawn through the lower part of the nose and the orifice of the ear.[2]

According to surveys,[3–6] occlusal plane orientation differs considerably among schools in Japan, the US, and Canada; however, the most widely used method in determining the plane of occlusion was the ala-tragus line method. Zarb et al[7] suggested anatomical landmarks that clinically determine the plane of occlusion. They said that the occlusal plane should be parallel to the hamular notch-incisive papilla plane, whereas other researchers have reported a close relationship between the ala-tragus line and occlusal plane.[6]

The use of a number of anatomical landmarks as guides from life or biometric guides for artificial tooth position has been suggested by many authors.[8–11] Anatomical landmarks suggested to clinically determine the position of the occlusal plane are the upper lip, corner of the mouth,[11] lateral margins of the tongue, two-thirds of the height of the retromolar pad, parallel to the ala-tragus (Camper's plane) and interpupillary lines,[6,7] parallel to the hamular notch-incisive papilla plane, and 3.3 mm below the parotid papilla.[12,13]

A common concept is that the occlusal plane should be parallel to a line drawn from the lowest point of the ala of the nose to the external auditory meatus or tragus of the ear.[14,15] There are differences in the literature concerning which part of the tragus to use, since some researchers believe in using the lower border of the tragus, others believe in using the middle part of the tragus, and still others believe in using the upper part.[6,7,16]

The occlusal plane of dentures must be oriented as closely as possible to the occlusal plane that existed in the natural dentition. By doing so, the tongue and cheeks will be more effective during deglutition and mastication, and speech and esthetics will be improved.[17] On the other hand, other researchers believe that reproducing the natural occlusal plane in complete dentures is not necessary due to conditions in natural dentitions differing from those of artificial dentures. They feel reproducing the natural occlusal plane offers no advantages for the extra care involved.[16,18–21] Therefore, what is considered normal arrangement of teeth could be modified to suit edentulous needs; however, it would seem reasonable that dentures should not depart too radically from what they are replacing.

Since 1931, cephalometric analysis has served as a valuable adjunct to dental research and diagnosis, although its clinical application has been directed largely toward orthodontics. Cephalometry is of special value to prosthodontics, in that it can be used to reestablish the correct position of lost structures such as the teeth. This can be achieved by identifying a predictable relationship between the teeth and other cranial landmarks not subjected to postextraction changes.

In this study, cephalometric analysis has been used to investigate the relationship between the natural occlusal plane and anatomical structure in the skull.[22]

MATERIALS AND METHODS

This study aims at determining the most reliable ala-tragus line as a guide for the orientation of the occlusal plane in complete dentures and the use of cephalometric landmarks to predict the occlusal plane orientation in edentulous patients. Prior to beginning the study, the research was approved by the Board Research Committee at the Faculty of Dentistry at the Jordan University of Science and Technology (JUST). Further approval was sought and received from the JUST Deanship of Research. This study included 51 fully dentate subjects with Angle's class I occlusion. The subjects were randomly selected. After clinical examination, four patients were excluded, because they either refused X-ray exposure, or because we were unable to locate the requested anatomical landmarks accurately.

This group of volunteers consisted of 47 young adults selected from fourth and fifth year dental students. The criteria for selection of these patients was the presence of 28 to 32 natural teeth in an ideal arch alignment, with Angle's class I molar relationship, a pleasing profile, and no history of orthodontic treatment.

Left lateral cephalograms were taken of the subjects by a standard technique with the mandible closed in maximum intercuspation. The dentulous occlusal plane was located as the line averaging the points of the posterior occlusal contact from the first permanent molar to the bicuspids to the most lingually placed incisor tooth.

A cephalometric radiograph was taken for each patient, using an Orthopantomograph model Orthophos-5 (Siemens,

Erlangen, Germany) with a focal film distance of 5 feet. Radiographs were obtained at 66 to 69 kVp and 15 to 16 mA according to the individual's physical status. Kodak T-MAT films (Eastman, Kodak, Rochester, NY) with Siemens special screens (Siemens) were used for conventional cephalometric radiography. An automatic processor with daylight loader (XR 24, Durr Dental, Bietigheim-Bissingen, Germany; 230 V and 50 to 60 Hz) was used with RP X-Omat (Kodak, Chalon-Sur-Saone, France) chemicals.

Barium sulfate creamy mix was applied to the teeth, one drop on the incisal edge of the left maxillary central incisor, and another drop painted to cover the mesio-palatal cusp of the left maxillary first molar. Another creamy mix of barium sulfate was painted on the skin on the left side of each patient's face in the shape of a triangle to mark required landmarks to be shown in the final radiograph. The apex of the triangle superiorly pointed to the lower border of the ala of the nose, and the other one was applied to mark the whole tragus of the ear. The apex of the painted triangle of the tragus pointed posteriorly to the tragus so that the lowest angle between occlusal plane and ala-tragus line at the superior, middle, and inferior border of the tragus could be identified.

Each subject was radiographed in standing position. Patients were asked to close in centric occlusion. The lips and the rest of the body were relaxed. Using the cephalostat, the patient's head was fixed bilaterally by the ear rod and anteriorly by a plastic stopper on the bridge of the nose. The cassette with the film inside was at the right side of the patient's face. The ear rods were inserted into the external auditory meatus with appropriate care to prevent the tragus from being forced anteriorly by direct pressure from the ear rods; however, displacement in this horizontal direction was considered unlikely to produce vertical distortion of the tragus point to an extent that would cause unacceptable error in the measurements. Each traced cephalogram was placed on the conventional viewing box. The cephalometric points used in this study are the following.

Ala (point A): The lowest point of the left ala of the nose represented by the superior apex of the triangular barium sulfate applied to the skin of the left side of the face.

Tragus (point T): The whole tragus of the left ear represented by the triangular barium sulfate applied to the skin of the face of the dentate and edentate subjects.

The cephalometric planes and lines used in this study are the following.

Ala-tragus line (Camper's plane): The line joining point A with point T.

Occlusal plane: The line connecting the lowest point of the incisal edge of the left maxillary central incisor with the lowest point of the mesio-palatal cusp of the left maxillary first molar.

For the purpose of comparison, angles rather than linear measurements were used, since angles can be compared directly in individuals of different sizes without the need

of an index. The angular measurements were recorded to the nearest degree. Measurements were done according to a method described by Jaccobson.[23] The angles to be studied, were as follows.

Camp I-OP: Angle between Camper's I (superior border of tragus) and occlusal plane.

Camp II-OP: Angle between Camper's II (middle border of tragus) and occlusal plane.

Camp III-OP: Angle between Camper's III (inferior border of tragus) and occlusal plane.

SPSS (SPSS, Inc., Chicago, IL) was used to calculate the mean and standard deviation of all angular measurements, age for the whole sample, and for both sex groups.

RESULTS

Subjects involved in this study included 47 dentate fourth and fifth year dental students (21 men, 26 women). Their age ranged from 21 to 34 years old.

Occlusal plane angle formed between the occlusal plane and Camper's plane had the lowest mean value in the angle formed with Camper's I, which represents the measure taken from the superior border of tragus of the ear with a score of 2.1°. The highest was measured in the angle formed with Camper's III, with score of 6.1°, while the mean angle formed with Camper's II was 3.2° (Table 1). The differences between the three planes in relation to the occlusal plane were found to be significant ($p < 0.001$) (Table 2).

DISCUSSION

An analysis of cephalometric lines and angles could provide useful information on the craniofacial skeleton and the orientation of the occlusal plane in dentulous and edentulous subjects. The plane of occlusion has been recognized as an essential functional part of the craniofacial skeleton.[24–27]

Angular variables were used in this study to illustrate variations in artificial occlusal plane (AOP) orientation in relation to other craniofacial planes and to determine the validity of the use of the ala-tragus line as a reference point for occlusal plane orientation. Complete dentures are constructed to function in the mouth in harmony with the masticatory system; therefore, the complete dentures should

TABLE 1 Angle between occlusal plane in the dentate group and Camper's I, II, and III

	Mean	Maximum	Minimum	Std. deviation	N
Camp I	2.0638°	12.00°	0.00°	2.11006°	47
Camp II	3.1574°	8.00°	0.00°	1.63318°	47
Camp III	6.1255°	11.00	2.00°	1.65352°	47

TABLE 2   **Significant difference between Camper's I, II, and III, by predicting the *p*-value (<0.001)**

95% Confidence interval of the difference						
Upper	Lower	Mean difference	Sig. (2-tailed)	df	t	
2.6834	1.4443	2.06383	.000	46	6.705	Camp I
3.6370	2.6779	3.15745	.000	46	13.254	Camp II
6.6110	5.6400	6.12553	.000	46	25.397	Camp III

be designed in accordance with all jaw movements and relations. Part of designing the complete denture is orienting the occlusal plane in the most acceptable cant for esthetics and function. Investigators have suggested various concepts and methods for the orientation of the occlusal plane in complete dentures based on morphologic studies on natural and artificial dentitions and on clinical experience.[6,16,28–30]

Historically, the assessment of a patient's occlusal line has been performed by comparing its inclination with selected craniofacial reference lines. The ala-tragus line was the most commonly used and widely taught method for the orientation of the plane of occlusion.[3,4]

In the literature, there is controversy in defining Camper's plane, which is considered the most popular plane used to orient the occlusal plane in edentulous patients. Definition of the Camper's line causes confusion, because the exact reference points are controversial. For example, the Glossary of Prosthodontic Terms[31] states that the Camper's line runs from the inferior border of the ala of the nose to the superior border of the tragus, while for Spratley[16] it runs from the center of the ala to the center of the tragus. Among seven of the most famous prosthodontic textbooks, only Boucher's provides a definition.[8] Two other textbooks[32,33] recommend the concept without defining it, while Basker et al,[34] Grant and Johnson,[35] and Neill and Naim[36] provide only pictorial representation, illustrating Camper's line as extending to a point, not at the superior border, but at the center of the tragus of the ear, corresponding to the definition of Ismail and Bowman,[30] which predates Boucher's definition. However, investigations into the clinical reliability of Camper's line serve only to compound the confusion, as Ismail and Bowman[30] compared the use of an ala-tragus line oriented to the middle of the tragus with the occlusal plane of natural teeth, and concluded that dentures constructed accordingly would have an occlusal plane set far too low posteriorly. This is contraindicated by Abrahams and Carey,[37] who concluded that the occlusal plane of complete dentures conforming to a line oriented to the superior border of the tragus results in the occlusal plane being leveled far too high posteriorly.

In the present study, we used three Camper's planes, based upon the superior, middle, and inferior part of the tragus; as Camper's plane I is the line extending from the inferior border of the ala of the nose to the superior border of the tragus of the ear, Camper's plane II is the line extending from the inferior border of the ala of the nose to the middle border of the tragus of the ear, and Camper's III is the line extending from the inferior border of the ala of the nose to the inferior border of the tragus of the ear. The lowest mean angle formed between Camper's I and the natural occlusal plane was 2.1°, Camper's II was 3.2°, and Camper's III was 6.1° (Table 1). Nissan et al,[38] on the other hand, recorded the angle formed between occlusal plane and Camper's line as 7.08°. Abrahams and Carey[37] reported the angle formed between the natural occlusal plane and Camper's plane to be 9.66°. Augsburger[28] found the angle of the occlusal plane deviated from Camper's plane by 3.2° to 7.85° in dentate patients of different facial types.

Van Niekerk et al[6] recorded a 2.45° angle between the occlusal plane of the complete denture and the ala-tragus line. Karkazis and Polyzois[22] did not find a correlation between Camper's plane and the occlusal plane of natural teeth (average 2.84°) or artificial teeth (average 3.25°); however, the inclination of the occlusal plane on complete dentures was similar to the natural occlusal plane. The difference between the average angle (2.0°) made by the occlusal plane and Camper's plane as found in the present study and that of other studies can be explained by the use of different points of measurement. Van Niekerk et al[6] used the inferior border of the tragus as the posterior border of the ala-tragus line, whereas Karkazis and Polyzois[22] used the center of the tragus as the posterior border of Camper's plane.

According to the findings of this study, Camper's I is the most suitable plane to orient the occlusal plane, forming a stop anteroposteriorly following the curve of the ramus of the mandible, and establishing a curve that would serve the artificial teeth to be set in a way to prevent any interferences that would dislodge the denture during protrusive movement, making the dentures more stable and ensuring satisfactory service. On the other hand, an investigation[30] has been carried out that compared the occlusal plane orientation before extraction of natural teeth and when artificial teeth were arranged so that the AOP paralleled the ala-tragus line. The results indicated that the natural occlusal plane was higher posteriorly than the AOP, which disagrees with what had been shown by Wylie,[39] Abrahams and Carey,[37] and Ow et al.[27] One can see the controversy regarding the position of the natural occlusal plane in relation to the AOP (determined by the use of the ala-tragus line). Moreover, in actual practice, the determination of the AOP by the ala-tragus line is taken only as an approximation and as the mean of the angle formed between the two planes. The ala-tragus line has proved to be a useful reference line for the initial orientation of the occlusal plane in complete dentures. Therefore, the ala-tragus line may be modified to be extended from the inferior part of the ala of the nose to the superior part of the tragus of the ear, instead of the mid- or inferior-tragus points. The differences between Camper's I, II, and III were tested and revealed a significant statistical difference (Table 2), which means that using Camper's I to orient the occlusal plane would make a significant difference in the esthetics and comfort of the complete denture.

The results of this study found that the superior border of the tragus is the most acceptable point to orient the occlusal plane, which complies with Boucher,[8] the Glossary of Prosthodontic Terms,[31] and Trapozzano.[40] On the other hand, this study does not agree with the findings of other studies. Van Niekerk[6] has suggested the use of the inferior part of the tragus rather than middle or superior, while Ismail and Bowman[30] suggested the use of the middle part of the tragus.

CONCLUSION

Within the limitations of this study, it can be concluded that the superior border of the tragus with the inferior border of the ala of the nose was most accurate in orienting the occlusal plane.

REFERENCES

1. Monteith BD: A cephalometric method to determine the angulation of the occlusal plane in edentulous patients. *J Prosthet Dent* 1985;54:81–87.
2. Karkazis HC, Polyzois GL: Cephalometrically predicted occlusal plane: implications in removable prosthodontics. *J Prosthet Dent* 1991;65:258–264.
3. Levin B, Sauer LJ: Results of a survey of complete denture procedure taught in American and Canadian dental schools. *J Prosthet Dent* 1969;22:171–177.
4. Ukai H, Yanagide S, Ratoh Y, et al: Examination into the questionnaire, "*Results of a survey of complete denture procedures taught in Japanese dental schools*" *Prac Prosthod* 1979;3:*324*.
5. Lundquist DO, Luther WW: Occlusal plane determination. *J Prosthet Dent* 1970;23:489–498.
6. van Niekerk FW, Miller VJ, Chem C, et al: The ala-tragus line in complete dentures prosthodontics. *J Prosthet Dent* 1985;53:67–69.
7. Zarb GA, Bolender CA, Carlsson GE: *Boucher's Prosthodontic Treatment for Edentulous Patients* (ed 11). St. Louis, Mosby, 1997.
8. Boucher CO: Complete denture prosthodontics—state of the art. *J Prosthet Dent* 1975;34:372–383.
9. Roraff AR: Arranging artificial teeth according to anatomic landmarks. *J Prosthet Dent* 1977;28:120–130.
10. Murray CG: Anterior tooth positions in prosthodontics. *Aust Dent J* 1977;22:113–119.
11. Hickey JC, Zarb GA, Bolender CL: *Boucher's Prosthodontic Treatment for Edentulous Patients* (ed 12) St. Louis, Mosby, 2004.
12. Rich H: Evaluation and registration of the H. I. P. plane of occlusion. *Aust Dent J* 1982;22:162–168.
13. Foley PF, Latta GH Jr: A study of the position of the parotid papilla relative to the occlusal plane. *J Prosthet Dent* 1985;53:124–126.
14. Anthony LP: *The American Textbook of Prosthetic Dentistry*. Philadelphia, Lea and Febiger, 1967.
15. Lammie GA: *Full Dentures*. Oxford, Blackwell, 1956.
16. Spartley MH: A simplified technique for determining the occlusal plane in full denture construction. *J Oral Rehab* 1980;7:31–33.
17. Kapur KK, Soman S: The effect of denture factors on masticatory performance. Part II the location of the food platform. *J Prosthet Dent* 1965;15:451–463.
18. Cocker WL: The occlusal plane. *Brit Dent J* 1925;46:463–464.
19. Kurth LE: The posterior occlusal plane in full denture construction. *J Am Dent Assoc* 1940;27:92–95.
20. Pound E: Modern American concepts in aesthetics. *Int Dent J* 1960;10:154–172.
21. Fish EW: *Principles of Full Denture Prostheses* (ed 6). London, Staples, 1964.
22. Karkazis HC, Polyzois GL: Cephalometrically predicted occlusal plane: implication in removable prosthodontics. *J Prosthet Dent* 1991;65:258–264.
23. Jaccobson A, Canfield PW: *Introduction to Radiographic Cephalometry*. Philadelphia, Lea and Febiger, 1985.
24. Kapur KK, Lestrel PE, Chauncey HH: Development of prosthodontic craniofacial standards: occlusal plane location. *J Dent Res* 1982;61:222. Abstract 391.
25. Ow RK, Keng SB, Djeng SK, et al: A radiographic interpretation of craniofacial reference lines in relation to prosthodontic plane orientation. *J Prosthet Dent* 1986;31:326–334.
26. Ow RK, Djeng SK, Ho CK: The relationships of upper facial proportions and the plane of occlusion to anatomic reference planes. *J Prosthet Dent* 1989;61:727–733.

27. Ow RK, Djeng SK, Ho CK: Orientation of the plane of occlusion. *J Prosthet Dent* 1990;64:31–36.

28. Augsburger RH: Occlusal plane relation to facial type. *J Prosthet Dent* 1953;3:53–65.

29. Hartono R: The occlusal plane in relation to facial types. *J Prosthet Dent* 1967;17:549–557.

30. Ismail YH, Bowman JF: Position of the occlusal plane in natural and artificial teeth. *J Prosthet Dent* 1968;20: 407–411.

31. Glossary of prosthodontic terms. *J Prosthet Dent* 2005;94: 10–92.

32. Sharry JJ: *Complete Denture Prosthodontics* (ed 3). New York, McGraw-Hill, 1974.

33. MacGregor AR: *Fenn, Liddlelow and Gimson's Clinical Dental Prosthetics* (ed 3). Oxford, Wright, Butterworth, 1983.

34. Basker RM, Davenport JC, *Tomlin HR: Prosthetic Treatment of the Edentulous Patient* (ed 1). London, Macmillan, 1976.

35. Grant AA, Johnson W: *An Introduction to Removable Denture Prosthetics*. Edinburgh, Churchill Livingstone, 1983.

36. Neill DJ, Naim RI: *Complete Denture Prosthetics*. Bristol, John Wright Sons, 1975.

37. Abrahams R, Carey PD: The use of ala-tragus for occlusal plane determination in complete dentures. *J Dent* 1979;7:339–341.

38. Nissan J, Barnea E, Zeltzer C: Relationship between the craniofacial complex and size of the resorbed mandible in complete denture wearers. *J Oral Rehab* 2003;30:1173–1176.

39. Wylie WL: The Naso-meatal line as guide for the determination of the occlusal plane. *J Dent Res* 1944;23:309–312.

40. Trapozzano V: Occlusal records. *J Prosthet Dent* 1955;5: 325–333.

21

PREDICTORS OF SATISFACTION WITH DENTURES IN A COHORT OF INDIVIDUALS WEARING OLD DENTURES: FUNCTIONAL QUALITY OR PATIENT-REPORTED MEASURES?

DAIANE CERUTTI-KOPPLIN, DDS, MSC, PHD,[1] ELHAM EMAMI, DDS, MSC, PHD,[2] JULIANA BALBINOT HILGERT, DDS, MSC, PHD,[1] FERNANDO NEVES HUGO, DDS, MSC, PHD,[1] ELKEN RIVALDO, DDS, MSC, PHD,[3] AND DALVA MARIA PEREIRA PADILHA, DDS, MSC, PHD[1]

[1]*Faculty of Dentistry, Universidade Federal do Rio Grande do Sul, Porto Alegre, Rio Grande do Sul, Brazil*
[2]*Faculty of Dentistry, Université de Montréal, Montreal, Canada*
[3]*Universidade Luterana do Brasil, Canoas - Rio Grande do Sul, Brazil*

Keywords
Denture quality; complete dentures; satisfaction; prognostic indicators

Correspondence
Daiane Cerutti-Kopplin, DDS, MSc, PhD,
Department of Dental Public Health,
Universidade Federal do Rio Grande do Sul,
Ramiro Barcelos Porto Alegre Rio Grande do
Sul, 974206031, Brazil.
E-mail: daianecerutti@hotmail.com

This study was supported in part by the Brazilian Ministry of Education, Coordination for the Improvement of Higher Education Personnel (CAPES).

The authors deny any conflicts of interest.

Accepted June 8, 2015

Published in *Journal of Prosthodontics* 2017; Vol. 26, Issue 3, pp. 196–200

doi: 10.1111/jopr.12383

ABSTRACT

Purpose: To examine the extent to which denture satisfaction can be determined by a measure of the denture's functional quality and by patient-reported measures.

Materials and Methods: This study used data obtained from 117 edentulous individuals with a mean age of 73.7 (SD = 5.6) years in southern Brazil. The edentulous individuals rated their levels of general satisfaction with their actual dentures, using a visual analog scale. Explanatory variables included the individual's information about ability to chew, ability to speak, esthetics, and sociodemographic factors. The dentures were evaluated using the validated 9-item Functional Assessment of Dentures instrument. Bivariate statistical analyses and Poisson regression models (prevalence ratio [PR]; 95% CI; $p < 0.05$) were used to test the association of explanatory variables with patients' general satisfaction with their complete dentures.

Results: There was a statistically significant association between patients' general satisfaction and stability of maxillary (rocking movement) (adjusted PR = 1.28; 95% CI: 1.07–1.52) and mandibular dentures (occlusal displacement) (adjusted PR = 1.68; 95% CI: 1.16–2.43), masticatory ability (adjusted PR = 1.54; 95% CI: 1.08–2.19), and the age of the mandibular denture (adjusted PR = 1.47; 95% CI: 1.10–1.97).

Conclusions: The results of this study indicated that measures of denture stability, masticatory ability, and age of dentures appeared to be determinants of patients' satisfaction with dentures.

Although conventional complete dentures have proven to be satisfactory to large numbers of patients,[1] many complete denture users are not satisfied with their prosthesis, regardless of its quality.[2] This issue is of great concern, since it may have an impact on patients' quality of life.[3,4]

Identification of correlates of satisfaction and clinical prediction of denture satisfaction have been described as a complex issue, since it can be influenced by a number of factors including anatomy, stability and retention of dentures, ability to chew, ability to speak, esthetics, psychological characteristics,[5–12] and patient adaptation to dentures.[13] The results of some studies, especially those using structural equation modeling, suggested that clinical factors such as technically high quality dentures[14] and adequate mandibular residual ridges[6] could be considered as indicators of complete denture success; however, most of these studies have been criticized due to limited clinical measures, nonvalid indicators of patients' denture experience, and failure to apply patient-reported measures in evaluations of complete dentures.[15–17]

In recent years there has been a shift to patient-based measures, as better methods for measuring patient-centered outcomes have been developed.[18–24] Moreover, according to a recent systematic review, patient satisfaction has been used as the primary outcome for the majority of removable prosthodontic clinical trials.[25] Furthermore, use of patient satisfaction as an outcome can facilitate the transfer of knowledge from research to clinical use; however, there is still no valid guideline for clinicians on the use of expert- and patient-based measures as prognostic tools for estimation of patient satisfaction with dentures.[26] Therefore, the main objective of this study was to examine the extent to which denture satisfaction could be determined by a measure of the denture's functional quality and by patient-reported measures.

MATERIALS AND METHODS

This study reports the results of cross-sectional analysis of data obtained from an ongoing cohort study in southern Brazil. The cohort has been followed since 2004 to assess the change in the oral health quality of life of study participants over time. Details regarding this cohort have been reported previously.[27,28] This analysis includes only data from completely edentulous elders (≥60 years old) wearing removable conventional dentures (92 women, 25 men). Dentate participants were excluded from the analysis. The State University of Campinas Institutional Review Board approved the study protocol. All study participants gave written informed consent.

Study Outcome, Measures, and Instruments

Overall patient satisfaction with existing complete dentures was considered as a study outcome. The level of satisfaction was measured with a 100 mm visual analog scale (VAS) anchored by the words "not at all satisfied" to "extremely satisfied."[29] Explanatory variables included both patient-reported and expert-based measures as well as socio-demographics, and variables related to history of tooth loss and denture use.

For patient-based measures, patients were asked about their experiences with their existing dentures using four validated 5-point Likert items:[30] Pain or discomfort, difficulty in speaking, difficulty in chewing, and esthetics. Responses were dichotomized into: "No problem (with complete denture)/Minimal problem" as adequate; and "Moderate problem/Considerable problem/Could not be worse" as inadequate.[31] The study participants were also asked about any change in their dietary habits due to problems with their dentures (dichotomous item).

Expert-based assessment of denture quality was conducted by the same prosthodontist using scores of the Functional Assessment of Dentures instrument (FAD).[32] The FAD includes the following criteria: (1) freeway space, (2) occlusion, (3i) maxillary retention (vertical pull), (3ii) maxillary retention (tongue control), (4i) maxillary stability (lateral displacement), (4ii) maxillary stability (pronounced rocking), (5i) mandibular stability (displacement), (5ii) mandibular stability (pronounced movement), and (5iii) mandibular stability (anteroposterior movement). The K-value for intrarater agreement ranged from 0.67 to 0.99, indicating substantial repro-ducibility to almost perfect reproducibility.[33]

Statistical Analysis

Descriptive statistics were used to examine the characteristics of the study participants. The median values of the equal interval or ordinal dependent and independent variables were used as cutoff points to determine binary forms of the data, and the natural binary divisions of the other categorical independent variables were applied, so that all variables were in the same format for analysis. Thus, individuals with VAS values ≥ 70 were considered to be satisfied.[34] The nine functional criteria were scored in a dichotomous manner as adequate or inadequate. Missing data and uncertain answer choices in the attitude items were excluded from further analysis. Pearson Chi-square (two-tailed) was used to test the association of the exploratory variables with the study outcome. Independent variables with results $p < 0.25$ from bivariate analyses were incorporated into the Poisson regression analysis.[35]

The adjusted prevalence ratios and their 95% confidence intervals (CI) were calculated to determine the strength of the association between exploratory variables and the outcome. The level of significance was established at $p < 0.05$. All analyses were carried out with SPSS v.20 (SPSS Inc., Chicago, IL).

RESULTS

The sample comprised 92 (78.6%) women and 25 (21.4%) men. The mean age of the sample population was 73.7 (SD 5.6) years, with a median of 73 years. Among the individuals, 94% reported elementary school as highest level of education, 60.7% lived in an urban area, most of them were married (70.1%), and 60.7% had a monthly income of less than two times the Brazilian minimum wage (± 540 USD). The average history of denture wearing was 35.9 years (SD = 11.6) (median = 40 years, ranging from 5.0 to 62); the median average age of the existing complete conventional dentures was 11.4 years (SD = 10.56) (median = 8 years, ranging from 0.5 to 46.5).

Tables 1 and 2 demonstrate the results of bivariate analyses on the association between explanatory variables and the study outcome. Seventy-six percent of the study participants were satisfied with their dentures, with a mean VAS satisfaction score of 70.5 (± 11.05). There was a statistically significant association between the age of individuals ($p < 0.05$) and adequacy of chewing ability ($p = 0.01$).

There was also a statistically significant association between the majority of expert-based FAD measures and the overall satisfaction with existing denture ($p < 0.05$). Among the FAD indicators, only the freeway space and the maxillary denture retention (tongue control) did not show a statistically significant association with overall satisfaction. After adjusting for independent variables ($p < 0.25$), only four variables remained statistically significant (Table 3): adequate chewing ability (adjPR 1.54, 95% CI 1.08–2.19; $p = 0.017$), age of existing denture (adjPR 1.47, 95% CI 1.1–1.97; $p = 0.008$), and adequate stability of the maxillary denture related to rocking movement (adjPR 1.28, 95% CI 1.07–1.52; $p = 0.005$) and of the mandibular denture in regard to occlusal displacement (adj PR 1.68, 95% CI 1.16–2.43; $p = 0.006$).

DISCUSSION

The main purpose of this cross-sectional analysis was to investigate the association of the patient- and expert-based measures with denture satisfaction. The results showed that both expert- and patient-based measures were associated with patient satisfaction. This association highlighted the importance of appropriate assessment of both measures. These findings were clinically relevant, as they may help clinicians predict the success of their complete denture treatment.

In this regard, by using the Functional Assessment of Dentures (FAD) instrument, it was ascertained what proportion of the individual's denture satisfaction was correlated with the clinician rating of the denture. The FAD is a valid instrument used by several investigators since 2002. This instrument can be easily used by clinicians or in practice-based studies because of feasibility, limited number of items, and clinical value. We also obtained the patients' rating of denture quality. In bivariate analysis, it was found that for most of the FAD items, adequacy of the denture was associated with higher prevalence of satisfaction; however, in multivariate analysis, only a few FAD items were associated with denture satisfaction.

The present results supported the findings of previous studies[14,23] that used multidimensional structural equation modeling to predict the success of patient adaptation to complete dentures; however, results were contradictory, with those studies using a unidimensional approach to assess successful outcome.[12,15,16,21] This may be explained by the

TABLE 1 Association of exploratory variables and perceived overall satisfaction

Bivariate analyses	Satisfied (%)	Dissatisfied (%)	p Value
Exploratory variables	Total	89 (76.1)	28 (23.9)
Age	N = 117		
<72 years	45 (38.5)	7 (6.0)	0.018
≥72 years	44 (37.6)	21 (17.9)	
Sex			
Female	71 (60.7)	21 (17.9)	0.591
Male	18 (15.4)	7 (6.0)	
Place of residency			
Urban	52 (44.4)	19 (16.2)	0.373
Rural	37 (31.6)	9 (7.7)	
Income			
≥1245.00 BRL (± 540 USD)	39 (33.3)	7 (6.0)	0.075
<1245.00 BRL (± 540 USD)	50 (42.7)	21 (17.9)	
Marital status			
Married/civil union	67 (57.3)	15 (12.8)	0.029
Single/divorced/ widowed	22 (18.8)	13 (37.1)	
Education			
≤Elementary school	82 (70.1)	28(23.9)	0.126
>Elementary school	7 (6.8)	0(0.0)	
Esthetics			
Adequate	82 (70.1)	23 (19.7)	0.129
Inadequate	7 (6.0)	5(4.3)	
Ability to speak			
Adequate	85 (72.6)	27 (23.1)	0.833
Inadequate	4 (3.4)	1 (0.9)	
Pain or discomfort			
Adequate	80 (68.4)	26 (22.2)	0.639
Inadequate	9 (10.1)	2(1.7)	
Ability to chew			
Adequate	78 (66.7)	17 (14.5)	0.001
Inadequate	11 (9.4)	11 (9.4)	
Need to alter food intake			
No	49 (41.9)	10 (8.5)	0.074
Yes	40 (34.2)	18 (15.4)	
Age of the maxillary denture			
>5 years	49 (41.9)	16 (13.7)	0.846
≤5 years	40 (34.2)	12 (10.3)	
Age of the mandibular denture			
>5 years	53 (45.3)	12 (10.3)	0.121
≤5 years	36 (30.8)	16 (13.7)	
Length of edentulism period			
>25 years	75 (64.1)	20(17.1)	0.129
≤25 years	12 (12.0)	8 (6.8)	

TABLE 2 Association of expert-based measures and perceived overall satisfaction: bivariate analyses

Expert-based measures (FAD items)	Satisfied (%)	Dissatisfied (%)	p Value
Total N = 117	89 (76.1)	28 (23.9)	
Freeway space			
Adequate	59 (50.4)	13 (11.1)	0.060
Inadequate	30 (25.6)	15 (12.8)	
Occlusion			
Adequate	78 (66.7)	19 (16.2)	0.015
Inadequate	11 (9.4)	9 (7.7)	
Maxillary denture retention (resistance to vertical pull)			
Adequate	84 (71.8)	20 (17.1)	0.001
Inadequate	5 (4.3)	8 (6.8)	
Maxillary denture retention (tongue control)			
Adequate	84 (71.8)	25 (21.4)	0.351
Inadequate	5 (4.3)	3 (2.6)	
Maxillary denture stability (lateral displacement)			
No pronounced displacement	42 (35.9)	4 (3.4)	0.002
Pronounced displacement	47 (40.2)	24 (20.5)	
Maxillary denture stability (rocking)			
No pronounced movement	50 (42.7)	5 (4.3)	<0.0001
Pronounced movement	39 (33.3)	23 (19.7)	
Mandibular denture stability (displacement occlusal)			
No pronounced displacement	76 (65.0)	14 (12.0)	<0.0001
Pronounced displacement	13 (11.1)	14 (12.0)	
Mandibular denture stability (lateral)			
No pronounced movement	33 (28.2)	4 (3.4)	0.024
Pronounced movement	56 (47.9)	24 (20.5)	
Mandibular denture stability (anterior-posterior)			
No pronounced movement	49 (41.9)	5 (4.3)	0.001
Pronounced movement	40 (34.2)	23 (19.7)	

difference between the modeling approach and the use of simple correlation analyses. As suggested by Fenlon and Sherrif,[13] Poisson multivariate regression was used to analyze the data in the present study. This statistical methodology allowed a robust control of variance, and represented a powerful analytical approach.[35] De Lucena et al[21] used the FAD instrument and did not show any association between patient- and expert-based assessment of dentures. These divergent results can be related to the difference in the

TABLE 3 Results of Poisson regression to the prevalence of overall satisfaction

| | | PR (CI 95%) | | |
| | | Unadjusted | Adjusted | |
Variables	Category			p Value
Income	≥1245.00 BRL (± 540 USD)	0.70 (0.61–0.82)	1.11 (0.91–1.27)	0.378
Ability to chew	No problem chewing	1.64 (1.07–2.52)	1.54 (1.08–2.19)	0.017
Age of the present mandibular denture	> 5 years	1.17 (0.95–1.46)	1.47 (1.1–1.97)	0.008
Maxillary denture stability (rocking)	No pronounced movement	1.44 (1.17–1.78)	1.28 (1.07–1.52)	0.005
Maxillary denture retention (resistance to vertical pull)	Adequate resistance	2.1 (1.05–4.20)	1.84 (0.93–3.61)	0.078
Mandibular denture stability (occlusal displacement)	Stays in place	1.75 (1.17–2.62)	1.68 (1.16–2.43)	0.006
Mandibular denture stability (anterior-posterior)	No anteroposterior movement	1.42 (1.16–1.75)	1.14(0.96–1.35)	0.145

population and in the FAD analysis, more specifically the use of total scoring rather than item analysis. In the present study, most of the nine FAD items were associated with patient satisfaction, except for freeway space and maxillary stability with tongue control (Table 2); however, in the regression model, seven of the nine FAD items lost their statistical significance, and the stability of the maxillary (rocking movement) and mandibular (occlusal displacement) prostheses were the only predictors for overall patient satisfaction.

In general, in this study, the majority of patients were satisfied with their complete denture. This fact was discussed in the review conducted by Carlsson and Omar,[26] who suggested that in developing countries, cultural factors might play a positive role in high prevalence of satisfaction. The high rate of satisfaction could also be explained by the fact that the study participants had long-term experience with dentures, and about half of the sample has used their existing dentures for more than 5 years. Celebic et al[10] reported that individuals with short experience with complete denture, or wearing their first set of dentures were less satisfied with their mandibular denture than those who had a long-term history of denture use; however, the available evidence on this issue was not conclusive and shows discrepancies, with some studies showing significant effect of the history of denture use[10,16] on patient satisfaction and others showing only a weak or no association.[15]

In the adjusted model, we did not find any statistically significant association between age of the patients and their level of satisfaction. This finding is in line with several studies[11,17,22] showing that the age of patients does not have a prognostic value in determination of successful denture therapy when the patients have been edentulous for a long time. Additionally, the lack of association between age and satisfaction may be due to the fact that the mean age of the sample population was homogeneously high (73.7 [SD 5.6] years), and it has been reported that overall satisfaction of individuals wearing dentures is broadly better at an increased age.[4]

There is a debate in the literature on the concept of using the denture-supporting tissues as a predictor of denture

satisfaction.[10,19] Clinically, a poor residual ridge will lead to lower stability and retention of the denture.[10] Therefore, it should be expected that denture stability, especially in the mandible, would lead to a higher rate of patient satisfaction. Our findings support this clinical expectation, as the stability of mandibular prostheses was significantly related to patient satisfaction. Although the median age of the existing dentures was 8 years, 61.5% of the sample had dentures with adequate freeway space. This can be explained by the fact that the study participants had been edentulous for more than 30 years with a significant effect on residual ridge resorption; however, since the bone loss was prior to the construction of the existing dentures, it is possible that the freeway space was adequate.[36]

In this study another predictor of patient satisfaction was the maxillary rocking movement in clinical examination. The maxillary rocking movement impairs the individual's ability to chew and can lead to patient dissatisfaction.[20] We also found that the ability to chew ($p < 0.05$) was the only item from a patient perspective that led to overall patient satisfaction. This result is aligned with the previous research,[29] which suggests that chewing ability is the most important factor in denture satisfaction. Over the last decade, there has been an emphasis on the use of patient-based measures and outcomes in prosthodontics research.[25] However, the majority of the published studies examined patient satisfaction with complete dentures, among patients with a range of experience and wearing dentures of various ages,[22,24] but not in the cohort of experienced denture wearers with old dentures.

This study has several limitations. First, the condition of oral mucosa and denture-bearing areas was not evaluated, and this should be considered as an important limitation of the present investigation. Another limitation is the use of cross-sectional analysis in the prediction models. Patient satisfaction can also be influenced by other factors such as patient expectation,[8] patient-dentist relationship, and psychological factors and personality traits,[7,9] which were not taken into account in this study

CONCLUSION

The results of this study showed that ability to chew, stability of the maxillary denture, and retention of the mandibular denture as well as the age of mandibular dentures contributed to patient satisfaction with dentures in a cohort of experienced denture wearers. These results indicate that although patientbased measures are essential to assess denture satisfaction, the importance of adequate denture conditions should not be underestimated.

REFERENCES

1. McNaugher GA, Benington IC, Freeman R: Assessing expressed need and satisfaction in complete denture wearers. *Gerodontology* 2001;18:51–57.

2. Carlsson GE: Facts and fallacies: an evidence base for complete dentures. *Dental Update* 2006;33:134–136, 8–40, 42.

3. Michaud PL, de Grandmont P, Feine JS, et al: Measuring patient-based outcomes: is treatment satisfaction associated with oral health-related quality of life? *J Dent* 2012;40: 624–631.

4. Pistorius J, Horn JG, Pistorius A, et al: Oral health-related quality of life in patients with removable dentures. *Schweiz Monatsschr Zahnmed* 2013;123:964–971.

5. al Quran F, Clifford T, Cooper C, et al: Influence of psychological factors on the acceptance of complete dentures. *Gerodontology* 2001;18:35–40.

6. Fenlon MR, Sherriff M, Walter JD: An investigation of factors influencing patients' use of new complete dentures using structural equation modelling techniques. *Community Dent Oral Epidemiol* 2000;28:133–140.

7. Critchlow SB, Ellis JS: Prognostic indicators for conventional complete denture therapy: a review of the literature. *J Dent* 2010;38:2–9.

8. Menassa M dGP, Audy N, Durand R, et al: Patients' expectations, satisfaction and quality of life with immediate loading protocol. *Clin Oral Implant Res* 2014 Nov 7. doi: 10.1111/clr.12515. [Epub ahead of print].

9. Perneger TV: Adjustment for patient characteristics in satisfaction surveys. *Int J Qual Health Care* 2004;16:433–435.

10. Celebic A, Knezovic-Zlataric D, Papic M, et al: Factors related to patient satisfaction with complete denture therapy. *J Gerontol A Biol Sci Med Sci* 2003;58:M948–M953.

11. Berg E, Johnsen TB, Ingebretsen R: Social variables and patient acceptance of complete dentures. A study of patients attending a dental school. *Acta Odontol Scand* 1985;43: 199–203.

12. Smith M: Measurement of personality traits and their relation to patient satisfaction with complete dentures. *J Prosthet Dent* 1976;35:492–503.

13. Fenlon MR, Sherriff M: Investigation of new complete denture quality and patients' satisfaction with and use of dentures after two years. *J Dent* 2004;32:327–333.

14. Fenlon MR, Sherriff M: An investigation of factors influencing patients' satisfaction with new complete dentures using structural equation modelling. *J Dent* 2008;36:427–434.

15. van Waas MA: The influence of clinical variables on patients' satisfaction with complete dentures. *J Prosthet Dent* 1990; 63:307–310.

16. Diehl RL, Foerster U, Sposetti VJ, et al: Factors associated with successful denture therapy. *J Prosthodont* 1996;5:84–90.

17. van Waas MA: Determinants of dissatisfaction with dentures: a multiple regression analysis. *J Prosthet Dent* 1990;64: 569–572.

18. Ebell MH, Siwek J, Weiss BD, et al: Strength of recommendation taxonomy (SORT): a patient-centered approach to grading evidence in the medical literature. *J Am Board Fam Pract* 2004;17:59–67.

19. Heydecke G, Klemetti E, Awad MA, et al: Relationship between prosthodontic evaluation and patient ratings of mandibular conventional and implant prostheses. *Int J Prosthodont* 2003;16:307–312.

20. Bilhan H, Erdogan O, Ergin S, et al: Complication rates and patient satisfaction with removable dentures. *J Adv Prosthodont* 2012;4:109–115.

21. De Lucena SC, Gomes SG, Da Silva WJ, et al: Patients' satisfaction and functional assessment of existing complete dentures: correlation with objective masticatory function. *J Oral Rehabil* 2011;38:440–446.

22. Kawai Y, Matsumaru Y, Kanno K, et al: The use of existing denture-satisfaction ratings for a diagnostic test to indicate prognosis with newly delivered complete dentures. *J Prosthodont Res* 2009;53:176–179.

23. Yamaga E, Sato Y, Minakuchi S: A structural equation model relating oral condition, denture quality, chewing ability, satisfaction, and oral health-related quality of life in complete denture wearers. *J Dent* 2013;41:710–717.

24. Fenlon MR, Sheriiff M, Walter JD: Agreement between clinical measures of quality and patients' rating of fit of existing and new complete dentures. *J Dent* 2002;30:135–139.

25. de Souza RF, Ahmadi M, Ribeiro AB, et al: Focusing on outcomes and methods in removable prosthodontics trials: a systematic review. *Clin Oral Implants Res* 2014;25: 1137–1141.

26. Carlsson GE, Omar R: The future of complete dentures in oral rehabilitation. A critical review. *J Oral Rehabil* 2010;37:143–156.

27. De Marchi RJ, Hugo FN, Hügert JB, et al: Association between number of teeth, edentulism and use of dentures with percentage body fat in south Brazilian community-dwelling older people. *Gerodontology* 2012;29:e69–e76.

28. Hilgert JB, Hugo FN, de Sousa Mda L, et al: Oral status and its association with obesity in Southern Brazilian older people. *Gerodontology* 2009;26:46–52.

29. Awad MA, Feine JS: Measuring patient satisfaction with mandibular prostheses. *Comm Dent Oral Epidemiol* 1998; 26:400–405.

30. Anastassiadou V, Katsouli S, Heath MR, et al: Validation of communication between elderly denture wearers and dentists: a

questionnaire on satisfaction with complete dentures using semi-structured interviews. *Gerodontology* 2004;21:195–200.

31. Zhang Q, Witter DJ, Bronkhorst EM, et al: Chewing ability in an urban and rural population over 40 years in Shandong Province, *China. Clin Oral Invest A* 2013;17:1425–1435.

32. Corrigan PJ, Basker RM, Farrin AJ, et al: The development of a method for functional assessment of dentures. *Gerodontology* 2002;19:41–45.

33. Viera AJ, Garrett JM: Understanding interobserver agreement: the kappa statistic. *Fam Med* 2005;37:360–363.

34. Kawai YAH, Takeo A, Kondoh T, et al: Determination of cutoff values on the 100-mm visual analogue scale to classify the satisfaction levels of complete denture wearers. *Prosthodont Res Pract* 2006;5:91–96.

35. Barros AJ, Hirakata VN: Alternatives for logistic regression in cross-sectional studies: an empirical comparison of models that directly estimate the prevalence ratio. *BMC Medical Res Methodol* 2003;3:21.

36. Tallgren A: The continuing reduction of the residual alveolar ridges in complete denture wearers: a mixed-longitudinal study covering 25 years 1972. *J Prosthet Dent* 2003;89:427–435.

22

ANALYSIS OF MASTICATORY CYCLE EFFICIENCY IN COMPLETE DENTURE WEARERS

Marcelo Coelho Goiato, DDS, MS, PHD, Alício Rosalino Garcia, DDS, MS, PHD, Daniela Micheline dos Santos, DDS, MS, PHD, and Paulo Renato Junqueira Zuim, DDS, MS, PHD
Department of Dental Materials and Prosthodontics, UNESP, São Paulo State University, Araçatuba, Brazil

Keywords
Efficiency; cycles; complete dentures

Correspondence
Marcelo Coelho Goiato, UNESP, Department of Dental Materials and Prosthodontics, São Paulo State University, José Bonifácio, 1193 Araçatuba, São Paulo 16050-050, Brazil. E-mail: goiato@foa.unesp.br

Accepted December 5, 2008

Published in *Journal of Prosthodontics* 2010; Vol. 19, Issue 1, pp. 10–3

doi: 10.1111/j.1532-849X.2009.00520.x

ABSTRACT

Purpose: This study assessed masticatory efficiency and duration of the masticatory cycle in 14 asymptomatic patients with severe bone resorption. All patients had worn complete dentures for over 10 years. Recall visits were scheduled at 5 months and 1 year after receiving new dentures.

Materials and Methods: Fourteen patients were evaluated in this study. The Research Diagnostic Criteria questionnaire and tests of the efficiency and duration of the mas-ticatory cycle were performed with artificial food before, 5 months after, and 1 year after new dentures were delivered. Masticatory efficiency was assessed using a sieve system; artificial food was ground for 35 masticatory cycles and monitored by the operator.

Results: Masticatory efficiency at 5 months was significantly improved for the 0.42-mm mesh. An improvement in masticatory efficiency and a reduction in mastication time were observed with the new dentures after 1 year.

Conclusion: The results of this study indicated that 5 months did not allow enough time to demonstrate improved muscular capacity and ability after receiving new dentures. After 1 year, the duration of the masticatory cycle was reduced, and masticatory efficiency was significantly improved.

Atrophy of denture-supporting tissues, poor adaptation, reduced masticatory efficiency, and psychosocial embarrassment are major complaints of edentulous patients wearing conventional dentures.[1] Such problems, even with the best possible prosthodontic care, have often been insurmountable with conventional denture techniques.[2] In addition, the complex neuro-muscular skills required to overcome the limitations of dentures diminish with aging.[2–5] Although there has been an increase in rehabilitation with osseointegrated implants,[6,7] treatment with conventional complete dentures still remains the most common treatment for edentulous patients.[1,8]

The loss of natural teeth leads to bone resorption, temporomandibular dysfunction,[8] and muscular hypotonicity, which may affect structures involved in mastication.[9] Furthermore, treatment success depends not only on management or preparation of the patient, but also on the clinical quality of the dentures.[10–14]

Food is generally eaten in mouthfuls, and the processing of a mouthful has been reported to involve a mastication sequence of 10 to 40 chewing cycles.[15,16] Some studies have reported findings in which subjects were generally represented by a point regarding age and number of cycles required to chew and swallow the model food with both natural dentition[17–20] and dentures.[4,18–25] Some researchers have reported that edentulous individuals, when provided with optimal complete dentures, presented with masticatory efficiency lower than in those with natural teeth, with fixed prostheses on natural teeth, or with osseointegrated oral implants.[18,26]

The aim of this study was to assess efficiency and duration of masticatory cycles in patients wearing dentures for 10 years in comparison to the evaluations performed 5 months and 1 year following fabrication and insertion of new dentures.

MATERIAL AND METHODS

Fourteen edentulous patients wearing maxillary and mandibular complete dentures for over 10 years were selected based on health history and clinical evaluations. All patients presented with reduced occlusal vertical dimension (OVD) with complete dentures showing worn teeth, alterations of anatomical occlusal form, and reduction in cuspal heights. Eight women, with a mean age of 74 years and six men, with a mean age of 71 years, were selected for the study. All patients presented with severe bone resorption in accordance with Ortman et al[27] particularly in the mandibular arch. Individuals presenting with diabetes, cardiovascular or articular alterations, hypertension, cancer, or history of temporomandibular disorders (TMD) were excluded from the study according to exclusionary criteria.

All patients were asymptomatic and presented no signs or symptoms of TMD, as defined by the Dworkin and Leresche Research Diagnostic Criteria (RDC) questionnaire.[28] The quesionnaires were administered by two examiners before the new dentures were inserted and again 5 and 12 months after denture insertion. Two examiners, calibrated according to RDC/TMD standards, performed the clinical evaluations in accordance with RDC/TMD standards.

The subjects with their old dentures were defined as the control group. Data from the control group were compared to the post-treatment data, which allowed within-subject comparsons. The selected subjects were informed about the treatment and signed an informed consent form in accordance with the recommendations of the Human Research Ethics Committee.

Clinical evaluations revealed the following conditions: severe decrease in lower face height yielding poor facial esthetics, inadequate fit of complete dentures, worn denture teeth, clinically perceptible deficiency in OVD, acquired protrusive maxillomandibular relationships secondary to resorption, or angular cheilitis.[29] The deficiencies in the preoperative OVD were corrected by adding increments of acrylic resin to the occlusal surfaces[30] of the teeth in the old mandibular dentures. The new complete dentures were made according to the procedure recommended by Zarb et al.[31]

The technique for denture fabrication consisted of preliminary impressions using stock trays and condensation silicone impression material (Zetaplus, Zhermack, Rovigo, Italy). The preliminary casts were fabricated to make custom trays for definitive impressions. Border molding was performed with heavy body condensation silicone (Zetalabor, Zhermack), and the definitive impressions were made with rubber base impression material (Pasta Lysanda Zincoenólica, Lysanda, São Paulo, Brazil) syringed around the borders of the trays until the trays were completely covered. The definitive impressions were poured with dental stone type IV (Durone, Dentsply, Rio de Janeiro, Brazil) to obtain the master casts.

The maxillary cast of each patient was mounted in a semiadjustable articulator (Whip Mix Corporation, Louisville, KY) using a face bow. OVD was established using the physiological rest positions associated with phonetic and esthetic techniques.[31]

Centric relation was established according to dynamic records based on physiological movements of the jaws, including opening, closing, and lateral movements performed by the patient.[31] These records were performed to position the mandibular casts on the articulators. Artificial teeth were selected, and bilateral balanced occlusion was obtained. The dentures were waxed, processed, finished, and polished for insertion and follow-up.[31] The new dentures showed improved facial esthetics, adequate fit, correct maxillomandibular relationships, and anatomical teeth with cusp inclination of 20°.

Mastication tests were performed using artificial food in accordance with Optocal ATF.[32] The food was fragmented as recommended by Slagter et al.[33] Each patient received an aliquot of artificial food fragments weighing a total of 3 g. The food was chewed for 35 cycles[15] and monitored by an examiner.

The patients were instructed to chew the artificial food with slight movements and not to swallow the food. The number of cycles was determined to be close to the moment of natural swallowing.[15] The cycles were monitored by an examiner and timed in seconds by a digital watch (Ikea, Hong Kong). Patients were allowed to select the chewing side. After mastication, the chewed particles were expelled into a set of four sieves. The prostheses were washed with water, and patients were asked to rinse the oral cavity to eliminate any remaining particles, expelling them into the same receptacles. At the end of the test, intraoral inspection was performed to certify that no residual food fragments remained in the oral cavity.

The particles contained in the sieve were washed with water and dried in an autoclave at 50°C for 1 hour. After drying, the sieve system was put into a vibrator for 60 seconds, and the food particles were separated according to granulometric meshes with openings of 2.0, 1.08, 0.42, and 0.20 mm, sequenced in decreasing order of size. Each mesh was weighed separately on an analytical balance (BEL Equipamentos Analítico, São Paulo, Brazil) with a precision of 0.001 g.[34,35]

The masticatory efficiency analysis was performed three times for each patient: (1) with the original denture, (2) 5 months following treatment, and (3) 1 year following treatment. Statistical analysis was performed by comparison of variance tests to compare masticatory cycles and efficiency, followed by the normal data distribution test, ANOVA, and Tukey's student range (HSD) ($p < 0.05$).

RESULTS

Denture replacement reduced the amount of artificial food retained in the 2.0-mm sieve at 5 months and 1 year after insertion of the new dentures. Food weight in the other sieve granulations (1.08, 0.42, and 0.20 mm) increased at 5 months, with further increase at 1 year (Table 1). With the original dentures, 9.93% of the material passed through the 2.0-mm sieve. With the new dentures, 14.2% passed through the 2.0-mm sieve at 5 months, and 21.4% passed through the 2.0-mm sieve at 1 year (Table 2). Five months postinsertion, masticatory efficiency was significantly improved for the small particles (0.42-mm mesh) (Table 1).

One patient reported difficulty in adapting to the new mandibular denture at the 5-month recall visit, without further improvement 1-year postinsertion. The time required to perform 35 masticatory cycles was significantly reduced only after 1 year with the new dentures (30.5 seconds), (Table 3); however, the mean amount of food that passed through the 2.0-mm sieve during masticatory cycles was statistically significant for all periods of evaluation.

DISCUSSION

In this study, there was no statistically significant improvement in masticatory efficiency and duration of masticatory cycles 5 months after denture replacement (Tables 1–3). Other authors have affirmed that patients with new dentures increased masticatory efficiency,[18,19,21,26] even with poor muscular adaptation and reduced electrical activity in the masticatory muscles.[1,8]

This small increase may be related to reestablishment of OVD[1] and presence of cusps;[6,22] however, this increase was not statistically significant–perhaps due to lack of muscular capacity and ability,[22] as well as the complex neuromuscular skills required to overcome the limitations of dentures.[1] These characteristics make occlusal adjustment of dentures difficult, perhaps permitting premature occlusal contacts that may destabilize the dentures and complicate mastication;[3] however, all but one of the patients presented significant improvement in masticatory efficiency following 1 year of treatment. This increased masticatory efficiency may have developed from muscular adaptation,[2,5,9] establishment of bilateral balanced occlusion,[18,19,21,26] presence of teeth with cusps,[6,22] and reestablishment of OVD and occlusal surfaces.[1] The new dentures with correctly positioned cusps facilitated intercuspation and perhaps required a lower amount of force to chew the food.[26] This could lead to greater chewing of food and a better quality diet.[15,16] The mean time to perform the 35 mastication cycles decreased with longer periods of new denture wear. These results are in agreement with those of Bakke et al,[10] Wilding,[11]

TABLE 1   Mean weight (g) and standard deviation (SD) of chewed artificial food retained in graduated sieve meshes before, after 5 months, and after 1 year of wearing new dentures (N = 14)

Period/mesh	Old dentures (SD)	After 5 months with new dentures (SD)	After 1 year with new dentures (SD)
2.00 mm	2.7008 ± 0.1633 A,a	2.5741 ± 0.1521 A,ab	2.358 ± 0.134 A,b
1.08 mm	0.1351 ± 0.0650 B,a	0.1822 ± 0.0601 B,a	0.234 ± 0.083 B,b
0.42 mm	0.0932 ± 0.0531 BC,a	0.1465 ± 0.0484 B,b	0.211 ± 0.067 B,c
0.20 mm	0.0700 ± 0.0557 C,a	0.0830 ± 0.0512 C,a	0.197 ± 0.00412 B,b

Different uppercase letters indicate statistically significant difference (5%) in rows (groups).
Different lowercase letters indicate statistically significant difference (5%) in columns (reading).

TABLE 2   Percentage means of ground artificial food passing through a 2.0-mm sieve before, after 5 months, and after 1 year of wearing new dentures

Period-granulation	With original dentures	After 5 months with new dentures	After 1 year with new dentures
First-2.0 mm	9.93%	14.20%	21.4%

TABLE 3   Mean time (seconds) and standard deviation (SD) of chewing cycles before, after 5 months, and after 1 year of wearing new dentures (N = 14)

Cycles/period	Time (SD)
Old denture	36.5 ± (0.52) A
After 5 months with new dentures	34.5 ± (0.45) A
After 1 year with new dentures	30.5 ± (0.40) B

Different letters indicate statistically significant difference (5%) in columns (reading).

Julien et al,[12] Christensen and Mohamed,[13] and Honma et al.[14] An additional possible explanation for improved masticatory efficiency may be explained by enhanced bilateral balanced occlusion obtained with the new dentures.

In the present study, the reduction in the number of cycles occurred mainly at the end of mastication. The reduction of cycles in this specific chewing period may have occurred due to a greater capacity of patients to chew food in the beginning of chewing[4,17,20,23–25] associated with adaptation to new dentures,[2,5,9] establishment of bilateral balanced occlusion,[18,19,21,26] and/or presence of teeth with cusps.[6,22]

Significant improvement in masticatory efficiency has been reported to occur after 5 months with implant over-dentures.[7] Geertman et al[7] speculated that this occurred due to improved adaptation and muscular capacity. The number of chewing strokes needed to pulverize the material was reduced more than with conventional dentures;[7] however, in this study, 5 months was not enough time to observe increased efficiency or change the number of masticatory cycles with the new complete dentures (Table 3).

Nevertheless, positive outcomes occurred in the majority of the patients, possibly due to reestablishment of the artificial tooth cusps with anatomic teeth and conventional balanced occlusion.[18,19,21,26] Further studies should clarify the association among masticatory efficiency and alterations in anatomical occlusal form.

CONCLUSION

In this study, patients experienced improved masticatory efficiency after 1 year with their new dentures. There were also significant decreases in particle size and number of masticatory cycles required to chew the test foods with the new complete dentures as compared to the original dentures. These results suggest that 5 months was not a long enough time to evaluate patient adaptation and functional capacity with new complete dentures.

REFERENCES

1. Goiato MC, Garcia AR, dos Santos DM: Electromyographic activity of the mandible muscles at the beginning and end of masticatory cycles in patients with complete dentures. *Gerontology* 2008;54:138–143.

2. Gunne HS, Bergman B, Enbom L, et al: Masticatory efficiency of complete denture patients. *Acta Odontol Scand* 1982;40:289–297.

3. Miralles R, Bull R, Manns A, et al: Influence of balanced occlusion and canine guidance on electromyographic activity of elevator muscles in complete denture wearers. *J Prosthet Dent* 1989;61:494–498.

4. Karkazis HC, Kossioni AE: Surface EMG activity of the masseter muscle in denture wearers during chewing of hard and soft food. *J Oral Rehabil* 1998;25:8–14.

5. Piancino MG, Farina D, Talpone F, et al: Surface EMG of jaw-elevator muscles and chewing pattern in complete denture wearers. *J Oral Rehabil* 2005;32:863–870.

6. Khamis MM, Zaki HS, Rudy TE: A comparison of the effect of different occlusal forms in mandibular implant overdentures. *J Prosthet Dent* 1998;79:422–429.

7. Geertman ME, Slagter AP, van't Hof MA, et al: Masticatory performance and chewing experience with implant-retained mandibular overdentures. *J Oral Rehabil* 1999;26:7–13.

8. Goiato MC, Garcia AR, Santos DM: Electromyographic evaluation of masseter and anterior temporalis muscles in resting position and during maximum tooth clenching of edentulous patients before and after new complete dentures. *Acta Odontol Latinoam* 2007;20:3–8.

9. Gunne HS, Wall A: The effect of new complete dentures on mastication and dietary intake. *Acta Odonto Scand* 1985;43:257–268.

10. Bakke M, Holm B, Jensen BL, et al: Unilateral, isometric bite force in 8-68-year-old women and men related to occlusal factors. *Scand J Dent Res* 1990;98:149–158.

11. Wilding RJ: The association between chewing efficiency and occlusal contact area in man. *Arch Oral Biol* 1993;38:589–596.

12. Julien KC, Buschang PH, Throckmorton GS, et al: Normal masticatory performance in young adults and children. *Arch Oral Biol* 1996;41:69–75.

13. Christensen LV, Mohamed SE: Bilateral masseteric contractile activity in unilateral gum chewing: differential calculus. *J Oral Rehabil* 1996;23:638–647.

14. Honma K, Kohno S, Honma W, et al: A study on the differences in function of free-sided and unilateral chewing. *Nihon Hotetsu Shika Gakkai Zasshi* 2005;49:459–468.

15. Woda A, Mishellany A, Peyron MA: The regulation of masticatory function and food bolus formation. *J Oral Rehabil* 2006;33:840–849.

16. Shinkai RS, Hatch JP, Rugh JD, et al: Dietary intake in edentulous subjects with good and poor quality complete dentures. *J Prosthet Dent* 2002;87:490–498.

17. Peyron MA, Blanc O, Lund JP, et al: Influence of age on adaptability of human mastication. *J Neurophysiol* 2004;92:773–779.

18. Wayler AH, Muench ME, Kapur KK, et al: Masticatory performance and food acceptability in persons with removable partial dentures, full dentures and intact natural dentition. *J Gerontol* 1984;39:284–289.

19. Fontijn-Tekamp FA, Slagter AP, Van Der Bilt A, et al: Biting and chewing in overdentures, full dentures, and natural dentitions. *J Dent Res* 2000;79:1519–1524.

20. Shikano Y: Clinical study of evaluation on masticatory function in complete denture wearers. A comparison of masticatory movements between normal natural dentition and complete denture wearers. *Nihon Hotetsu Shika Gakkai Zasshi* 1990;34:318–332.

21. Michael CG, Javid NS, Colaizzi FA, et al: Biting strength and chewing forces in complete denture wearers. *J Prosthet Dent* 1990;63:549–553.

22. Brills N: Reflexes, registrations and prosthethic therapy. *J Prosthet Dent* 1957;7:341–360.

23. Lucas PW, Luke DA: Methods for analysing the breakdown of food in human mastication. *Arch Oral Biol* 1983;28:813–819.

24. Rissin L, House JE, Manly RS, et al: Clinical comparison of masticatory performance and electromyographic activity of patients with complete dentures, overdentures, and natural teeth. *J Prosthet Dent* 1978;39:508–511.

25. Van Der Bilt A, Ottenhoff FA, Van Der Glas HW, et al: Modulation of the mandibular stretch reflex sensitivity during various phases of rhythmic open close movements in humans. *J Dent Res* 1976;76:839–847.

26. Slagter AP, Bosman F, Van Der Glas HW, et al: Human jaw-elevator muscle activity and food comminution in the dentate and edentulous state. *Arch Oral Biol* 1993;38:195–205.

27. Ortman LF, Hausmann E, Dunford RG: Skeletal osteopenia and residual ridge resorption. *J Prosthet Dent* 1989;61:321–325.

28. Dworkin SF, LeResche L: Research diagnostic criteria for temporomandibular disorders: review, criteria, examinations and specifications, critique. *J Craniomandib Disord* 1992;6:301–355.

29. Wagner AG: Complete dentures with an acquired protrusive occlusion. *Gen Dent* 1989;37:56–57.

30. Mays KA: Reestablishing occlusal vertical dimension using a diagnostic treatment prosthesis in the edentulous patient: a clinical report. *J Prosthodont* 2003;12:30–36.

31. Zarb G, Bolender C, Eckert S, et al: *Prosthodontic Treatment for Edentulous Patients (ed 12).* St. Louis, Mosby, 2004.

32. Olthoff LW, Van Der Bilt A, de Boer A, et al: Comparison of force deformation characteristics of artificial and several natural foods for chewing experiments. *J Texture Stud* 1986;7: 275–289.

33. Slagter AP, Van Der Glas HW, Bosman F, et al: Force-deformation properties of artificial and natural foods for testing chewing efficiency. *J Prosthet Dent* 1992;68:790–798.

34. Gavião MB, Raymundo VG, Sobrinho LC: Masticatory efficiency in children with primary dentition. *Pediatr Dent* 2001;23:499–505.

35. Gavião MB, Raymundo VG, Rentes AM: Masticatory performance and bite force in children with primary dentition. *Braz Oral Res* 2007;21:146–152.

23

SHORT-TERM ASSESSMENT OF THE OHIP-14 SCALE ON DENTURE WEARERS USING ADHESIVES

Gregory Polyzois, DDS, DR.DENT, MSCD,[1] Panagiotis Lagouvardos, DDS, DR.DENT,[2] Christos Partalis, DDS, MSC,[1] Panagiotis Zoidis, DDS, MS, DR.DENT,[1] AND Hector Polyzois, MPHARM[3]

[1]Department of Prosthodontics, Dental School, University of Athens, Athens, Greece
[2]Department of Operative Dentistry, Dental School, University of Athens, Athens, Greece
[3]School of Pharmacy and Biomolecular Sciences, University of Brighton, United Kingdom

Keywords

Quality of life; OHIP-14; new complete dentures; denture adhesive

Correspondence

Dr. Gregory Polyzois, Department of Prosthodontics, Dental School of Athens, 2 Thivon Str, Goudi 115 27, Athens, Greece. E-mail: grepolyz@dent.uoa.gr

The authors deny any conflicts of interest.

Accepted April 30, 2014

Published in Journal of Prosthodontics 2015; Vol. 24, Issue 5, pp. 373–80

doi: 10.1111/jopr.12227

ABSTRACT

Purpose: The purpose of this study was to assess differences of the Oral Health Implant Profile-14 (OHIP-14) scale over a month and determine association with gender, supporting tissues (KIS), and denture base (KID) among patients wearing complete dentures using denture adhesives.

Materials and Methods: Sixteen denture wearers, candidates for a new set of complete dentures, were selected. OHIP-14 scores were recorded at the beginning of the study, 6 weeks after fitting of the new set (T_0), 15 days (T_1), and finally 30 days (T_2) after daily use of a denture adhesive as instructed. The KIS and KID were clinically examined and rated according to the Kapur Index. Statistical analyses were based on repeated-measures ANOVA, Mann-Whitney test, regression analysis, and Friedman test at a = 0.05.

Results: The OHIP-14 scale was found to have a high reliability (alpha = 0.847) and a high test-retest consistency (ICC = 0.889); however, domain 1 had the lowest item-total correlation (rho = 0.144) and item 7 a negative one (rho = -0.414). Trend analysis indicated a significant negative linear trend over time (slope = -3.156, $p = 0.002$), while repeated-measures ANOVA showed differences in OHIP-14 between T_2 and T_1 ($p = 0.003$) or T_0 ($p = 0.005$) intervals. OHIP-14 groups were found to be positively associated with KIS ($p = 0.010$) and negatively with KID ($p = 0.047$) groups, but not with gender ($p = 0.272$).

Conclusions: The study shows that OHIP-14 has a high internal reliability and consistency when applied to new denture wearers, and its score decreases if denture adhesives are used for at least 15 days. Low KIS and high KID contributes to this trend. Some OHIP-14 items are more associated than others with the total score trend over time.

Edentulism is a debilitating and irreversible condition and a major health problem affecting millions of people around the world, negatively influencing oral function, social life, and daily activities.[1,2] It is managed, not always successfully, by the provision of conventional complete dentures. Rehabilitation with conventional complete dentures is a great challenge, and anatomic, clinical, technical, and psychogenic factors determine treatment success.[3–5] In view of this, it might be expected that tooth loss and the wearing of conventional complete dentures could have an impact on overall quality of life (QoL). Evidence shows the negative effect of edentulism and conventional complete denture therapy on oral health quality of life (OHQoL).[1,6–11]

Maladaptive conventional denture patients can benefit from implant-supported dentures that improve oral comfort and OHQoL.[12–14] Despite the positives, implant therapy cannot be available to all edentulous patients for various economic or patient-related factors. In such cases, few techniques or remedies remain to aid the maladaptive denture patient. Use of the neutral zone concept, altered occlusal forms, and denture adhesives have been proposed.[15]

Denture adhesives are available globally, and used by millions of denture wearers as an over-the-counter approach to improve denture retention and stability and to prevent food particles migrating under the dentures, thereby causing discomfort.[16] They are accepted as useful adjuncts to denture treatment and aftercare when properly used, as reported by prosthodontic academia and a recent publication of the American College of Prosthodontists on guidelines for the care and maintenance of complete dentures.[17,18]

The relevant literature reflects the clinical indications and benefits for use of denture adhesives in well-made and -fitting dentures, for instance, when well-made complete dentures do not satisfy a patient's perceived expectations for retention and stability.[18–23] A number of recognized objective methods have been used to evaluate the effectiveness of denture adhesives, including the Kapur Index,[23,24] occlusal force,[20–23] electromyography, and kinesiography,[25] or masticatory parameters.[26]

In addition to objective measures, self-perceived patient-based outcomes with the use of denture adhesives have confirmed increased comfort, confidence, and satisfaction with complete dentures.[23,27] In 2010, Nicolas et al[28] studied the effect of denture adhesives on OHQoL involving 14 complete denture patients for 6 months. In this study, patient QoL was assessed at three intervals: denture insertion and 3 and 6 months following insertion. At 3 months, patients were provided with denture adhesives until the 6-month assessment. They were assessed by means of Geriatric Oral Health Assessment Index (GOHAI), and the results indicated that denture adhesives improved both the patients' OHQoL and their ability to manage their dentures.

Several measurements to assess OHQoL have been developed over the past three decades as a result of increased concern about the impact of oral health status on a person's QoL. GOHAI, Subjective Oral Health Status Indicators, Oral Health Impact Profile-49 (OHIP-49), Oral Health Impact Profile-14 (OHIP-14), Dental Impact on Daily Living, and Oral Impact on Daily Performances are considered instruments of choice to assess OHQoL in the elderly.[29]

The current literature contains a number of reports using the OHIP-14 to assess OHQoL among complete denture wearers depending on prosthetic and patient-related factors.[11,30–33] However, we were unable to find any studies that correlated OHIP-14 and the use of denture adhesives among patients wearing new complete dentures. The objective of this study was to assess a possible trend and differences of the OHIP-14 scale over a 1-month period and any association of OHIP-14 with gender, quality of supporting tissues (KIS), and quality of denture base groups (KID) among patients wearing complete dentures with denture adhesives. We hypothesised a zero OHIP-14 trend over time, no significant differences of OHIP-14 scores among time intervals, and no association of gender, KIS, and KID with the OHIP-14 scale.

MATERIALS AND METHODS

Participants

For the purpose of this study, 16 volunteers (8 women, 8 men), edentulous on both arches and seeking denture treatment, were selected. Their median age was 65 years, and their median time of denture wearing was 15 years. A priori, within-factors sample size determination, using G*Power software (G*Power v.3.1.5, Kiel, Germany) indicated a total size of 16 participants, in a repeated-measures ANOVA design (effect size = 0.25, a = 0.05, $p(1-\beta) > 0.85$).

All the participants were seen in the Comprehensive Care Clinic of Athens Dental School, where they were examined and placed on a predoctoral student waiting list. Inclusion criteria were as follows: (1) fully edentulous with existing complete dentures in both arches for at least 1 year before the study, (2) adequate cognitive ability for understanding, answering questions, and completing a form, (3) no medical issues that would preclude participants from understanding the questionnaire, (4) absence of serious health problems that would prohibit attendance for scheduled appointments, (5) no known history of temporomandibular joint problems, and (6) full compliance with the study's protocol and objectives. All participants were informed of the aims and procedures of the study, and consent was obtained regarding their voluntary participation. Ethical approval from the institutional review board at the Dental School of Athens was obtained prior to the study.

Study Procedures

Before the start of the study, each patient received a new set of complete dentures according to the standard protocol used in the Division of Removable Prosthodontics. All the prosthetic treatments were performed by senior-year students under the close supervision of two faculty specialists in removable prosthodontics (GP, PZ). This protocol includes preliminary and definitive impressions with modeling compound (Sybron/Kerr, Romulus, MI) and zinc oxide eugenol (SS White; Prima Dental Group, Gloucester, UK) paste after border molding (custom trays), respectively, maxillomandibular registrations and their transfer to a semi-adjustable articulator (Hanau H2; Whip Mix Corp, Louisville, KY) using a mounting jig and a centric relation record (Exabite II NDS; GC Europe N.V, Leuven, Belgium). The denture bases were designed with a postdam seal, anatomic acrylic teeth (SR-Vivodent PE; Ivoclar Vivadent AG, Schaan, Liechtenstein) in a bilateral balanced occlusal scheme and fabricated with a standard heat-cured acrylic (Paladon 65; Heraeus Kulzer GmbH, Hanau, Germany). After fabrication, a clinical remounting was used to refine occlusion, dentures were tested on the patients for accuracy, adjustments were made, and the dentures were delivered with appropriate cleaning and wearing instructions.

Also, the functional quality of old or new dentures and supporting tissues were clinically examined and scored by a single examiner (CP) using the Kapur Index, a scale that evaluates retention and stability of dentures and denture-supporting tissues, based on categorical criteria commonly used in clinical practice.[24] Stability and retention were assessed using a 3- and 4-point scale, respectively, with a maximum sum score of 10 for each set of dentures. Dentures with a Kapur Index (KID) > 6 were considered of high functional quality (KID-H) and up to 6 of low quality (KIS-L). Participants' median KID score of their old dentures was 2, but this increased to 7 with the new dentures. Supporting tissues' quality was rated with a maximum sum score of 20 for maxilla plus mandible. Tissues with a

Kapur Index (KIS) score > 13 were considered of high quality (KIS-H) and below 14 of low quality (KIS-L). The median KIS score of our sample was 13.

The new dentures were delivered to the patients, who were asked to wear them for 6 weeks, during which all the necessary adjustments were made as required. After this adaptation/adjustment period, and once patients were free of any soreness or discomfort, the study commenced by recording patient's responses to the questionnaire and giving them instructions for when and how to apply the denture adhesive. The participants were instructed to use a denture adhesive (Corega Neutral; Stafford Miller Ltd., Waterford, Ireland) daily for 16 hours for a 1-month period. The application of cream adhesive on both dentures was done according to manufacturer's instructions ("strip method") and reapplied every 8 hours.

Oral Health Quality of Life

OHQoL was measured with the OHIP-14-GR (Greek-validated version of the OHIP-14).[34] A trained examiner applied the questionnaire during a face-to-face interview. This consisted of 14 items divided in 7 domains (functional limitation, pain, psychological discomfort, physical disability, psychological disability, social disability, and handicap). For each OHIP-14 item, participants were asked how frequently they had experienced the impact of that item. Responses were made on a 5-point Likert scale: 0 "never," 1 "hardly ever," 2 "occasionally," 3 "fairly often," 4 "very often." OHIP-14 total scores, ranging from 0 to 56 points, were obtained by summing the responses on all 14 questions (items). Higher scores imply poorer OHQoL and thus, lower satisfaction of the denture wearer. OHIP-14 total scores were also classified into a low and a high group. We hypothesized that an OHIP-14 total score up to 14 (if all items received a 'never' or 'hardly ever' vote) was considered low, while scores greater than 14 were considered high. Data were collected at baseline before the use of denture adhesive (T_0), 15 days (T_1), and 30 days (T_2) after the application of denture adhesive.

Statistical Analysis

Before validation of the OHIP-14 scale, internal and test-retest reliability of the scale was evaluated. Internal reliability or consistency was measured by Cronbach's alpha at baseline (T_0), which captures the extent of agreement among all subsets (domains) and items. Alpha values >0.80 indicate a reliable scale, although values >0.70 indicate an acceptable scale. Reliability for OHIP-14 minus item was also measured to estimate any improvement of the scale's reliability after removal of an item. Test-retest reliability was measured by intraclass correlation coefficient (ICC) using repeated measures data of OHIP-14 at T_0, T_1, and T_2 time intervals.

To determine the validity of the OHIP-14 scale for assessing differences in OHIP-14 total scores among time intervals, a repeated-measures ANOVA (within factors effects) was used. The analysis was based on Log transformed by natural logarithms OHIP-14 values and Bonferroni post hoc multiple comparisons test. The scale's ability to differentiate groups with known differences (discriminant validity) was evaluated by the association of gender, KIS, and KID groups with OHIP-14 low and high groups, using Mann-Whitney nonparametric tests. Evaluation of the amount and rate of change of the OHIP-14 scale over time, as well as between gender, KIS, or KID groups was based on linear regression analyses and comparisons of the respective regression lines.

Finally, to estimate the impact of each item on the OHIP-14 over time, the difference in individual scores of each item among time intervals was evaluated by Friedman's nonparametric test. Differences in item and domain scores over time and between gender, KIS, and KID groups were also evaluated using Wilcoxon tests. All tests were performed by SPSS statistical package (SPSS 15.0; SPSS Inc., Chicago, IL) at a significance level of $\alpha = 0.05$.

RESULTS

Scale Reliability

Reliability analysis of the scale's internal consistency showed a Cronbach's alpha value of 0.847, indicating a strong internal reliability of the scale. Since alpha values for almost all items after item removal were lower than 0.847, the inclusion of these items in the additive scale was supported, with the exception of item 7 (Table 1). Cronbach's alpha for the scale's domain groups (Table 1) also indicated that if domain 1 was deleted, the scale's reliability is improved. Test-retest reliability analysis showed a value of ICC = 0.889 with a 95% confidence interval of 0.744 to 0.958, indicating a high consistency of the repeated measures.

Scale Validity

Mean OHIP-14 total scores with their standard deviation for gender, KIS, and KID groups are shown in Table 2. For most participants, a decrease in OHIP-14 total score over time was recorded (Fig 1). Trend analysis indicated a very significant negative linear trend of OHIP-14 score with time (slope = −3.156, $p = 0.002$, Obs.Power 0.950). Repeated-measures ANOVA showed significant differences for within-factor effects (F = 11.01, $p = 0.001$, Obs.Power = 0.944), located by Bonferroni multiple comparisons test between T_0 or T_1 and T_2 ($P_{T0-T2} = 0.005$, $P_{T1-T2} = 0.003$). These results indicate that the OHIP-14 scale is able to detect changes over time and to measure the effects of denture adhesives.

TABLE 1 Reliability analysis of OHIP-14 item-total at baseline (T_0)

OHIP-14 item	Corrected item-total correlation	Squared multiple correlation	Cronbach's alpha if item deleted
Domain 1	0.144	0.348	0.881
Q1	0.221	0.799	0.851
Q2	0.106	0.974	0.856
Domain 2	0.738	0.694	0.804
Q3	0.730	0.990	0.819
Q4	0.662	0.972	0.825
Domain 3	0.639	0.545	0.818
Q5	0.569	0.881	0.832
Q6	0.521	0.934	0.835
Domain 4	0.420	0.419	0.847
Q7	−0.414	0.990	0.899
Q8	0.790	0.985	0.814
Domain 5	0.825	0.898	0.803
Q9	0.272	0.997	0.847
Q10	0.940	0.997	0.812
Domain 6	0.768	0.892	0.811
Q11	0.838	0.999	0.819
Q12	0.493	0.998	0.843
Domain 7	0.869	0.764	0.774
Q13	0.945	0.999	0.803
Q14	0.648	0.990	0.827

Mann-Whitney tests for differences between the scale's subgroups (discriminant validity evaluation) in respect to their classification into one of the two OHIP-14 groups, showed differences between low and high KIS and KID groups (Table 3). Spearman's rho rank correlation coefficients also indicated similar associations (Table 3). These findings indicate that the OHIP-14 scale is able to identify

TABLE 2 Mean OHIP-14 total scores of gender, KIS, and KID groups at T_0, T_1, and T_2 time intervals

	n		T_0	T_1	T_2
Females	8	Mean	13.25	11.50	9.38
		SD	10.88	8.47	7.73
Males	8	Mean	14.37	8.50	5.62
		SD	10.11	6.09	2.20
KIS-high	8	Mean	18.37	12.37	9.37
		SD	12.64	9.22	7.65
KIS-low	8	Mean	9.25	7.25	5.62
		SD	3.77	3.99	2.44
KID-high	8	Mean	11.90	8.80	5.70
		SD	8.96	5.88	2.21
KID-low	8	Mean	17.00	12.00	10.50
		SD	12.08	9.46	8.69
Overall	16	Mean	13.81	10.00	7.50
		SD	10.17	7.29	5.82

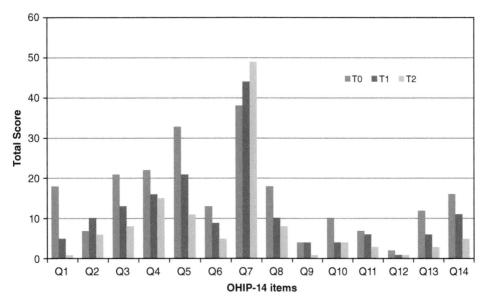

FIGURE 1 OHIP-14 items total score at T_0, T_1, and T_2 time intervals.

TABLE 3 Mann-Whitney and Spearman's rho test results for gender, KIS, and KID group pairs (n = 24)

	Mann-Whitney		Spearman's	
Group pairs	U-test*	p-value	rho*	p-value
Females/males	139.50	0.272	−0.160	0.277
KIS-low/KIS-high	91.50	0.010	0.374	0.009
KID-low/KID-high	112.00	0.047	−0.289	0.046

*Based on OHIP-14 groups.

differences in OHIP-14 score groups between KIS and KID subgroups.

Regression analysis of the OHIP-14 scale with gender, KIS, and KID groups (N = 48), is shown in Figures 2 to 4 and Table 4. Figure 2 shows that male and female trend lines start both at about the same OHIP-14 score, but the males' line is steeper than females'. This means that females are more reluctant to accept improvements in OHIP-14 than males. Coefficient of determination for both sexes was low ($R_{\mathrm{m}}^2 = 0.231, R_{\mathrm{f}}^2 = 0.033$), but the males' slope was found

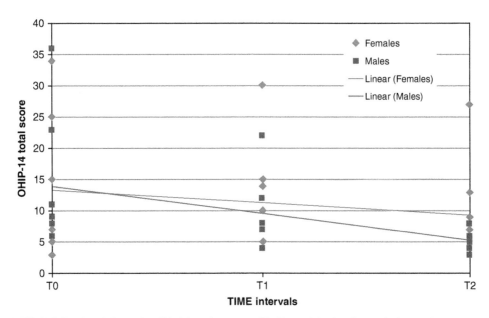

FIGURE 2 Trend lines of OHIP-14 total scores at T_0, T_1, and T_2 time intervals for gender groups.

TABLE 4   Slope, trend, and coefficient of determination for gender, KIS, and KID groups

Group	n	Slope	Trend	R^2
Females	24	−1.94	13.31	0.033
Males	24	−4.38	13.88	0.231*
KIS-low	24	−1.81	9.31	0.172*
KIS-high	24	−4.50	17.88	0.132
KID-low	18	−3.25	16.42	0.075
KID-high	30	−3.10	11.90	0.151*

*Significant at the 0.05 level 2-tailed.

to be statistically significantly different from 0 ($p_f = 0.394$, $p_m = 0.018$), indicating that a linear regression equation can be used cautiously in males, but not in females, to predict changes over time. When an exponential line was fitted to the males' data, the coefficient of determination improved ($R_m^2 = 0.313$), showing that this equation is a better predictor of changes over time for males. Figure 3 shows that KIS-H trend line starts at a higher OHIP-14 score than KIS-L line, but it is steeper than KIS-L and ends close to KIS-L. This means that the amount and rate of change in OHIP-14 was greater in KIS-H than in KIS-L group. This change was found to be significant ($p = 0.012$); however, both coefficients of determination were poor ($R_L^2 = 0.172$, $R_H^2 = 0.132$), showing that their value to predict changes over time is poor. Figure 4 shows that trend line of KID-L starts at a higher OHIP-14 score than KIS-H, and both have almost the same slope. Since both coefficients of determination were poor ($R_L^2 = 0.075$, $R_H^2 = 0.151$), we can conclude that the amount and rate of change was the same in both groups, and their

value to predict changes over time is poor. The above evaluation is only indicative for the OHIP-14 score trend over time of the involved groups, and more data from several time intervals are needed to establish a more definite image of their trend.

Friedman test results for differences among time interval scores within items, are shown in Table 5. Only four items (1, 5, 10, 13) present a significant difference, indicating close association with total score change over time.

Wilcoxon test results between pairs of gender, KIS, and KID groups, at T_0, T_1, and T_2 time intervals are shown in Table 6. Item scores for the OHIP-14 scale given by the participants were different between males and females at the T_1 and T_2 intervals, between low and high KIS at all intervals, and between low and high KID groups at the T_0 interval only. It means that the association of OHIP-14 items with KIS groups is evident throughout all time intervals, with gender groups at T_1, T_2, intervals and with KID groups at baseline (T_0) only.

DISCUSSION

The study rejected the hypothesis of a zero trend of OHIP-14 scale over time in denture wearers with adhesives and the hypothesis of no differences among time intervals. Results led us to accept the hypothesis of no association of gender with OHIP-14 scale, but rejected that KIS and KID have no association with OHIP-14.

The strong internal reliability of the scale found in this study indicates its ability to be used as an instrument to measure the impact of oral health on the QoL of denture wearers with or without adhesives and with a high

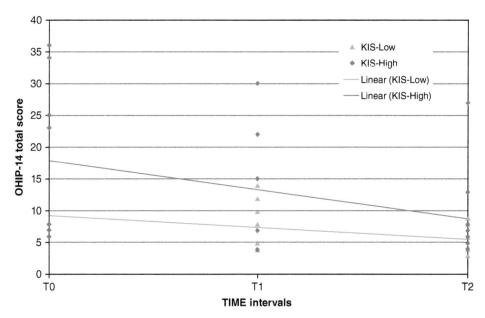

FIGURE 3   Trend lines of OHIP-14 total scores at T_0, T_1, and T_2 time intervals for KIS groups.

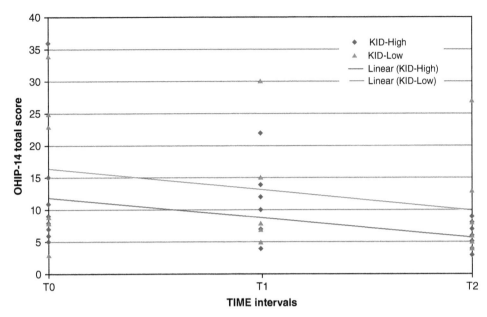

FIGURE 4 Trend lines of OHIP-14 total scores at T_0, T_1, and T_2 time intervals for KID groups.

TABLE 5 Friedman's test results for differences among time intervals within each item

Question	x^2	p
Q1	13.42	0.001
Q2	2.00	0.368
Q3	4.22	0.121
Q4	2.80	0.332
Q5	19.14	0.000
Q6	1.37	0.504
Q7	1.00	0.614
Q8	4.00	0.135
Q9	2.80	0.247
Q10	7.62	0.022
Q11	2.00	0.368
Q12	2.00	0.368
Q13	7.44	0.024
Q14	5.03	0.081

TABLE 6 Wilcoxon test* for differences in item scores betweer pairs for gender, KIS, and KID groups at T_0, T_1, and T_2 time intervals

	T_0	T_1	T_2
Females-males	0.695	0.013	0.003
KIS-low/KIS-high	0.021	0.027	0.035
KID-low/KID-high	0.042	0.176	0.791

*Based on item scores (n = 14).

consistency of their responses to the questionnaire. Its strong test-retest reliability also shows an ability to be used for repeated measurements over time; however, the study revealed that domain 1 and item 7 are the weak points of the Greek version of the OHIP-14 scale used in the study and need to be rephrased or removed and revalidated to increase scales reliability even further.

The decrease of OHIP-14 score just 15 days after the use of an adhesive in both dentures indicates that this short period is capable of revealing the effect of denture adhesives on OHIP-14. Veyrune et al[10] reported an improvement in the OHQoL measure (GOHAI) following the fitting of new dentures not sooner than 12 weeks, indicating a long denture adaptation process. This study indicates a definite improvement in 2 weeks after use of an adhesive, implying that adhesives do help the improvement of OHQoL in patients with new complete dentures and may be used to shorten new dentures' adaptation period.

Improvement of OHQoL after using adhesives was also shown by Nicolas et al[28] after 3 months, using the GOHAI scale. The improvement shown in our study, a short time after using an adhesive, may also be attributed to the adaptation effect of new dentures; however, this part is rather small considering that new dentures were allowed to adapt for 6 weeks before the use of an adhesive and that adhesives have an immediate action on the fitting of new dentures. Nicolas et al[28] investigated the adaptation effect in their study and also showed that the improvement in the GOHAI scale was mainly an effect of denture adhesives.

In this study, gender was found to have no association with OHIP-14 groups and may not play a significant role in the trend of OHIP-14 scores over this short period of time.

Mastrogeorgopoulou and Anastasiadou[34] also reported no association, reasoning that OHIP-14 can be safely applied to both sexes; however, there seems to be a tendency for higher scores in females with the use of adhesive, findings that have been presented by others[11,33,35,36] and is explained by the fact that women have higher complaints than men about several oral health conditions and for this reason are more reluctant to admit improvements.

The study rejected the hypothesis of no association of KIS with OHIP-14, since it was found that low KIS groups present low OHIP-14 scores and vice versa. Despite this, high KIS groups have a stronger negative trend than low KIS groups, which show a rather flat trend line. A possible explanation for this is that good supporting tissues may offer a quicker and greater improvement over time by using denture adhesives in new dentures than poor supporting tissues.

The null hypothesis for KID groups was also rejected, since low KID groups were associated with low OHIP-14 groups. This can be explained by the fact that low-quality dentures are more prone to improvement by the applying adhesives than those of high quality.

Finally, the study revealed that items with significant differences among time intervals were 1b, 2a, 2b, 3a, and 5b. These questions concern problems with taste, pain, eating, self-consciousness, and relaxation when wearing dentures with adhesives, and it seems that these may partly explain the OHIP-14 trend.

Although results were sufficiently documented, the problem of sample size remains a concern due to differences within participants and the difficulty of homogenizing individuals, especially when costly devices are to be constructed and delivered. Multivariate analyses do not resolve the problem, since sample subgroups of interest also have the same problem. The clinical relevance supported by the findings of the study was that the use of an adhesive for a short period by denture wearers, regardless of gender, could improve denture adaptation and satisfaction.

CONCLUSION

The study shows that OHIP-14 has a high internal reliability and consistency when applied to new denture wearers, and its score decreases if denture adhesives are used for at least 15 days. A low Kapur Index for denture-supporting tissues and high Kapur Index for denture base quality contribute to this trend. Some OHIP-14 items are more associated than others with the total score trend over time.

REFERENCES

1. Emami E, de Souza RF, Kabawat M, et al: The impact of edentulism on oral and general health. *Int J Dent* 2013; doi: 10.1155/2013/498305. Epub May 8, 2013.

2. Heydecke G, Thomason JM, Lund JP, et al: The impact of conventional and implant supported prostheses on social and sexual activities in edentulous adults. Results from a randomized trial 2 months after treatment. *J Dent* 2005;33:649–657.

3. Carlsson GE, Omar R: The future of complete dentures in oral rehabilitation. A critical review. *J Oral Rehabil* 2010;37:143–156.

4. Fenlon MR, Sherriff M, Newton JT: The influence of personality on patients' satisfaction with existing and new complete dentures. *J Dent* 2007;35:744–748.

5. al Quran F, Clifford T, Cooper C, et al: Influence of psychological factors on the acceptance of complete dentures. *Gerodontology* 2001;18:35–40.

6. Hugo FN, Hilgert JB, de Sousa Mda L, et al: Oral status and its association with general quality of life in older independent-living south-Brazilians. *Community Dent Oral Epidemiol* 2009;37:231–240.

7. Nitschke I, Müller F: The impact of oral health on the quality of life in the elderly. *Oral Health Prev Dent* 2004;2 Suppl 1: 271–275.

8. Fiske J, Davis DM, Francce C, et al: The emotional effects of tooth loss in edentulous people. *Br Dent J* 1998;184:90–93.

9. Heydecke G, Tedesco LA, Kowalski C, et al: Complete dentures and oral health-related quality of life – do coping styles matter? *Community Dent Oral Epidemiol* 2004;32: 297–306.

10. Veyrune JL, Tubert-Jeannin S, Dutheil C, et al: Impact of new prostheses on the oral health related quality of life of edentulous patients. *Gerodontology* 2005;22:3–9.

11. Perea C, Suárez-García MJ, Del Río J, et al: Oral health-related quality of life in complete denture wearers depending on their socio-demographic background, prosthetic-related factors and clinical condition. *Med Oral Patol Oral Cir Bucal* 2013;18: e371–e380.

12. Feine JS, Carlsson GE, Awad MA, et al: The McGill Consensus Statement on overdentures. Mandibular two-implant overdentures as first choice standard of care for edentulous patients. Montreal, Quebec, May 24–25, 2002. *Int J Oral Maxillofac Implants* 2002;17:601–602.

13. Feine JS, Lund JP: Treatment outcomes of fixed or removable implant-supported prostheses in the edentulous maxilla. *J Prosthet Dent* 2000;84:372–373.

14. Torres BL, Costa FO, Modena CM, et al: Association between personality traits and quality of life in patients treated with conventional mandibular dentures or implant-supported overdentures. *J Oral Rehabil* 2011;38:454–461.

15. Cooper LF: The current and future treatment of edentulism. *J Prosthodont* 2009;18:116–122.

16. Duqum I, Powers KA, Cooper L, et al: Denture adhesive use in complete dentures: clinical recommendations and review of the literature. *Gen Dent* 2012;60:467–477.

17. Slaughter A, Katz RV, Grasso JE: Professional attitudes toward denture adhesives: a Delphi technique survey of academic prosthodontists. *J Prosthet Dent* 1999;82:80–89.

18. Felton D, Cooper L, Duqum I, et al: Evidence-based guidelines for the care and maintenance of complete dentures: a

publication of the American College of Prosthodontists. *J Prosthodont* 2011;20 Suppl 1:S1–S12.

19. Grasso JE: Denture adhesives. *Dent Clin North Am* 2004;48:721–733.

20. Pradíes G, Sanz I, Evans O, et al: Clinical study comparing the efficacy of two denture adhesives in complete denture patients. *Int J Prosthodont* 2009;22:361–367.

21. Polyzois G, Lagouvardos P, Frangou M, et al: Efficacy of denture adhesives in maxillary dentures using gnathodynamometry: a comparative study. *Odontology* 2011;99:155–161.

22. Polyzois G, Partalis C, Lagouvardos P, et al: Effect of adaptation time on the occlusal force at denture dislodgement with or without denture adhesive. *J Prosthet Dent* 2014;111:216–221.

23. Munoz CA, Gendreau L, Shanga G, et al: A clinical study to evaluate denture adhesive use in well-fitting dentures. *J Prosthodont* 2012;21:123–129.

24. Kapur KK: A clinical evaluation of denture adhesives. *J Prosthet Dent* 1967;18:550–558.

25. Grasso J, Gay T, Rendell J, et al: Effect of denture adhesive on retention of the mandibular and maxillary dentures during function. *J Clin Dent* 2000;11:98–103.

26. Fujimori T, Hirano S, Hayakawa I: Effects of a denture adhesive on masticatory functions for complete denture wearers consideration for the condition of denture-bearing tissues. *J Med Dent Sci* 2002;49:151–156.

27. Kelsey CC, Lang BR, Wang RF: Examining patients' responses about the effectiveness of five denture adhesive pastes. *J Am Dent Assoc* 1997;128:1532–1538.

28. Nicolas E, Veyrune JL, Lassauzay C. A six-month assessment of oral health-related quality of life of complete denture wearers using denture adhesive: a pilot study. *J Prosthodont* 2010;19:443–448.

29. Hebling E, Pereira AC: Oral health-related quality of life: a critical appraisal of assessment tools used in elderly people. *Gerodontology* 2007;24:151–161.

30. Palac A, Bitanga P, Capkun V, et al: Association of cephalometric changes after 5 years of complete dentures wearing and oral health-related quality-of-life. *Acta Odontol Scand* 2013;71:449–456.

31. Forgie AH, Scott BJ, Davis DM: A study to compare the oral health impact profile and satisfaction before and after having replacement complete dentures in England and Scotland. *Gerodontology* 2005;22:137–142.

32. Scott BJ, Forgie AH, Davis DM: A study to compare the oral health impact profile and satisfaction before and after having replacement complete dentures constructed by either the copy or the conventional technique. *Gerodontology* 2006;23:79–86.

33. Chen YF, Yang YH, Chen JH, et al: The impact of complete dentures on the oral health-related quality of life among the elderly. *Dent Sci* 2012;7:289–295.

34. Mastrogeorgopoulou C, Anastassiadou V: The contribution of the Greek version of OHIP-14 in cross-cultural adaptation. *Stoma* 2011;39:183–188.

35. Ulinski KG, do Nascimento MA, Lima AM, et al: Factors related to oral health-related quality of life of independent Brazilian elderly. *Int J Dent* 2013; doi: 10.1155/2013/705047. Epub Mar 6, 2013.

36. Khalifa N, Allen PF, H Abu-bakr NH, et al: Psychometric properties and performance of the oral health impact profile (OHIP-14s-ar) among Sudanese adults. *J Oral Sci* 2013;55:123–132.

24

COMPARISONS OF PATIENT SATISFACTION LEVELS WITH COMPLETE DENTURES OF DIFFERENT OCCLUSIONS: A RANDOMIZED CLINICAL TRIAL

Mohhamadjavad Shirani, dds,[1] Ramin Mosharraf, dds, msc,[2] and Mohammadkazem Shirany, bsc[3]

[1]Dentist, Dental Students' Research Committee, School of Dentistry, Isfahan University of Medical Sciences, Isfahan, Iran
[2]Associate Professor, Dental Materials Research Center, Department of Prosthodontics, School of Dentistry, Isfahan University of Medical Sciences, Isfahan, Iran
[3]PhD student, Department of Statistics, University of Michigan, Ann Arbor, MI

Keywords
Patient satisfaction; complete denture; balanced dental occlusion; lingualized occlusion

Correspondence
Dr. Ramin Mosharraf, Associate Professor, Dental Material Research Center and Department of Prosthodontics, School of Dentistry, Isfahan University of Medical Sciences, Hezar-Jarib Ave, Isfahan, 8174673461 Iran.

E-mail: mosharraf@dnt.mui.ac.ir

Financial support was provided from Isfahan University of Medical Sciences (grant number 190052).

This trial was registered in ClinicalTrials.gov and IRCT as "NCT01493232" and "IRCT201110097749N1," respectively.

The authors declare no potential conflicts of interest.

Accepted July 10, 2013

Published in *Journal of Prosthodontics* 2014; Vol. 23, Issue 4, pp. 259–66

doi: 10.1111/jopr.12101

ABSTRACT

Purpose: There is a lack of evidence to recommend a particular type of posterior occlusal form for conventional complete dentures. The type of posterior occlusal scheme can affect complete denture stability, retention, and patient satisfaction. The objective of this study was to compare patient satisfaction to three types of complete denture occlusion using a randomized, crossover controlled trial.

Materials and Methods: Three sets of complete dentures were made for each of 15 patients (mean age = 58.87 ± 15.02 years). They received (1) fully bilateral balanced occlusion (BBO), (2) lingualized occlusion, and (3) buccalized occlusion (BO) denture sets in random order. After wearing each set for 6 weeks, patient satisfaction was assessed using a 19-item version of the Oral Health Impact Profile for Edentulous Patients (OHIP-EDENT). Each question was scored on a 1 to 5 scale for patients' problems with dentures (for these ordinal variables, 1 = "never" and 5 = "very often"). These items were first analyzed by Friedman tests and then by Wilcoxon rank tests for 80% test power at the 0.05-alpha level (d = 0.7).

Results: BO resulted in lower avoidance of particular foods and physical disability scores than fully BBO.

Conclusions: With the caution of small sample size, the results of this study provide evidence that use of BO can improve food avoidance and physical disability aspects of patient satisfaction with complete dentures.

A patient's quality of life is greatly affected by his/her satisfaction with complete dentures.[1] Support, retention, and stability are fundamental considerations for a successful prosthesis.[2–4] More patient problems are associated with mandibular conventional complete dentures (CCDs),[1,5] particularly in female patients.[6,7] The stability and retention of mandibular dentures are important factors related to patient satisfaction with CCDs.[8] Meticulous preparation of impressions and polishing and balancing occlusal surfaces improve retention and stability.[2,9]

Unfavorable tongue positions, CCD design defects, unhealthy mucosal conditions, and excessive denture wearing times will increase patient complaints.[10–13] Because of the effects of masticatory postarticulation forces on denture retention and stability, dentures must be adjusted perfectly.[14] Bonwill described how the teeth should be adjusted to obtain balanced occlusion without interference.[15] Occlusal harmony is important for patient comfort. Thus, occlusal adjustments by both laboratory remounts and clinical procedures can increase patient comfort.[16]

It has been stated that dentures with lingualized occlusion (LO) are more stable. Thus, it is the occlusion of choice for patients with severe ridge resorption.[14] Greater chewing ability has been reported for patients with LO or fully bilateral balanced occlusion (FBBO) dentures compared to monoplane occlusion dentures.[17] Clough et al[18] in a crossover randomized clinical trial found that LO was superior to monoplane occlusion in terms of chewing ability and patient comfort. Similar conclusions were reached for better chewing efficacy and patient preferences for LO and FBBO than for monoplane occlusion.[19] Patients reported greater denture retention satisfaction with LO than with FBBO.[20] At the Dental Hospital of Manchester, Sutton and McCord[21] fabricated three sets of dentures for 45 patients and followed up each set for 8 weeks. Patients reported greater satisfaction with LO dentures than with monoplane occlusions, particularly with regard to sore spots, and also reported that FBBO provided better masticatory function than did a 0° occlusal form. Perfect physiology of restorations in terms of biomechanical concepts in occlusion provide for better stomatognathic system health.[22]

In light of the previously cited studies, although LO and FBBO provide relatively better CCD satisfaction, some patients still have problems with dentures, particularly mandibular problems. Further, the necessity for complete dentures is not likely to decrease in the near future, and investigators should pay close attention to improving

CCDs.[23] In this study, we sought to present and evaluate a new occlusal Scheme [14,18,21,24–27] for the first and to compare patient satisfaction with it to LO and FBBO. Buccalized occlusion (BO) provides for simple occlusal adjustments and less occlusal interference and surface contacts between maxillary and mandibular teeth. Consequently, there should be fewer mandibular denture loadings and dislodgings because of its movements, and possibly greater CCD retention without unpleasant dark spaces between maxillary and mandibular buccal cusps in centric positions. Our null hypothesis was that there would be no difference in patient satisfaction with complete dentures fabricated with either a fully bilateral balanced, lingualized, or buccalized occlusion.

MATERIALS AND METHODS

Patient satisfaction with complete dentures with different types of occlusions was compared in a crossover randomized clinical study. For each patient, three sets of complete dentures were made using different posterior occlusal schemes: FBBO, LO, and BO in a completely balanced manner. Fifteen patients used these sets in a random order. After wearing each set for a 6-week period, patient satisfaction was recorded. The Isfahan Regional Bioethics Committee granted ethical approval for our study protocol.

For cluster sampling, after selection of five prosthodontists, we enrolled edentulous patients of their students, in the Torabinejad Dental Research Center. The inclusion criteria were as follows: having ideal maxillomandibular relationships (cl I and mild cl II, cl III Skeletal base classification); absence of severely resorbed ridges; and completely edentulous for at least 3 months. These patients also had to provide written informed consent. Exclusion criteria were uncontrolled systemic disease, mental problems, and unwillingness to remain in the study. Uncooperative patients before tooth selection were not allowed to continue in the study.

A list was prepared with 15 rows, for which the types and order of dentures were determined randomly in three categories in front of each number. Patients were arranged randomly in this list using a random number generator created with a calculator when tooth size and color were selected. Five patients were assigned to each intervention category. One intervention group first received FBBO, then LO, and finally BO. A second group received LO, BO, and

FBBO, respectively, and the third group received BO, FBBO, and LO, in that order.

Clinical procedures were performed by dental students. All clinical and laboratory procedures that appeared to be similar (duplicating definitive casts, making a record base, verifying records, LO and BO set arrangements, denture waxing, remounting and occlusal adjustments, finishing and polishing, denture insertion, and recall appointments) were performed by one student and observed by one experienced prosthodontist (MR).

The denture fabrication process consisted of making a preliminary impression with irreversible hydrocolloid (Iralgin; Golchay, Tehran, Iran) and pouring with type II stone (Dental Stone; Pars Dandan, Tehran, Iran), making a special autopolymerizing resin (Acropars; Marlik, Tehran, Iran) tray, border molding with a modeling plastic impression compound (Impression Compound; Kerr, Salerno, Italy), making a zinc oxide eugenol (Luralite; Kerr) definitive impression, boxing it, and pouring the final cast with type III stone (Dental Stone). Each final cast was duplicated three times using reversible hydrocolloid (Grun, Hinrigel, Germany). After recording the maxillo-mandibular relationship with the modeling plastic impression compound on wax rims (Modeling Wax; Dentsply, Hoorn, UK) over an autopolymerizing baseplate, final casts were mounted[28] with an average value articulator (Free Plan; Pars Dandan), and an anatomic 30° tooth set was selected (Teeth Mold; Myerson, Laventille, Trinidad & Tobago) with the same size and color for each of the three sets.

All students arranged an FBBO set with anterior teeth and attempted to fit it in. An FBBO (Figs 1 to 3) was defined as the bilateral, simultaneously anterior, and posterior occlusal contact of teeth in centric and eccentric positions.[29] After final tooth adjustment and registering the verifying records by one experienced prosthodontist for all patients, two other sets of eight maxillary and mandibular incisors in the articulator were arranged by putty index (Speedex; Coltene,

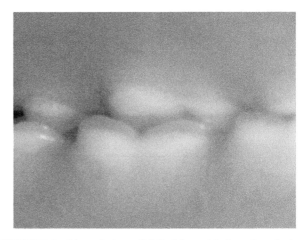

FIGURE 2   Lingual view of fully bilateral balanced occlusion.

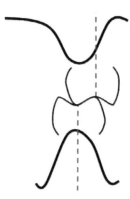

FIGURE 3   Fully bilateral balanced occlusion.

Alstatten, Switzerland) so that the position of the anterior teeth would be similar for each three sets in each of the 15 patients, and posterior mandibular teeth were articulated against the FBBO maxillary teeth. An LO (Figs 4 to 6) tooth arrangement was described not only by articulation of the

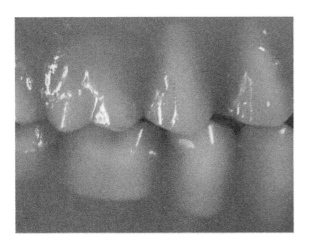

FIGURE 1   Buccal view of fully bilateral balanced occlusion.

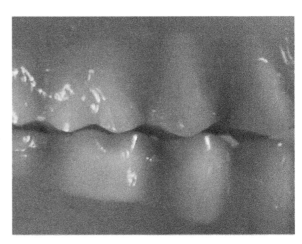

FIGURE 4   Buccal view of lingualized occlusion.

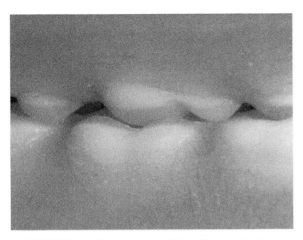

FIGURE 5   Lingual view of lingualized occlusion.

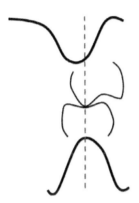

FIGURE 6   Lingualized occlusion.

maxillary palatal cusps with the opposing mandibular occlusal surfaces but also by maxillary buccal cusps, which were not allowed to contact the mandibular teeth in centric or eccentric positions. The contacts at the balanced side were between maxillary palatal and mandibular buccal cusps.[26] When BO (Figs 7 to 9) sets were to be arranged, mandibular

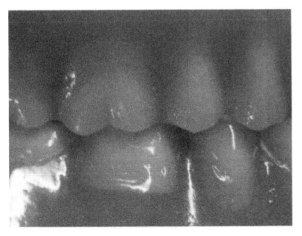

FIGURE 7   Buccal view of buccalized occlusion.

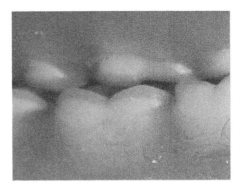

FIGURE 8   Lingual view of buccalized occlusion.

posterior teeth were primarily moved and tilted somewhat to the lingual until mandibular buccal cusp tips were located against the mandibular ridge crest. After grinding the lingual slopes of the maxillary buccal cusps, they were arranged in position so that buccal cusps were about 0.5 mm higher than palatal cusps. Finally, the four remaining cuspids were positioned. After tooth arrangement was complete, denture sets were waxed.

They were flasked and processed by the same flasking procedure (Flask; Ash, Plymouth, UK), wax was removed, a thin foil substitute was painted, packed with resin (Ivoclar Vivadent, Schaan, Liechtenstein, Germany), cured by machine (Type 5518; Kavo, Warthausen, Germany), anddeflasked. These procedures were performed by one technician. Dentures were remounted using an average articulator value by remounting casts, and occlusal adjustments were made to achieve BO. Buccal slopes of lingual cusps and lingual slopes in buccal cusps were reduced for mandibular teeth of LO sets. BO was adjusted with all mandibular buccal cusps articulating to opposite surfaces of maxillary posterior teeth, all maxillary palatal cusps were reduced about 0.5 mm, and there was no contact between these and mandibular teeth in centric and eccentric positions. The contacts were settled to be between maxillary palatal and mandibular buccal cusps for the balancing side.

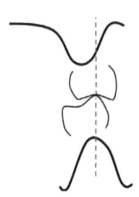

FIGURE 9   Buccalized occlusion.

Finishing and polishing were performed using laboratory carbide burs (Carbide Bur; Renfert, Hinzingen, Germany), super-flex and soft-flex abrasive paper (Schleifpapier; Matador Wasserfest, Leipzig, Germany), and pumicing (White Pumice; Hess Pumice, Malad City, ID) with a prepared rag wheel.

Patients were blinded to the dentures they wore. A 4-hour period between changes in dentures between two sets was set as a wash-out period.[30] During the study, only one set of dentures was retained by the patients at a time until all three sets were delivered. After wearing each set for a 6-week period, according to the predetermined list, patient satisfaction was evaluated by interview using the Oral Health Impact Profile for Edentulous Patients (OHIP-EDENT) questionnaire. Interviews were conducted by one impartial interrogator for all patients. In previous studies, the 14-, 19-, 20-, and 49-question versions of this questionnaire were presented.[1,21,31] Due to the length of the 49-item version of the OHIP-EDENT, it is not applicable in the clinical setting.[1] The extra item in the 20-question version in contrast with the 19-question version is an item about unclear speech, whose influence can already be observed in the discomfort items as 'self-conciousness'. On the other hand, the 14-question version may change the efficacy of the instrument.[31] For this study, a 19-question version (of 49 items) of the OHIP-EDENT was used. Each question was scored on a 1-to-5 scale. For these ordinal variables, 1 = "never" and 5 = "very often." Each question was weighted.[1] The 19 questions pertained to seven domains as follows: functional limitation, physical pain, psychological discomfort, physical disability, psychological disability, social disability, and handicap. When the domain's scores were to be calculated, the weights for each item were considered. After translating this questionnaire, content validity was verified by two experienced prosthodontists, and face validity was investigated in a pilot study. Cronbach's alpha ($\alpha = 0.906$) and the intraclass correlation coefficients were determined to confirm test reliability.

Based on previous similar studies, 14 patients with each method were required for 80% test power to identify significant differences in median values at the 5% level (d = 0.7); however, because of three comparison groups, considering Bonferroni adjustment, $p < 0.0167$ ($0.05/3 = 0.0167$) was deemed to be significant. One patient was added to divide them into three equal groups. The alpha level was verified in all tests at 0.05. Data analysis was performed using SPSS version 16.0 statistical software (SPSS, Inc., Chicago, IL) by a statistician blinded to the study patients and treatments. Data were first compared by Friedman tests. Then a Wilcoxon test was used to compare the paired results for the different groups.

Thirty-six patients were initially examined by an experienced prosthodontist, out of which 30 were selected for this study. These patients were asked to provide written informed consent within 1 week; 20 signed these informed consent forms. Three patients refused to continue participating before tooth selection during the clinical procedures. Two were excluded due to noncooperation. One left during the study because of incompatibility with the first set of dentures, and another patient was entered instead. Finally, 15 patients (8 males, 7 females) completed the 18-week follow-up period.

RESULTS

Figure 10 shows a flow chart for the patients throughout this study. First, p-values from Friedman tests between the three denture sets were determined for each question (Table 1). Then, those questions with $p \leq 0.1$ were examined by Wilcoxon signed rank tests (Table 2). The frequencies, mean values, and standard deviations of the identified items from Table 2 are shown in Table 3. FBBO was scored significantly higher for uncomfortable eating than LO, and also higher for avoiding particular foods than both LO and BO. FBBO was scored significantly lower for uncomfortable dentures than LO. No other significant differences were found after comparing the other items.

Each domain score's median was calculated using the weights noted in Table 1, and the total score was also calculated for each set (Table 4). Table 5 shows the p-values for these scores derived from Wilcoxon signed rank tests. FBBO had a significantly higher score for physical disability than BO. Cronbach's alpha values for the FBBO, LO, and BO denture sets were 0.864, 0.896, and 0.924, respectively.

DISCUSSION

The null hypothesis of our study was that there would be no differences in patient satisfaction with complete dentures made with either a fully bilateral balanced, lingualized, or buccalized occlusion; this hypothesis was rejected. With FBBO, patients had more unpleasant eating experiences than with LO, and a greater tendency to avoid eating some foods than with LO and BO. The reason for these differences may have been worse masticatory performance with FBBO than BO with regard to a more occlusal contact surface that causes more dislodging of dentures on eccentric movements and force to penetrate the cusps into foods.[14] The inability to perform activities was described as "physical disability."[1,31]

Clough et al[18] fabricated dentures for 30 patients in a crossover randomized clinical trial. The dentures were worn for a 3-week period and then exchanged. They found that LO was superior to monoplane occlusion in terms of chewing ability, patient comfort, and esthetics. In 2007, Sutton and

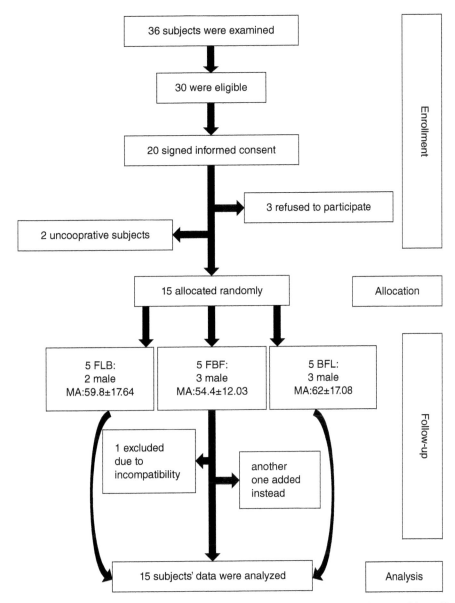

FIGURE 10 Diagram of trial phases. F: Fully bilateral balanced occlusion. L: Lingualized occlusion. B: Buccalized occlusion. MA: Mean Age ± Standard deviation (years).

McCord[21] prepared three sets of dentures for 45 patients and followed up each set for 8 weeks. Patients reported greater satisfaction with LO dentures than with monoplane occlusions, particularly with regard to sore spots, and also reported that FBBO provided better masticatory function compared with a 0° occlusal form.

Masticatory efficiency was evaluated using objective food tests and a subjective questionnaire by Khamis et al.[19] They found patient preference for the FBBO and LO as opposed to monoplane occlusion by their improved ability to chew hard foods with no differences between these two (FBBO, LO). Similar conclusions were reached for better masticatory

efficiency for LO[18] and FBBO than monoplane occlusion.[21] However, Kydd[27] found no differences between complete dentures when assessed for masticatory efficiency for these three occlusal schemes. Furthermore, Matsumaru[14] suggested that patients with severely resorbed ridges treated with FBBO present decreased masticatory efficiency in contrast with LO, while Kimoto et al[20] reported no significant differences between these two.

The findings of this study were similar to those of previous trials that compared LO and FBBO.[18,21] FBBO is not obligatory for a successful complete denture. Only simple occlusal adjustments are needed for LO and BO.

TABLE 1   OHIP-EDENT and *p*-values from the Friedman test

Domain	Question	Weight	Items	*p*-value
FL	1	1.253	Chewing problems	0.06[a]
FL	2	1.181	Food catching	0.54
P1	3	1.213	Pain in mouth	0.06[a]
P1	4	0.998	Uncomfortable eating any food	0.008[a]
P1	5	1.264	Sore spots	0.02[a]
FL	6	1.472	Fitting improperly	0.12
P1	7	1.002	Uncomfortable denture	0.009[a]
P2	8	2.006	Worried about dental problems	0.42
P2	9	1.902	Self-conscious due to denture	0.60
D1	10	1.266	Avoid eating some foods	0.001[a]
D1	11	1.351	Unable to eat	0.65
D1	12	0.952	Interrupted meals	0.17
D2	13	1.393	Upset because of denture problems	0.36
D2	14	1.437	Embarrassed by denture problems	0.60
D3	15	1.572	Avoid going out	0.13
D3	16	2.555	Less tolerant with family	0.03[a]
D3	17	1.236	Irritable with other people	0.47
H	18	1.545	Dislike other peoples' company	1
H	19	1.567	Lower life satisfaction	0.77

FL = functional limitation.
P1 = physical pain.
P2 = psychological discomfort.
D1 = physical disability.
D2 = psychological disability.
D3 = social disability.
H = handicap.
[a]Items with $p < 0.1$ for analysis in the next step (Table 2).

Additionally, LO and BO present less occlusal interference and surface contacts between maxillary and mandibular teeth and, consequently, fewer mandibular denture loadings and dislodgings on lateroprotrusion movements.[16,24] Therefore FBBO presents worse masticatory performance,[8,14,26] a distinct FBBO disadvantage. With BO in centric position, occlusal forces are transferred to ridge crests because of the direction of resorption in which the mandibular crest is moved buccally rather than toward the maxilla in molar regions.[30] BO increased retention and stability, and it can be used successfully in patients with a more buccally inclined posterior mandibular ridge crest than one inclined toward the

maxilla. A new BO was perceived to be successful, although the investigators proposed that the occlusal design for patients should be selected based on the conditions of their ridges.

The limitations of this study included the small number of patients, restrictions for performing the clinical procedures, a short wash-out period, and assistance by multiple students;

TABLE 2   *p*-values from the Wilcoxon signed rank test

Question	FBBO vs. LO	FBBO vs. BO	LO vs. BO
1	0.050	0.111	0.527
3	0.167	0.167	1
4	0.013[a]	0.031	0.257
5	0.124	0.112	0.564
7	0.014[a]	0.157	0.046
10	0.010[a]	0.006*	1
16	0.063	0.317	0.102

[a]Significant at $p < 0.0167$.

TABLE 3   Frequencies, mean values, and standard deviations of questions 4, 7, and 10

Question	Frequencies					Mean	Std dev
	1	2	3	4	5		
4 FBBO	5	6	0	2	2	2.33	1.44
4 LO	13	1	0	0	1	1.33	1.04
4 BO	11	2	1	0	1	1.53	1.12
7 FBBO	12	1	1	0	0	1.33	0.72
7 LO	8	5	0	2	0	1.73	1.03
7 BO	11	2	1	1	0	1.47	0.91
10 FBBO	5	5	2	2	1	2.27	1.28
10 LO	11	2	2	0	0	1.40	0.73
10 BO	11	5	0	2	0	1.40	0.73

1 = never; 2 = hardly ever; 3 = occasionally; 4 = fairly often; 5 = very often.

TABLE 4 Weighted median values of domains and sum scores

Domain	FBBO	LO	BO
Fl	9.13	7.81	8.77
P1	7.95	6.68	5.47
P2	3.90	3.90	5.81
D1	6.10	4.52	3.56
D2	2.83	2.83	2.83
D3	5.36	5.36	5.36
H	3.11	3.11	3.11
Sum	41.10	35.92	34.57

TABLE 5 Domains' *p*-values from the Wilcoxon signed rank test (*significant at $p < 0.0167$)

Domain	FBBO vs. LO	FBBO vs. BO	LO vs. BO
Fl	0.020	0.093	0.413
P1	0.034	0.041	0.497
P2	1	0.305	0.222
D1	0.114	0.009*	0.313
D2	0.593	0.285	0.891
D3	0.028	1	0.041
H	0.715	0.593	0.564
Sum	0.048	0.026	0.27

Example: Fl = (1.253 × question 1 score) + (1.181 × question 2 score) + (1.472 × question 6 score).
Sum score = FL + P1 + P2 + D1 + D2 + D3 + H.

however, the students were instructed similarly, and in addition, all steps should be similar when performed by one student. Another limitation was the lack of prefabricated tooth molds for BO. Perhaps tooth grinding and loss of tooth glaze biased the results by enticing patients. The short duration of follow-up and no matching for age and gender were also limitations. Bias was minimized by close attention to simulation during denture fabrication, insertion, and the follow-up period, and by randomly allocating patients according to a predetermined list. The effect of intervention was increased by one mounting procedure with a single record, one verifying record, indices for teeth arrangement, and insertions by the same person. Future patient-oriented investigations on comparing patient satisfaction with dentures should be made based on maxillomandibular relationships and locations of ridge crests after designing BO tooth molds with smaller mandibular posterior teeth, particularly lingual parts for preserving neutral zones.

CONCLUSION

With the caution of our small sample size, the results of this study provided proof of principle that in patients within ideal maxillomandibular relationships with mild and moderately resorbed ridges, FBBO scored significantly higher for uncomfortable eating and avoiding particular foods than LO. Also, FBBO scored significantly higher for avoiding particular foods and physical disability than BO. Furthermore, FBBO scored significantly lower for uncomfortable dentures than LO.

ACKNOWLEDGMENTS

The authors gratefully acknowledge the Isfahan Regional Bioethics Committee for ethical approval, and Dr. Behnaz Ebadian.

REFERENCES

1. Adam RZ: Do complete dentures improve the quality of life of patients? Department of Restorative Dentistry, Faculty of Dentistry and World Health Organisation (WHO) Oral Health Collaborating Centre, University of the Western Cape, 2006.

2. Jacobson T, Krol A: A contemporary review of the factors involved in complete denture retention, stability, and support. Part I: retention. *J Prosthet Dent* 1983;49:5–15.

3. Jacobson T, Krol A: A contemporary review of the factors involved in complete dentures. Part III: support. *J Prosthet Dent* 1983;49:306–313.

4. Jacobson T, Krol A: A contemporary review of the factors involved in complete dentures. Part II: stability. *J Prosthet Dent* 1983;49:165–172.

5. Celebic A, Knezovic-Zlataric D: A comparison of patient's satisfaction between complete and partial removable denture wearers. *J Dent* 2003;31:445–451.

6. Divaris K, Ntounis A, Marinis A, et al: Patients' profiles and perceptions of complete dentures in a university dental clinic. *Int J Prosthodont* 2012;25:145–147.

7. Pan S, Awad M, Thomason JM, et al: Sex differences in denture satisfaction. *J Dent* 2008;36:301–308.

8. Fenlon MR, Sherriff M: An investigation of factors influencing patients' satisfaction with new complete dentures using structural equation modelling. *J Dent* 2008;36:427–434.

9. Patil PG: Conventional complete denture for a left segmental mandibulectomy patient: a clinical report. *J Prosthodont Res* 2010;54:192–197.

10. Bohnenkamp DM, Garcia LT: Phonetics and tongue position to improve mandibular denture retention: a clinical report. *J Prosthet Dent* 2007;98:344–347.

11. Brunello DL, Mandikos MN: Construction faults, age, gender, and relative medical health: factors associated with complaints in complete denture patients. *J Prosthet Dent* 1998;79:545–554.

12. Nikawa H, Makihira S: Research projects related to complete dentures published in 2008 by members of the Japan Prosthodontic Society. *J Prosthodont Res* 2009;53:103–106.

13. Turker SB, Sener ID, Ozkan YK: Satisfaction of the complete denture wearers related to various factors. *Arch Gerontol Geriatr* 2009;49:e126–e129.

14. Matsumaru Y: Influence of mandibular residual ridge resorption on objective masticatory measures of lingualized and fully bilateral balanced denture articulation. *J Prosthodont Res* 2010;54:112–118.

15. Engelmeier RL: Early designs for the occlusal anatomy of posterior denture teeth: part III. *J Prosthodont* 2005;14:131–136.

16. Shigli K, Angadi GS, Hegde P: The effect of remount procedures on patient comfort for complete denture treatment. *J Prosthet Dent* 2008;99:66–72.

17. Sutton A, Worthington H, McCord J: RCT comparing posterior occlusal forms for complete dentures. *J Dent Res* 2007;86: 651–655.

18. Clough HE, Knodle JM, Leeper SH, et al: A comparison of lingualized occlusion and monoplane occlusion in complete dentures. *J Prosthet Dent* 1983;50:176–179.

19. Khamis MM, Zaki HS, Rudy TE: A comparison of the effect of different occlusal forms in mandibular implant overdentures. *J Prosthet Dent* 1998;79:422–429.

20. Kimoto S, Ghunji A, Yamakawa A, et al: Prospective clinical trial comparing lingualized occlusion to bilateral balanced occlusion in complete dentures: a pilot study. *Int J Prosthodont* 2006;19:103–109.

21. Sutton A, McCord J: A randomized clinical trial comparing anatomic, lingualized, and zero-degree posterior occlusal forms for complete dentures. *J Prosthet Dent* 2007;97:292–298.

22. Racich MJ: Orofacial pain and occlusion: Is there a link? An overview of current concepts and the clinical implications. *J Prosthet Dent* 2005;93:189–196.

23. Carlsson GE, Omar R: The future of complete dentures in oral rehabilitation. A critical review. *J Oral Rehabil* 2010;37: 143–156.

24. Becker CM, Swoope CC, Guckes AD: Lingualized occlusion for removable prosthodontics. *J Prosthet Dent* 1977;38: 601–608.

25. Farias-Neto A, Carreiro Ada F: Complete denture occlusion: an evidence-based approach. *J Prosthodont* 2013;22:94–97.

26. Phoenix RD, Engelmeier RL: Lingualized occlusion revisited. *J Prosthet Dent* 2010;104:342–346.

27. Kydd WL: The comminuting efficiency of varied occlusal tooth form and the associated deformation of the complete denture base. *J Am Dent Assoc* 1960;61:465–471.

28. Heydecke G, Vogeler M, Wolkewitz M, et al: Simplified versus comprehensive fabrication of complete dentures: patient ratings of denture satisfaction from a randomized crossover trial. *Quintessence Int* 2008;39:107–116.

29. The glossary of prosthodontic terms. *J Prosthet Dent* 2005;94: 10–92.

30. Zarb GA, Bolender CL: *Prosthodontic Treatment for Edentulous Patients (ed 12).* St. Louis, Mosby, 2004, p. 259.

31. Allen PF, Locker D: A modified short version of the oral health impact profile for assessing health-related quality of life in edentulous adults. *Int J Prosthodont* 2002;15: 446–450.

25

FACTORS ASSOCIATED WITH SUCCESSFUL DENTURE THERAPY

ROBERTA L. DIEHL, DDS,[1] ULRICH FOERSTER, DDS,[2] VENITA J. SPOSETTI, DMD,[3] AND TERESA A. DOLAN, DDS, MPH[4]

[1]Assistant Professor, Department of Community Dentistry, From the University of Florida College of Dentistry, Gainesville, FL
[2]Assistant Clinical Professor, Department of Operative Dentistry, From the University of Florida College of Dentistry, Gainesville, FL
[3]Associate Professor, Department of Prosthodontics, From the University of Florida College of Dentistry, Gainesville, FL
[4]Associate Professor, Department of Community Dentistry, From the University of Florida College of Dentistry, Gainesville, FL

Keywords
Denture success; complete dentures; patient satisfaction

Correspondence
Robert L. Diehl, DDS, Department of Community Dentistry, Box 100404, JHMHC, University of Florida, Gainesville, FL 32610.

Supported by the Bureau of Health Professions, DHHS, PHS, grant D31-PE94000.

Preliminary results of this research were presented at the International Association of Dental Research, Geriatric Oral Research Group: abstract 1533 on March 12, 1993, in Chicago, IL, and abstract 1429 on March 11, 1994, in Seattle, WA.

Published in *Journal of Prosthodontics* 1996; Vol. 5, Issue 2, pp. 84–90

ABSTRACT

Purpose: The purpose of this investigation was to evaluate complete denture patients at pretreatment and postinsertion, 6 months and 18 months after denture delivery in order to develop an explanatory model of successful denture therapy to better understand patient acceptance of complete dentures.
Materials and Methods: Sixty complete-denture patients treated at a dental student clinic were followed through denture therapy and for 18 months thereafter. Subjects were examined and completed pretreatment questionnaires and posttreatment interviews. Three outcome measures of denture success were tested, and factors considered substantive in achieving a successful denture outcome were examined using multivariate analyses.
Results: At post-insertion, 76.7% of subjects were satisfied with their dentures, 74.6% said their expectations were met, and 66.7% said they adjusted easily to their new dentures; reports at 6 and 18 months were similarly high. Logistic regression findings suggest that psychological and interpersonal factors are more important determinants of denture satisfaction than anatomic or clinical factors.

Conclusions: Subject characteristics including age, gender, race, income level, education, marital status, and maxillary and mandibular anatomy were not significantly associated with denture success as defined by the three outcome measures used in this study. Although these variables may represent important co-factors in the patient's acceptance of dental services and may affect the way a patient perceives dental care outcomes, statistically significant relationships were not found within our sample. Psychosocial variables, such as pretreatment expectations, satisfaction with the dental care received, and mental health showed a stronger relationship to a successful outcome.

With advances in dental research, technology, and education, many older Americans have retained their natural teeth longer than their predecessors. Yet more than 40% of adults over age 65[1] as well as many younger adults are edentulous and in need of complete denture therapy. The placement of implants to reestablish lost function and esthetics has increased substantially in recent years. Despite this advancement, implant dentistry may not be recommended for a significant number of adults because of medical, physiological, psychological, and/or financial constraints. Conventional complete denture therapy will remain an important and essential tool in restoring the oral function of edentulous adults in the foreseeable future.

Despite the large volume of literature regarding patient satisfaction with complete denture therapy, there is little consensus among authors as to reliable predictors of denture success. Kalk and deBaat[2] examined patient complaints and satisfaction 5 years after denture treatment. Well-fitting, well-functioning dentures, the absence of pain, and a socially acceptable appearance were reported to contribute most to patient satisfaction. Conversely, Vervoon et al[3] report no significant association between denture success and denture quality, or between denture complaints and denture quality. They suggest that other aspects of care, perhaps dentist-patient interactions, may be most responsible for denture success. Seiffert et al[4,5] suggest that the patient's personality and relationship with the dentist play a substantial role in overall success. They found psychological attributes to be as important to success as a patient's anatomical features and the skill involved in complete denture therapy. They also report that patient satisfaction with complete dentures is based on an interplay of psychological, biological, anatomic, and constructional factors. Davis et al[6] examined the dilemma of providing dentures to patients with unrealistic expectations of dental care. A patient's pretreatment expectations may influence treatment outcomes, and treatment failures may result from mismatched perceptions and expectations of the patient and the dentist.[6]

There are numerous other reports[7–36] in the literature evaluating many variables concomitant with an individual's acceptance of complete dentures. Because individual patients have unique experiences, expectations, emotions, adaptive abilities, and physical attributes, the task of predicting denture success is complex. Often, there are factors beyond a dentist's control that will affect a patient's ability to achieve a successful denture outcome.

The purpose of this investigation was to develop an explanatory model for successful denture therapy in a group of edentulous adults. At postinsertion, 6 and 18 months after the delivery of new dentures, we examined three outcome measures assessing a successful denture outcome: (1) the patient's satisfaction with the denture; (2) the actualization of the patient's pretreatment expectations; and (3) the patient's ability to adjust to new dentures.

MATERIALS AND METHODS

Adults over the age of 21 undergoing complete denture therapy at the University of Florida College of Dentistry's predoctoral dental clinic were invited to participate in the investigation. Eighty-three of 91 patients agreed to participate for an initial response rate of 91.2%. Patients were excluded from the study if treatment involved overdenture therapy or implant placement before denture fabrication. Informed consent was given by all participants before treatment. Patients were enrolled and baseline data were collected between April 1992 and February 1993. Of the original 83 patients enrolled, 1 patient died, 17 patients had not completed denture therapy before the conclusion of the enrollment period, and 5 patients were lost to follow-up. Findings from the remaining 60 patients are presented in this report. Data collected at each point during the study were coded numerically to ensure participant anonymity.

Upon enrollment, each participant completed a self-administered baseline questionnaire, followed by a brief, noninvasive examination of the mouth performed by one of three investigators. Examiners participated in a calibration exercise in which standardized, written criteria were used to evaluate edentulous patients not involved in the study. Discrepancies in clinical assessment were reviewed, and additional patients were then examined. Interexaminer reliability was determined to be adequate for the purpose of this study.

Denture therapy was completed by student dentists under the direction of faculty in the Department of Prosthodontics.

Upon completion of denture treatment, participants were re-evaluated by an investigator on the date of denture delivery or during a subsequent adjustment appointment. Approximately 1 month after the final denture adjustment, the 60 patients were contacted by telephone and a post-insertion interview was completed. To measure denture success over time, patients were again interviewed by telephone at 6 and 18 months after denture delivery. Fifty-two and 46 patients, respectively, cooperated for the follow-up portions of the investigation. An attrition analysis showed that patients remaining in the study at 18 months reported fewer denture problems at 6 months (mean denture problem scale score: 7.6 vs. 12.7, t-test, $P = 0.04$) than those who dropped out of the study. There were no statistically significant differences between groups in terms of age, race, gender, education and income levels, previous denture use, mental health index, satisfaction, ability to adjust, and expectations being met.

Questionnaire Content

Baseline and follow-up questionnaires were designed after a thorough review of the literature. Demographic information obtained at baseline included age, gender, educational level, marital status, and income. Participants also were asked to rate overall general and dental health as either excellent, very good, good, fair, or poor.

Five multi-item scales were developed and used in the analysis of denture success. A summaiy of the information requested, the parameters examined by each scale, and the data collection points are summarized in Table 1. Identical scales were used at baseline, post-insertion (at 6 and 18 months) with the exception of a seven-item expectation scale, which measured baseline (pretreatment) expectations for comfort, fit, chewing ability, appearance, and speaking ability.

Remaining scales include a six-item denture rating scale in which participant's rated existing complete dentures, if applicable, as well as the new dentures at follow-up based on comfort, fit, chewing ability, appearance, and speaking ability. The eight-item denture problem scale evaluated discomfort, lack of retention, cheek biting, inability to chew, food entrapment, and speech impairment. The seven-item satisfaction scale, a short form of the Rand Dental Satisfaction Questionnaire[37] measured patient satisfaction with the care, cost, convenience, pain management, and interpersonal aspects of treatment. The five- item Rand Mental Health Inventory[37] measured levels of anxiety, depression, behavioral/emotional control, general positive affect, and emotional ties of the participants.

The scales for denture rating, denture problems, expectations, satisfaction with recent dental care, and mental health incorporated items with Likert-type responses into multiitem summary scales. The mean scores, standard deviations, and range of each scale at post-insertion 6- and 18-month follow-

TABLE 1 Baseline, Postinsertion, and 6- and 18-month Follow-up Questionnaire Items and Scales

	Base-line	Post-insertion	6 mo	18 mo
Demographie Information age, gender, education, marital status, and income	X			
Expectations of New Dentures (expectation scale) comfort, fit, chewing ability, appearance, speaking ability	X			
General and Dental Health Rating self-raings of overall general physical and dental health (excellent, very good, good fair, or poor)	X	X	X	X
Rating of Complete Dentures (denture rating scale) comfort, fit, chewing ability, appearance, speaking ability	X	X	X	X
Denture Problems Experienced (denture problem scale) discomfort, lack of retention, cheek biting, inability to chew, food entrapment, speech impairment	X	X	X	X
Satisfaction With Dental Services (satisfaction scale: short form of the Rand Dental Satisfaction Questionnaire) satisfaction with care, cost, convenience, pain management, interpersonal aspects of satisfaction	X	X	X	X
Mental Health Inventory (mental health scale: short form of the Rand Mental Health Inventory) anxiety, depression, behavioral/emotional control, general positive affect, emotional ties	X	X	X	X

up are presented in Table 2. Reliability or internal consistency of the scales used in this study were evaluated using the Cronbach's coefficient a. Values ranged from .73 to .89, which are within an acceptable range for this investigation.

Examination Content

Baseline data recorded on the study participants included the number of prior complete dentures, age of existing complete dentures, time since most recent extraction, and existing denture quality based on esthetics, phonetics, vertical dimension of occlusion, occlusal plane, centric occlusion/centric relation, retention, stability, post-palatal seal, borders, and hygiene. Mouth moisture was rated as either favorable, xérostomie, or excessive based on visual assessment. The number of intraoral lesions or pathological conditions, and an intraoral anatomy rating based on favorable or unfavorable

TABLE 2   The Number of Items, Means, Standard Deviations, and Ranges For Each Scale Used in the Analysis

Scale	No. of Items	Mean	SD	Range
Expectation* (scored 0–14)				
baseline	7	12.5	1.9	7–14
Denture rating‡ (scored 6–30)				
post–insertion	6	19.9	5.8	7–30
6 month		20.6	6.4	6–30
18 month		20.9	7.1	7–30
Denture problem‡ (scored 0–24)				
post–insertion	8	6.3	4.7	0–22
6 month		8.2	5.7	0–24
18 month		7.5	5.0	0–22
Satisfaction§ (scored 0–100)				
post–insertion	7	78.0	11.6	37.5–100
6 month		75.9	12.7	31.3–93.8
18 month**				
Mental health¶ (scored 0–100)				
post–insertion	5	51.0	7.0	35.6–71.9
6 month		48.7	6.7	31.7–64.5
18 month		58.0	5.4	41.4–73.0

**Data not collected at 18 months.
*Expectation: a higher score indicates a high level of expectation for the new denture.
†Denture rating: a higher score indicates a positive rating of the new denture.
‡Denture problem: a higher score indicates more problems associated the new denture.
§Satisfaction: a higher score indicates more satisfaction with dental care.
¶Mental Health: a higher score indicates better mental health.

features of the maxilla and mandible regarding ridge/palatal shape and height, vestibular depth, tongue position, inter-ridge distance, skeletal jaw relationship, and muscular coordination also were recorded.

Statistical Analysis

Questionnaire and clinical examination data were entered and verified using Excell (Microsoft Corp, Richmond, WA) for Macintosh (Apple Computer Inc, Cupertino, CA) and analyzed using SPSS (SPSS Inc, Chicago, IE) statistical software. Frequency distributions of all baseline and follow-up items were calculated and reviewed. Bivariate associations were tested using χ^2 square statistic or t tests where appropriate. Spearman Correlation Coefficients of outcome measures and explanatory' variables were determined. Forward stepwise logistic regression models were developed for each of the dichotomous outcomes of interest: (1) the

patient's satisfaction with the denture; (2) the actualization of the patient's pretreatment expectations; and (3) the patient's ability to adjust to new dentures. The parameters of each model were estimated using the maximum likelihood method, and for each outcome a "best" model was developed by including only variables that were significant at $P < .05$. Direct estimation of each event or outcome occurring was calculated and reported, and "goodness of fit" indicating how well each model classified the observed data was used to assess each logistic regression model.

RESULTS

Subjects' mean age at baseline was 60.5 years, and ranged from 27 to 88 years. More than 40% of the sample reported an annual income of less than $10,000. About one third (32%) of the sample had less than a high school education, 35% were high- school graduates, and 33% completed some college and/or trade school. The sample was 60% female, 81% white and 55% married, and 45% had worn one or more sets of complete dentures previously (Table 3).

At baseline, 41% of the subjects had their remaining teeth extracted within 1 year of starting denture therapy, and 55% of the patients had no prior denture history. Anatomical features of the maxilla were rated favorably for 71% of the patients; mandibular anatomy was rated favorably for

TABLE 3   Participant Characteristics at Baseline

Age (yr)	
Mean	60.5
Range: 27–88 (SD, 13.7)	
Annual income	
<$10,000	42.9%
$10–20,000	33.9%
>$20,000	23.2%
Sex	
Male	40.0%
Female	60.0%
Marital status	
Married	55.0%
Not married	45.0%
Education	
<HS	31.7%
HS graduate	35.0%
>HS	33.3%
Race	
White	81.4%
Other	18.6%
Prior complete denture use	
None	55.0%
≥IC/C	45.0%

Note: n = 60.

42%. Most subjects (85%) had favorable inter-ridge distance, skeletal jaw relationship, and overall coordination; 88% had adequate mouth moisture.

About half (56%) of the participants with denture experience were dissatisfied with their existing dentures, and 75% of all subjects felt they had average or better than average bone and gums. Patients' pretreatment expectations of their new dentures, as well as their perceived adaptive ability, were high. Responses to a seven-item expectation scale at baseline indicated that expectations were generally high (mean = 12.5, SD = 1.9). Sixty-three percent of participants expected a new mandibular complete denture to "fit perfectly and not move." More than 70% expected improvement in comfort, fit, and chewing ability with the new dentures.

At post-insertion, 75% of the sample reported pretreatment expectations had been met; 29% of the participant's rated their new dentures as good, 31% as very good, and 29% as excellent. The three outcome measures of denture success were also rated favorably by the majority of the sample at post-insertion and subsequent follow-up interviews (Table 4), despite reporting denture problems similar to those noted at baseline. At post-insertion 6 and 18 months, respectively, 65%, 71%, and 69% of participants reported the new dentures were uncomfortable; 77%, 71%, 80% indicated that the lower denture became loose during eating, speaking, or yawning; and 48%, 41%, 41% reported no improvement in comfort, fit or chewing ability.

Of those patients satisfied with the new dentures at post-insertion, 85% were satisfied at 6 months and 86% were satisfied at 18 months. Of those whose expectations were met at post-insertion, 89% responded positively at 6 months and 83% responded positively at 18 months. Of those who adjusted easily at post-insertion, 88% adjusted easily at 6 months, and 94% adjusted easily at 18 months. At each time

TABLE 4   Outcome Measures of Successful Denture Therapy Measured Postinsertion and at 6- and 18-month Follow-Up

	PI (n = 60)	6 mo (n = 52)	18 mo (n = 46)
Satisfied?[*] (% yes)	76.7	71.2	71.7
Expectations met?[†] (% yes)	74.6	71.2	71.7
Adjusted easily?[‡] (% yes)	66.7	73.1	78.3

Note: Frequency distribution.
[*]"In general, are you satisfied with your new dentures?"
[†]"Were the expectations you had for your new dentures before beginning your denture treatment met?"
[‡]"Some people may adjust more easily or quickly than others to new eyeglasses or dentures. Compared to other people like yourself, would you say: (a) you adjusted easily to your new dentures; (b) it took a little time, but you are now adjusted to your new dentures; (c) you are still not adjusted; (d) you don't think you'll ever adjust to your new dentures." The responses were dichotomized as a, b = adjusted easily (yes) and c, d = did not adjust easily (no).

period, participants with no history of prior denture use were generally more satisfied with their new dentures, adjusted more easily to the new dentures, and reported their pretreatment expectations had been met.

At post-insertion at 6 and 18 months, the participants' gender, race, income level, education, and marital status were not statistically associated with satisfaction, expectations, and adjustment. The number of intraoral lesions, chronic medical conditions, adequate mouth moisture, and maxillary and mandibular anatomy to the three outcomes also were not statistically significant. However, at post-insertion, age was associated with denture satisfaction and ability to adjust. Subjects less than 60 years of age were more satisfied with and adjusted more easily to new dentures than those persons over age 60 ($\chi^2 = P < 0.05$). Persons less than 60 years of age reported more pretreatment expectations being met at the completion of care, but the finding was not statistically significant.

Logistic Regression Analysis

Three stepwise logistic regression models were used to identify variables significantly associated with each of the three outcomes measures. Independent variables tested in each model were age, an intraoral rating as either favorable or unfavorable, prior denture use (yes/no), and the scales developed to evaluate patient expectations, satisfaction, mental health/well-being, and denture problems. Although anatomy was not statistically significant using χ^2 square testing, it was included in the regression models because of the possible effects of severely atrophic ridges on denture success. The denture rating scale was not used in the regression models because of its collinearity with the denture problem scale. Results of the three post-insertion explanatory regression models are shown in Table 5.

The first model correctly classified 93% of subjects in terms of their satisfaction with their new dentures. Significant independent variables included in the model were the satisfaction scale, the denture problem scale, and prior denture use. Patients more satisfied with the quality of their care in terms of cost, convenience, pain management, and satisfaction with the treating student dentist were more likely to be satisfied with their dentures. Subjects experiencing more difficulties with comfort, fit, chewing ability, appearance, and speaking ability with their new dentures were less likely to be satisfied. Patients with no prior denture use were more satisfied after denture treatment. This finding is consistent with the trend noted in bivariate analyses of outcome measures over time and subjects' prior denture use.

The second model correctly classified 86% of those subjects in terms of their ability to adjust to their dentures. Significant variables in the model were the satisfaction and denture problem scales, along with the mental health inventory, which evaluated the participants' level of anxiety,

TABLE 5   Stepwise Logistic Regression Models For Three Outcomes of Interest: Were Participant's Satisfied With Their New Dentures? (yes/no); Were Their Expectations Met? (yes/no); and Did They Adjust Easily to New Dentures? (yes/no)

Logistic Regression Models and Variables	Parameter Estimates	SE	df	P	Percent of Sample Conectly Classified fig the Model	Goodness of Fit	Variables Not Entering Model
Satisfied?					93.1%	0.92	Age
Constant	3.03	4.50	1	0.08			Anatomy
Prior dentures (yes/no)	4.83	0.62	1	0.03			Expectation scale
Satisfaction scale	6.73	0.06	1	0.01			Mental Health scale
Denture Problem scale	7.26	0.14	1	0.01			
Adjust easily?					86.2%	0.88	Age
Constant	2.86	3.93	1	0.09			Anatomy
Satisfaction scale	3.94	0.04	1	0.05			Prior denture use
Mental Health scale	4.06	0.02	1	0.04			Expectation scale
Denture Problem scale	6.40	0.12	1	0.01			
Expectations met?					80.7%	0.99	Age
Constant	10.76	5.50	1	0.001			Anatomy
Satisfaction scale	11.57	0.08	1	0.001			Prior denture use
							Expectation scale
							Mental Health scale
							Denture Problem scale

depression, behavioral/emotional control, general positive affect, and emotional ties.

The third model correctly classified 81% of the participants as to whether their pretreatment expectations had been met after care. The model contained only the satisfaction scale. Perhaps more notable was the fact that the expectation scale did not enter the model, which may be indicative of the sample's high expectations before care. Variables that failed to enter any regression models were age, anatomy, and the expectation scale.

The three logistic regression models also were tested using data collected at 6 months. In each model, only the satisfaction scale was a significant independent variable. These results suggest that after the initial adjustment phase of wearing a new denture, important variables associated with subject satisfaction are appreciation of the care received, cost of service, convenience in accessing care, and successful interpersonal relationship with the treating dentist.

DISCUSSION

As the literature of the past 40 years has shown, the task of predicting denture success is complex. The purpose of this investigation was to develop an explanatory model of successful denture therapy to better understand a patient's acceptance of complete dentures. Postinsertion, 6 and 18 months after denture therapy, we evaluated variables that may be considered substantive in achieving a successful denture outcome. Subject characteristics including age,

sex, race, income level, education, marital status, and maxillary and mandibular anatomy were not associated with denture success as defined by the outcome measures used in this study. Although these variables represent important cofactors in the patient's acceptance of dental services and may affect the way a patient perceives dental care outcomes, statistically significant relationships could not be found within our sample.

Logistic regression findings postinsertion and at 6 months suggest that psychological and interpersonal factors are more important determinants of denture satisfaction than anatomic or clinical factors. Regression models tested at postinsertion suggest that persons who are well adjusted emotionally, have a positive self-image, and are not depressed should adjust to new dentures with greater ease. Results at postinsertion and at 6 months also suggest that patient satisfaction with the care received, the cost of service, convenience in accessing care, and a successful interpersonal relationship with the treating dentist are as important as the comfort, fit, and function of dentures. The presence of less-than-ideal maxillary and/or mandibular anatomy does not appear to significantly alter the patient's ability to achieve a successful denture outcome.

The majority of participants remained satisfied with their new dentures over time despite reporting denture problems similar to those noted at baseline. This general trend in subject satisfaction might be attributed to the provision of dental services at a university-based clinic. Many patients develop an amicable relationship with their student dentist during the rather long course of treatment and may be reluctant to voice dissatisfaction with services provided. Patients may perceive the dental college to be a center of excellence capable of providing superior care that is unequaled in the private sector. Although patients may still report difficulties such as discomfort, nonretentive lower complete dentures, and little improvement in comfort, fit, and chewing ability, the patient may feel their student dentist exceeded the accepted standard of care because of the close supervision of attending dental faculty.

Denture problems that remained at postinsertion suggest that the adjustment phase of wearing new complete dentures was longer than the 1-month period after the participant's last adjustment appointment. It is interesting to note that 78% of subjects reported they adjusted easily to their new dentures at 18 months, yet only 67% responded positively postinsertion. Denture problems reported at all follow-up interviews may have continued for this group because of limited scheduling, patient reassignment upon graduation of senior dental students, and the logistical problems associated with accessing care at a university clinic. Older and rural patients may have experienced even greater difficulty in returning to the university clinic for necessary adjustment appointments as quickly or easily as they might have in the private sector.

In assessing the results of this study, several limitations are acknowledged. Despite our efforts to ensure the confidentiality of subjects' responses, some participants may have been reluctant to speak against their student dentist during the follow-up interviews, thus introducing bias. It is also acknowledged that subjects lost through attrition reported higher denture problem scores at 6 months than those who remained with the study. Because our university-based population is a unique group composed of generally older, low-income, rural-dwelling white females, the generalizability of these findings may only be extended to similar populations. Further research efforts would include a larger, more diverse community sample, possibly treated in the private sector.

REFERENCES

1. National Institute of Dental Research. Oral Health of United Slates Adults: The national survey of oral health in US employed adults and seniors: 1985–1986, national findings; National Institutes of Health NIH publication no. 87–2868, Hyattsville, MD, August 1987, US Dept, of Health and Human Services, Public Health Service.

2. Kalk W, deBaat C: Patient complaints and satisfaction 5 years alter complete denture treatment. *Community Dent Oral Epidemiol* 1990;18:27–30.

3. Vervoon JM, Duinkerke AS, Luteijn F, et al: Assessment of denture satisfaction. *Community Dent Oral Epidemiol* 1988;16:364–367.

4. Seiffert I, Langer A, Michman J: Evaluation of psychologic factors in geriatric dental patients. *J Prosthet Dent* 1962;12: 516–523.

5. Langer A, Michman J, Seiffert I: Factors influencing satisfaction with complete dentures in geriatric patients. *J Prosthet Dent* 1961;11:1019–1031.

6. Davis EL, Albino JE, Tedesco LA, et al: Expectations and satisfaction of denture patients in a university clinic. *J Prosthet Dent* 1986;55:59–63.

7. Sharp GS: Treatment for low tolerance to dentures. *J Prosthet Dent* 1960;10:47–52.

8. Yoshizumi DT: An evaluation of factors pertinent to the success of complete denture service. *J Prosthet Dent* 1964;14: 866–878.

9. Bolcndcr CL, Swoopc CC, Smith DE: The Cornell Medical Index as a prognostic aid for complete denture patients. *J Prosthet Dent* 1969;22:20–29.

10. Carlsson GE, Otterland A, Wennstom A: Patient factors in appreciation of complete dentures. *J Prosthet Dent* 1967;17: 322–328.

11. Silverman S, Silverman S, Silverman B: Self-image and its relation to denture acceptance. *J Prosthet Dent* 1976;35: 131–141.

12. Smith M: Measurement of personality traits and their relation to patient satisfaction with complete dentures. *J Prosthet Dent* 1976;35:492–503.

13. Ramsey WO: The relation of emotional factors to prosthodontic service. *J Prosthet Dent* 1970;23:4–10.

14. Koper A: Human factors in prosthodontic treatment. *J Prosthet Dent* 1973;30:678–679.

15. Heartwell CM: Psychologic considerations in complete denture prosthodontics. *J Prosthet Dent* 1970;24:5–10.

16. Levin B, Landesman HM: A practical questionnaire for predicting denture success or failure. *J Prosthet Dent* 1976;35: 124–130.

17. Berg E: A 2-year follow-up study of patient satisfaction with new complete dentures. *J Dent* 1988;16:160–165.

18. Magnusson T: Clinical judgment and patients' evaluation of complete dentures five years after treatment. A follow-up study. *Swed Dent J* 1986;10:29–35.

19. Bergman B, Carlsson GE: Clinical long-term study of complete denture wearers. *J Prosthet Dent* 1985;53:56–61.

20. Chamberlain BB, Razoog ME, Robinson E: Quality of care: compared perceptions of patient and prosthodontist. *J Prosthet Dent* 1984;52:744–746.

21. Berg E, Johnsen TB, Ingebretsen R: Psychological variables and patient acceptance of complete dentures. *Acta Odontol Scand* 1986;44:17–22.

22. Kotkin H: Diagnostic significance of denture complaints. *J Prosthet Dent* 1985;53:73–77.

23. Chamberlain BB, Chamberlain KR: Depression: A psychologic consideration in complete denture prosthodontics. *J Prosthet Dent* 1985;53:673–675.

24. Tau S, Lowental U: Some personality determinants of denture preference. *J Prosthet Dent* 1980;44:10–12.

25. Giddon DB, Hittleman E: Psychologic aspects of prosthodontic treatment. *J Prosthet Dent* 1980;43:374–379.

26. Marbach JJ: Psychosocial factors for failing to adapt to dental prostheses. *Dent Clin N Am* 1985;29:215–233.

27. Weinstein M, Schuchman J, Lieberman J, et al: Age and denture experience as determinants in patient denture satisfaction. *J Prosthet Dent* 1988;59:327–329.

28. Vervoorn JM, Duinkerke AS, Luteijn F, et al: Assessment of denture satisfaction. *Community Dent Oral Epidemiol* 1988;16:364–367.

29. Friedman N, Landesman H, Wexler M: The influence of fear, anxiety, and depression on the patient's adaptive responses to complete dentures. Part I. *J Prosthet Dent* 1987;58: 687–689.

30. Friedman N, Landesman H, Wexler M: The influence of fear, anxiety, and depression on the patient's adaptive responses to complete dentures. Part II. *J Prosthet Dent* 1988;59:45–48.

31. Friedman N, Landesman H, Wexler M: The influence of fear, anxiety, and depression on the patient's adaptive responses to complete dentures. Part III. *J Prosthet Dent* 1988;59: 169–173.

32. Smith JP, Hughes D: A survey of referred patients experiencing problems with complete dentures. *J Prosthet Dent* 1988;60: 583–586.

33. Vervoorn JM, Duinkerke AS, Luteijn F, et al: Relative importance of psychologic factors in denture satisfaction. *Community Dent Oral Epidemiol* 1991;19:45–47.

34. van-Waas MA: Determinants of dissatisfaction with dentures: a multiple regression analysis. *J Prosthet Dent* 1990;64:569–572.

35. van-Waas MA: The influence of psychologic factors on patient satisfaction with complete dentures. *J Prosthet Dent* 1990;63: 545–548.

36. van-Waas MA: The influence of clinical variables on patient satisfaction with complete dentures. *J Prosthet Dent* 1990;63: 307–310.

37. Brook RH, Ware JE, Davies-Avery A, et al: Overview of adult status measures fielded in Rand's Health Insurance Study. *Med Care* 1979;17(suppl):1–131.

PART V

ESTHETIC CONSIDERATIONS

26

PERCEPTION OF ESTHETIC IMPACT OF SMILE LINE IN COMPLETE DENTURE WEARERS BY DIFFERENT AGE GROUPS

Matheus Melo Pithon, dds, ms, phd,[1] Leandro Pereira Alves, ds,[1] Matheus da Costa Prado, ds,[1] Rener Leal Oliveira, ds,[1] Matheus Souza Campos Costa, ds,[1] Raildo da Silva Coqueiro, dds, ms, phd,[1] João Milton Rocha Gusmão, dds, ms, phd,[1] and Rogério Lacerda Santos, dds, ms, phd[2]

[1]Department of Health I, Southwest Bahia State University UESB, Jequié, Bahia, Brazil
[2]Department of Health and Technology Rural, Federal University of Campina Grande, Patos, Paraíba, Brazil

Keywords
Esthetics; complete dental prosthesis; smile

Correspondence
Matheus Melo Pithon, Southwest Bahia State University—Health I, Av. Otavio Santos 395 sala 705 Centro Odontomedico Dr. Altamirando da Costa Lima Vitória da Conquista Bahia 45020750, Brazil.
E-mail: matheuspithon@gmail.com

The authors deny any conflicts of interest.

Accepted March 25, 2015

Published in *Journal of Prosthodontics* 2016; Vol. 25, Issue 7, pp. 531–35

doi: 10.1111/jopr.12355

ABSTRACT

Purpose: To evaluate esthetic perceptions based on tooth exposure when smiling of patients wearing complete dentures by evaluators in different age groups.

Materials and Methods: Alterations were made to a front view photograph of a smiling patient wearing complete maxillary and mandibular dentures. Alterations in the smile line were simulated to increase or decrease tooth exposure (increments of 0.5 mm). For this purpose, image manipulation software was used. After manipulation, images were printed on photo paper, attached to a questionnaire, and distributed to individuals in three age groups (n = 150). To evaluate the esthetic perception for each image, a visual analog scale was used, with 0 representing least attractive, 5 representing attractive, and 10 representing very attractive. Differences between examiners were analyzed using the Mann-Whitney test. All statistical analyses were performed with a degree of confidence of 95%.

Results: Two evaluators did not observe any differences between images. The images given the best and worst scores were E and O (alterations of 2 and 7 mm), respectively, in the 15- to 19-year-old group, B and O (alterations of 0.5 and 7 mm), respectively, in the 35- to 44-year-old group, and A and M (no alteration and 6 mm alteration), respectively, in the 65- to 74-year-old group. When the images were presented together (images 1 and 2), the unaltered image was selected by individuals of different age groups as the best, and the image with a change of 7 mm was selected as the worst.

Conclusion: In this study, complete dental prostheses with smile lines that coincided with the cervical margins of the anterior teeth were the most acceptable. Less exposure of the maxillary teeth when smiling corresponded with decreased attractiveness.

An attractive smile has been considered to be an important component of facial harmony.[1,2] A pleasing appearance has been considered a factor of great relevance in social interaction, and evidence has suggested that an attractive smile plays a significant role in decisions made by the public.[3]

The esthetic appearance of a smile has been shown to be affected by, among other factors, the position of the lips and their curvature and relationship with the maxillary anterior teeth.[3] In the analysis of the smile, this parameter, also known as the smile line or tooth exposure when smiling, is calculated as the difference between the height of the lip line and the tooth exposure.[4,5]

The goal of treatment with complete dentures has been described as the achievement of a smile that is esthetically and functionally[6,7] as close as possible to the smile obtained with natural teeth.[8] Therefore, when planning a complete denture, a careful and detailed analysis must be made of all the anatomic and prosthetic components to achieve an esthetically and functionally ideal smile.[8]

Facial beauty has been reported to be a subjective concept; thus, the precise diagnosis and consequent formulation of an optimal treatment plan involves a high degree of difficulty and complexity.[9–11] The mouth may be considered the most dynamic part of the face, and the placement of a denture may result in pleasant or unpleasant facial features.[12] The denture may occupy much or little vertical height in the smile line.[13] Therefore, adequate planning according to the patient's age and gender is necessary.

In this context, this study aimed to evaluate the perception of the esthetic appearance of smiles in images with different degrees of maxillary anterior tooth exposure using complete dental prostheses by systematically altering the photographs.

MATERIALS AND METHODS

The study was conducted with approval from the Research Ethics Committee. This study was conducted using a front view intraoral photograph of a 65-year-old patient with complete maxillary and mandibular dentures. The photograph, in which the teeth, gingiva, and lips were exposed, was obtained with a digital camera (Canon Rebel XTI; Canon, Tokyo, Japan) mounted on a tripod with lighting control and a fixed focal length of 50 cm.

Once the original photograph was obtained, the images were manipulated using a software program (Adobe Photoshop CS3; Adobe Systems Inc., San Francisco, CA). Changes were made only in the maxillary denture; the same mandibular position was maintained. With the intention of simulating alterations in the smile line of the teeth in the maxillary denture, the initial image was digitally manipulated to simulate the progressive upward and downward displacement of the maxillary teeth. Fifteen images were thus obtained, including the original. The manipulated images underwent progressive alterations of 0.5 mm (Fig 1).

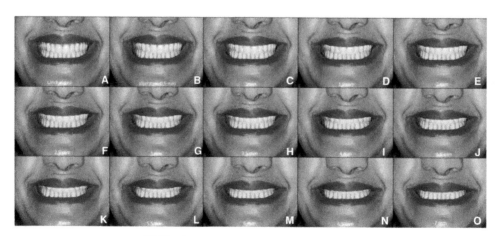

FIGURE 1   Images evaluated in this study.

After the images were obtained, they were randomly numbered and printed all together on photo paper. On another sheet, the order and numbering of these images were randomly rearranged. Upon being shown these images, the evaluators were asked to state whether they were able to differentiate the images and to select which images they thought were the most and least attractive. The second sheet, with all the printed images in a different order, served to verify the reliability of the responses obtained using the first sheet.

Finally, the 15 images were printed individually and were randomly presented to the evaluators along with an attached visual analog scale (VAS). This stage enabled the evaluators to attribute scores to the esthetic appearance of each particular image. On this scale, the score 0 corresponded to a minimally attractive image, 5 to an attractive image, and 10 to a very attractive image. The evaluators had a maximum of 60 seconds to analyze each image.

The evaluations were performed by 150 laypersons from three population groups, individuals aged 15 to 19 years, 35 to 44 years, or 65 to 74 years, as recommended by the WHO/FDI.[9] Before the study began, a pilot study was conducted to verify the sample size required. The sample size calculation was performed using nQueryAdviser (v.6.01; Solution Statistics, York, Ireland). Based on a 5% ($\alpha = 0.05$) significance level, the sample size was calculated to achieve a statistical power of 80%. The sample size calculation revealed that 40 to 120 individuals would be needed for each group. In this study, the evaluations were conducted with 50 evaluators in each age group.

Included individuals were healthy and were not missing any of their permanent teeth. Evaluators were excluded from the study if they had any visual deficiencies or had difficulty in understanding and completing the questionnaires.

The frequencies of replies provided by the participants in each age group (15 to 19, 35 to 44, and 65 to 74 years) were compared using the chi-square test. In cases in which the expected frequency was less than five (n < 5), Fisher's exact test was used. The point scores awarded to each photograph were compared using the Kruskal-Wallis test, and comparisons between pairs were performed using the Mann-Whitney test. The mean score awarded to each photograph by each group was calculated, and Spearman correlation coefficients were determined to evaluate the similarity between perceptions based on age group. The level of significance was set at 5% ($\alpha = 0.05$). The data were tabulated and analyzed using BioEstat (v.5.0; Belém-PA, Brazil).

RESULTS

Of the 150 participants, 68% were women, but the sex distribution differed between the age groups, with men accounting for only 10% of the participants in the 65- to

TABLE 1   **Demographic data of study participants per group**

Features	Age group (years)		
	15 to 19 (n = 50)	35 to 44 (n = 50)	65 to 74 (n = 50)
Sex			
Male	21 (42.0%)	22 (44.0%)	5 (10.0%)
Female	29 (58.0%)	28 (56.0%)	45 (90.0%)

74-year-old group (Table 1). Table 2 presents the research participants' perceptions of the differences and their preferences recorded for images 1 and 2. Among the participants who noted differences between the photographs, there was a significant difference among the groups in terms of the least preferred image but not the most preferred image.

The mean scores awarded to each photograph are shown in Table 3. Image O (alteration of 7 mm) was awarded the worst score by individuals in the 15 to 19 and 35 to 44 age groups; however, individuals in the age range of 65 to 74 years attributed the worst score to image M (alteration of 6 mm). Only the scores awarded to photographs E and O were significantly different between the age groups. The correlations between the scores given by the three age groups were significant and strong (r > 0.9).

DISCUSSION

The three main determinants of the acceptability of a prosthetic treatment are comfort, function, and esthetics.[6,7] Among these determinants, esthetics demand that various factors be considered, such as social and cultural beliefs.[14] The edentulous patient seeks to have an esthetically satisfactory denture and to have a pleasant smile that is as close as possible to the original smile and is appropriate for his or her age.[15]

The smile line is defined as the line between the curvature of the maxillary anterior teeth and the curvature of the top edge of the bottom lip.[16] Some authors define the smile line as the "arch of the smile," emphasizing that the ideal shape of the incisal edges of the maxillary anterior teeth creates a convex arch.[17] Reestablishing the patient's ideal smile line is one of the goals of any dental treatment, whether it is achieved using orthognathic surgical procedures or restorative procedures, as is the case with prosthetic rehabilitation in edentulous patients. Various studies[9,11,18,19] have evaluated esthetic preferences related to the smile line in orthodontic and/or surgical patients. Until now, however, there have been no published scientific studies evaluating this esthetic component in patients who wear complete dentures. Based on this premise, this study aimed to evaluate the perception of the esthetic appearance of the smile in cases

TABLE 2 Participants' perception with respect to differences and their preferences as regards image 1 and 2

Answers	Age group (years)			p-value	Answers	Age group (years)			p-value
	15 to 19	35 to 44	65 to 74			15 to 19	35 to 44	65 to 74	
Differences perceived—n (%)		Image 1			Differences perceived—n (%)		Image 2		
Yes	49 (98.0)	49 (98.0)	50 (100.0)	1.000[‡]	Yes	47 (94)	50 (100)	50 (100.)	0.107[‡]
No	1 (2.0)	1 (2.0)	0 (0.0)		No	3(6)	0(0)	0(0)	
Most liked Image*—n (%)					Most liked image*—n (%)				
A - unchanged	12 (24.5)	21 (42.9)	15 (30)	<0.398[‡]	A - alteration 3 mm	2 (4.3)	1 (2)	2 (4)	< 0.062[†]
B - alteration 0.5 mm	6 (12.2)	9 (18.4)	5(10)		B —1 mm	5 (10.6)	9 (18)	5(10)	
C-1.0 mm	3 (6.1)	4 (8.2)	5(10)		C—5.5 mm	3 (6.4)	0 (0)	5(10)	
D—1.5 mm	1 (2)	3 (6.1)	5(10)		D—2 mm	3 (6.4)	2 (4)	6 (12)	
E—2.0 mm	5 (10.2)	3 (6.1)	4 (8)		E—7 mm	5(10.6)	1 (2)	3 (6)	
F—2.5 mm	1 (2)	1 (2)	1 (2)		F—2.5 mm	1 (2.1)	1 (2)	5(10)	
G—3.0 mm	1 (2)	0 (0)	0 (0)		G—4.5 mm	0 (0.0)	2 (4)	1 (2)	
H—3.5 mm	2 (4.1)	2 (4.1)	0 (0)		H—0.5 mm	7 (14.9)	11 (22)	4 (8)	
I—4 mm	1 (2)	2 (4.1)	2 (4)		I—5 mm	0 (0)	1 (2)	3 (6)	
J—4.5 mm	4 (8.2)	0 (0)	3 (6)		J—3.5 mm	4 (8.5)	1 (2)	2 (4)	
K—5.0 mm	1 (2)	0 (0)	1 (2)		K—4 mm	0(0)	1 (2)	0 (0)	
L—5.5 mm	1 (2)	0 (0)	0 (0)		L—1.5 mm	2 (4.3)	2 (4)	1 (2)	
M—6.0 mm	1 (2)	1 (2)	3 (6)		M—6 mm	0(0)	0 (0)	3 (6)	
N—6.5 mm	1 (2)	1 (2)	3 (6)		N—6.5 mm	2 (4.3)	1 (2)	3 (6)	
O—7.0 mm	9 (18.4)	2 (4.1)	3 (6)		O—unchanged	13 (27.7)	17 (34)	7 (14)	
Least liked image*—n (%)					Least liked image*—n (%)				
A - unchanged	9 (18.4)	1 (2)	3 (6)	0.001[†]	A - alteration 3 mm	1 (2.1)	0 (0)	1 (2)	0.024[‡]
B - alteration 0.5 mm	5 (10.2)	0 (0)	2 (4)		B—1 mm	2 (4.3)	2 (4)	2 (4)	
C—1.0 mm	2 (4.1)	2 (4.1)	4 (8)		C—5.5 mm	6(12.8)	0 (0)	2 (4)	
D—1.5 mm	0 (0)	0 (0)	2 (4)		D—2 mm	0 (0)	0 (0)	2 (4)	
E—2.0 mm	1 (2)	2 (4.1)	1 (2)		E—7 mm	15 (31.9)	16 (32)	9 (18)	
F—2.5 mm	0 (0)	2 (4.1)	4 (8)		F—2.5 mm	0 (0)	2 (4)	3 (6)	
G—3.0 mm	0 (0)	3 (6.1)	4 (8)		G—4.5 mm	3 (6.4)	2 (4)	1 (2)	
H—3.5 mm	0 (0)	4 (8.2)	3 (6)		H—0.5 mm	1 (2.1)	3 (6)	6 (12)	
I—4.0 mm	0 (0)	0(0)	2 (4)		I—5 mm	2 (4.3)	4 (8)	2 (4)	
J—4.5 mm	1 (2)	2 (4.1)	4 (8)		J—3.5 mm	0(0)	2 (4)	2 (4)	
K—5.0 mm	4 (8.2)	2 (4.1)	7 (14)		K—4 mm	2 (4.3)	2 (4)	8 (16)	
L—5.5 mm	1 (2)	2 (4.1)	5(10)		L—1.5 mm	1 (2.1)	1 (2)	0 (0)	
M—6.0 mm	4 (8.2)	3 (6.1)	0 (0)		M—6 mm	1 (2.1)	5(10)	2 (4)	
N—6.5 mm	5 (10.2)	9(18.4)	2 (4)		N—6.5 mm	8(17)	11 (22)	6 (12)	
O—7.0 mm	17 (34.7)	17 (34.7)	7 (14)		O—unchanged	5 (10.6)	0 (0)	4 (8)	

*Answered only by individuals who perceived differences between the images.
[†]Chi -square test.
[‡]Exact Fisher test.
n = number of participants.

of different degrees of tooth exposure in patients wearing complete dental prostheses.

In the present study, an original photograph was manipulated with the aid of a software program, Adobe Photoshop CS3. Various published studies have used this methodology.[6,7] This method makes it possible to standardize the image and change only the property one wishes to evaluate. Another potential method involves the use of various patients with different smile lines; however, this approach may make it difficult to make comparisons. To verify that the evaluators were able to perceive the differences between the images, all the images were presented simultaneously, and then the evaluators were asked whether they observed differences between the images. The results obtained for the first image,

in which all the photographs were presented together, suggested that almost all the individuals, irrespective of age group, perceived differences between the images when they were able to compare the photographs directly. In this first case, they were also asked to select which images they considered the most and least attractive. The responses were significantly different among the groups with respect to the least-preferred image but not regarding the most preferred image. The original image (A, no alteration, 0 mm) was the most accepted image in all the groups. That is, 24.5% of the 15- to 19-year-old group, 42.9% of the 35- to 44-year-old group, and 30.0% of the 65- to 74-year-old group considered the best image to be the one in which the original esthetic and functional profile was

TABLE 3 Mean scores (standard deviation) attributed to photographs by the study participants, according to age group

Photograph	Age group (years)			
	15 to 19	35 to 44	65 to 74	p-value*
Image A (unchanged)	6.74(2.2)	7.13 (2.1)	6.75 (3.1)	0.679
B (0.5 mm)	6.60 (1.7)	7.23 (2.0)	5.83 (3.0)	0.054
C (1.0 mm)	6.31 (1.8)	6.84 (1.8)	6.16 (2.7)	0.355
D (1.5 mm)	6.93 (1.9)	6.67 (2.0)	6.26 (2.4)	0.499
E (2.0 mm)	7.05 (1.6)[a]	6.53 (2.0)[a,b]	5.79 (2.4)[b]	0.030
F (2.5 mm)	6.33 (2.2)	6.14 (2.0)	5.74 (2.6)	0.558
G (3.0 mm)	6.02 (1.9)	5.77 (1.8)	5.74 (2.8)	0.845
H (3.5 mm)	5.77 (2.0)	5.60 (1.8)	5.69 (2.5)	0.889
I (4.0 mm)	5.48 (2.4)	5.13 (2.0)	5.30 (2.6)	0.705
J (4.5 mm)	5.50 (2.9)	4.88 (2.2)	5.22 (2.6)	0.548
K (5.0 mm)	5.28 (2.8)	4.44 (1.9)	5.13 (2.7)	0.271
L (5.5 mm)	4.47 (2.3)	4.09 (2.0)	4.56 (2.8)	0.585
M (6.0 mm)	4.72 (2.4)	3.88 (2.2)	4.39 (2.7)	0.155
N (6.5 mm)	3.94 (2.4)	3.64 (2.3)	4.44 (2.8)	0.292
O (7.0 mm)	3.44 (2.7)[a]	3.26 (2.6)[a]	4.50 (2.6)[b]	0.026

*The scores of points were compared by means of the Kruskal-Wallis test.
[a,b]Values with different superscript letters are significantly different (Mann-Whitney test).

respected. Regarding the least attractive image, there was perfect agreement in the two younger groups: 34.7% of these individuals chose the image with 7 mm of tooth exposure (displacement of the smile line). This image or the image with a 5 mm displacement was chosen as least attractive by 14% of the individuals in the 65 to 74 age group.

When the image order was randomized, the original image (O, complete maxillary tooth exposure) was preferred by 27.7% of the 15- to 19-year-old group, 34% of the 35- to 44-year-old group and 14% of the 65- to 74-year-old group, thus constituting a consensus opinion. With regard to the least attractive image, agreement was once again established. For 31.9% of the individuals between 15 and 19 years old, 32% of those between 35 and 44 years old, and 18% of those 65 years of age or older, the image with a 7 mm displacement of the smile line was the least attractive.

These results corroborate those of other studies, which affirm that certain factors, such as age, influence the perception of esthetics of the smile.[9,17,20,21] In this study, there was agreement in the images chosen as the most and least attractive. Nevertheless, there was a significant difference among the age groups in the percentage of individuals who chose each image.

In the second part of the study, the 14 individually printed images were evaluated for attractiveness with the aid of a VAS. This method consists of an absolute scoring scale from 0 to 10, in which 0 represents "hardly attractive," 5 represents "attractive," and 10 represents "very attractive." The VAS analyses indicated that there were differences in the esthetic evaluations made by the different age groups. The images with displacements of 2 or 0.5 mm and the original image were scored as the most attractive by the 15- to 19-year-old, 35- to 44-year-old, and 65- to 74-year-old groups, respectively. All the groups were capable of defining the most and least attractive photographs. There was a strong positive correlation between the three age groups, suggesting agreement between the scores and the image preferences.

Notably, 90% of the evaluators in the 65- to 74-year-old group were women. Women pay more attention to detail when making evaluations related to the esthetic appearance of teeth, and this phenomenon may have caused this group to rank the unaltered image as the best.[22,23]

A limitation of this study was the fact that only exhibition of the incisors of the maxillary anterior teeth was diminished. In addition, the gingival margins of the maxillary anterior teeth and exposure of the mandibular teeth were not altered. It is worth emphasizing the importance of these alterations in future studies, because with these images, the visualization would be closer to reality.

One of the effects of aging on an individual's face is reduced exposure of the teeth and smile line. To rehabilitate an adult individual with the smile line of a younger individual, or vice versa, may introduce an esthetic conflict that is easily perceptible by any layperson. The results obtained in the present study revealed the need to respect the esthetic characteristics appropriate for the patient's age, thereby preventing negative esthetic effects.

CONCLUSION

This study provided the following conclusions:

1. Complete dental prostheses that present a smile line coinciding with the cervical lines of the teeth were the most acceptable.
2. Less exposure of the maxillary teeth corresponded with reduced attractiveness.

REFERENCES

1. Heravi F, Rashed R, Abachizadeh H: Esthetic preferences for the shape of anterior teeth in a posed smile. *Am J Orthod Dentofacial Orthop* 2011;139:806–814.
2. Kattadiyil MT, Goodacre CJ, Naylor WP, et al: Esthetic smile preferences and the orientation of the maxillary occlusal plane. *J Prosthet Dent* 2012;108:354–361.
3. Passia N, Blatz M, Strub JR: Is the smile line a valid parameter for esthetic evaluation? A systematic Literature review. *Eur J Esthet Dent* 2011;6:314–327.

4. Vander Geld P, Oosterveld P, VanHeck G, et al: Smile attractiveness. Self-perception and influence on personality. *Angle Orthod* 2007;77:759–765.

5. Peck S, Peck L: Selected aspects of the art and science of facial esthetics. *Semin Orthod* 1995;1:105–126.

6. De Lucena SC, Gomes SG, Da Silva WJ, et al: Patients' satisfaction and functional assessment of existing complete dentures: correlation with objective masticatory function. *J Oral Rehabil* 2011;38:440–446.

7. Scott BJ, Hunter RV: Creating complete dentures that are stable in function. *Dent Update* 2008;35:259–62, 65–7.

8. Sellen PN, Jagger DC, Harrison A: Methods used to select artificial anterior teeth for the edentulous patient: a historical overview. *Int J Prosthodont* 1999;12:51–58.

9. Pithon MM, Bastos GW, Miranda NS, et al: Esthetic perception of black spaces between maxillary central incisors by different age groups. *Am J Orthod Dentofacial Orthop* 2013;143:371–375.

10. Pithon MM, Santos AM, Campos MS, et al: Perception of laypersons and dental professionals and students as regards the aesthetic impact of gingival plastic surgery. *Eur J Orthod* 2014;36:173–178.

11. Pithon MM, Santos AM, Viana de Andrade AC, et al: Perception of the esthetic impact of gingival smile on laypersons, dental professionals, and dental students. *Oral Surg Oral Med Oral Pathol Oral Radiol* 2013;115:448–454.

12. Vezzetti E, Marcolin F: 3D landmarking in multiexpression face analysis: a preliminary study on eyebrows and mouth. *Aesthetic Plast Surg* 2014;38:796–811.

13. Lombardi RE: A method for the classification of errors in dental esthetics. *J Prosthet Dent* 1974;32:501–513.

14. Conny DJ, Tedesco LA, Brewer JD, et al: Changes of attitude in fixed prosthodontic patients. *J Prosthet Dent* 1985;53:451–454.

15. Waliszewski M: Restoring dentate appearance: a literature review for modern complete denture esthetics. *J Prosthet Dent* 2005;93:386–394.

16. Ackerman JL, Proffit WR, Sarver DM: The emerging soft tissue paradigm in orthodontic diagnosis and treatment planning. *Clin Orthod Res* 1999;2:49–52.

17. Roden-Johnson D, Gallerano R, English J: The effects of buccal corridor spaces and arch form on smile esthetics. *Am J Orthod Dentofacial Orthop* 2005;127:343–350.

18. Murakami T, Fujii A, Kawabata Y, et al: Relationship between orthodontic expertise and perception of need for orthodontic treatment for mandibular protrusion in Japan. *Acta Med Okayama* 2013;67:277–283.

19. Livas C, Delli K: Subjective and objective perception of orthodontic treatment need: a systematic review. *Eur J Orthod* 2013;35:347–353.

20. Rodrigues Cdc D, Magnani R, Machado MS, et al: The perception of smile attractiveness. *Angle Orthod* 2009;79:634–639.

21. Soh J, Chew MT, Wong HB: A comparative assessment of the perception of Chinese facial profile esthetics. *Am J Orthod Dentofacial Orthop* 2005;127:692–699.

22. Cazzato V, Siega S, Urgesi C: "What women like": influence of motion and form on esthetic body perception. *Front Psychol* 2012;3:235.

23. Demas PN, Braun TW: Esthetic facial surgery for women. *Dent Clin North Am* 2001;45:555–569.

27

ASSESSMENT OF THE ABILITY TO RELATE ANTERIOR TOOTH FORM AND ARRANGEMENT TO GENDER

Fernanda Ferreira Jassé, dds, ms,[1] Josiane Vilhena Corrêa, dds,[2] Andréa Ferreira Santos da cruz, dds, ms,[2] Mauro José Pantoja Fontelles, dds, ms, phd,[2] Andiara Ribeiro Roberto, dds, ms,[1] José Roberto Cury Saad dds, ms, phd,[1] and Edson Alves de campos, dds, ms, phd[1]

[1]Department of Restorative Dentistry, University of Estadual Paulista—UNESP, Araraquara School of Dentistry, Araraquara, Brazil
[2]Department of Dental Prostheses, Pará Federal University, Belém, Brazil

Keywords
Esthetics; tooth shape; dentogenic theory

Correspondence
Fernanda Ferreira Jassé, Department of Dentistry, São Paulo State University, Rua Humaitá 1680 Araraquara, São Paulo 14801-903, Brazil.

E-mail: fernandajasse@hotmail.com.

Accepted August 7, 2011

Published in *Journal of Prosthodontics* 2012; Vol. 21, pp. 279–82

doi: 10.1111/j.1532-849X.2011.00822.x

ABSTRACT

Purpose: This study evaluated the assumption that there are morphological differences between the natural anterior dentition of men and women. The goal of the study was to determine the gender of patients based on the appearance of the anterior teeth in photographs.
Materials and Methods: Laymen and observers from different specialties were asked to determine the gender of individuals based on the shape and arrangement of anterior teeth. Forty anterior dentition photographs of dental students of both genders (20 women, 20 men) between 18 and 26 years old were selected, coded, and randomly arranged in an album. The albums were delivered to five groups of observers: general practitioners (recently graduated dentists), prosthodontists, orthodontists, restorative dentists (specialists in cosmetic and restorative dentistry), and laymen (control group). The observers evaluated the photographs twice at 1-week intervals.
Results: The average correctly identified values in women and men were 57.6% and 58.8%, respectively. There was no statistical difference between observers and between each group of professionals and the laymen group ($p > 0.05$). An intraobserver agreement was not observed between the evaluations (kappa $= -0.01$).
Conclusion: The results of this limited study indicated that it was not possible to differentiate gender by viewing photographs of anterior teeth.

Esthetic dentistry is an issue of importance for dentists and patients.[1–6] From economic, social, and sexual points of view, the desire to look attractive is no longer considered a sign of vanity. In a competitive world, an esthetic appearance is a necessity.[7,8] Given that the face is the most exposed part of the body, and the mouth is one of its most prominent features, teeth have become perhaps even more important.[7,9]

Currently, dentistry is widely practiced on patients with preserved natural dentitions,[10] despite the need for partial or total replacement of missing teeth. With advancements in techniques, materials, and knowledge, such as adhesive procedures, dental whitening, microabrasion, and cosmetic remodeling, dentists are able to modify the shape, color, size, and position of teeth predictably and efficiently.[7] Current restorative techniques enable clinicians to perform dental alterations previously possible only with dentures.[4]

When anterior teeth need to be restored, secondary to neglect, trauma, or esthetics, features inherent in the natural dentition may be of great value to achieve individualized and attractive restorations.[3,11] However, if all teeth are missing, and records relative to the original dentition are not available, other criteria will have to be used. These criteria may have been previously used for complete dentures and are now found to be useful for anterior dental restorations as well.[4] In this context, the maxillary central incisors are generally considered to be the most dominant teeth in the human dentition, and therefore the most important in terms of esthetics.[11]

Concerning the tooth shape, a century ago, Williams[12] suggested that a correlation existed between the shape of the inverted face and the shape of maxillary central incisors, a theory that became known as the "law of facial harmony." The contours of maxillary incisors were classified into three categories: triangular, ovoid, and square. In 1955, Frush and Fisher[13] proposed the so-called "dentogenic theory," which stated that gender, personality, and age could be used as guidelines for tooth selection, arrangement, and characterization to "enhance the natural appearance of the individual."[14] These authors believed that delicacy, smoothness, and softness, described as female characteristics, could be reflected in prostheses for women, and that vigor and courage should be reflected in prostheses for men.[15] According to this theory, femininity was characterized by teeth with oval shapes and rounded edges, while masculinity was expressed with more square-shaped teeth.[16] Besides the shape, arrangement of teeth could also influence perceptions of femininity or masculinity, so that positioning lateral incisors in certain positions either softened or produced ruggedness depending on a patient's gender. The same occurred with positioning the long axis of canines: for women, the necks of canines would be more prominent than the incisal edges, and anteriorly, only the mesial half would be visible.[17] The dentogenic theory has been taught in dental schools for decades and has been adopted by generations of dentists as a major esthetic principle.[2,4]

The purpose of this article was to evaluate the assumption that there are morphological differences between the natural anterior dentition of men and women. The null hypothesis was that there would be no significant difference in dental professionals' abilities to correctly identify the gender of individuals by viewing intraoral photographs. To this aim, judges from different specialties, as well as laymen, attempted to determine gender, based on overall morphology and arrangement of anterior teeth.

MATERIALS AND METHODS

Forty dental students (20 men, 20 women) were selected from consenting persons in the College of Dentistry of Pará Federal University. The criteria used for selection were ages between 18 and 26 years, no missing teeth or any type of anterior tooth restorations, and no history of prior orthodontic treatment. The study was approved by the Research Bioethics Committee of the School of Dentistry of Pará Federal University (process no. 050/2006).

An intraoral photograph was taken of each student with a Dimage Z6 digital camera (Konica Minolta Photo Imaging, Mahwah, NJ). Plastic lip retractors (Expandex; Indusbello, Londrina, Brazil) were used to retract the lips. Images exposed only the labial surfaces of the occluded anterior teeth; lips were not visible in the photographs. For standardization of the images, the camera was attached to a tripod positioned at a 90° angle relative to the ground, 1 m between the middle of the chair where students sat and the middle of the tripod. The camera height was adjusted to the student's mouth level. The anterior teeth were framed in the camera display. The natural head position was adopted by asking students to sit in an upright position, looking into their own eyes through a mirror positioned behind the camera. Photographs were printed in color (size $10 \times 15\,cm^2$), coded, and organized randomly in an album.

Photographs were analyzed by 15 judges: three orthodontists (Ortho), three restorative dentists (Res—specialists in cosmetic and restorative dentistry), three prosthodontists (Pro), three recently graduated general practitioners (Gen), and three laymen (not graduated in dentistry—control group). Each judge was directed to evaluate the photographs and identify the gender of patients and to describe the criteria used in the choice. These data were logged in a table with numbers corresponding to those in the album. After this initial evaluation, the process was repeated a week later, with the images in a different order to test reproducibility of the results of the first identifications.

All data were stored in a databank using the software program Microsoft Excel, version 2002 (Microsoft Co., Redmond, WA). Since nonparametric data were obtained, kappa and chi-squared tests were used for statistical analysis. This was complemented by the use of the odds ratio (OR). A 5% level of significance was adopted.

TABLE 1   **Reliability and validity of the method**

Judge	Kappa	% of correct responses in phase 1	% of correct responses in phase 2	% of correct and consistent responses between phases
Ortho 1	0.02	62.5	60.0	65.5
Ortho 2	−0.02	52.5	55.0	54.5
Ortho 3	−0.05	52.5	57.5	57.0
Res 1	−0.07	47.5	55.0	52.0
Res 2	0.07	72.5	65.0	76.0
Res 3	0.10	60.0	50.0	57.0
Pro 1	−0.10	57.5	67.5	66.0
Pro 2	0.05	52.5	47.5	50.0
Pro 3	−0.05	55.0	60.0	62.5
Gen 1	0.02	60.0	57.5	61.0
Gen 2	−0.15	55.0	70.0	68.0
Gen 3	0.02	62.5	60.0	67.0
Layman 1	0.02	57.5	55.0	62.0
Layman 2	−0.05	52.5	57.5	57.5
Layman 3	−0.10	60.0	70.0	82.6
Average%	−0.01	57.3	59.1	62.5

RESULTS

Reliability and Validity

Table 1 identifies kappa values, the proportion of correct responses in the two phases, and the proportion of correct responses in agreement between phases for each judge. Kappa values were estimated to measure agreement between the first and second phases. These values measured the degree of agreement beyond what would be expected solely by chance. The overall kappa value was −0.01, which suggested nonexistent agreement or disagreement (i.e., less than chance concordance). There were no statistically significant differences between judges ($p > 0.05$). On analyzing the correct and coincident responses for the same judge in the two phases, a minimum percentage of 50% was observed for Pro 2 and maximum of 82.6% for layman 3, with an average of 62.5%. On comparing the rate of correct and erroneous responses between groups of professionals through the chi-squared test, no statistically significant differences were found ($p > 0.05$). The same occurred when the layman group (control group) was compared with each group of professionals.

Photographic Evaluation

In the first phase, from a total of 40 photographs, the gender of only one woman and one man was determined correctly by more than 90% of the evaluators. In contrast, photographs of one man and two women were erroneously identified by more than 85% of the participants. In the second phase, two photographs of men were correctly determined by more than 90% of the evaluators, whereas one woman was incorrectly identified by more than 85% of the participants. Figures 1 and 2 are examples of photographs classified correctly by a majority of judges as "female" and "male," respectively. Figures 3 and 4 are examples of images classified incorrectly by a majority of judges as "female" and "male," respectively. The photographs of male patients were correctly selected 58.8% of time; females were correctly identified 57.6%.

Regarding the criteria used for gender identification by the professionals, the predominate criteria noted were

- For women: rounded shapes; disproportionate sizes between central and lateral incisors; diastemas; short teeth; and inclinations of canines and lateral incisors.
- For men: square shapes; flat incisal edges; long, broad, and large teeth; incisal wear; and inclination of canines.

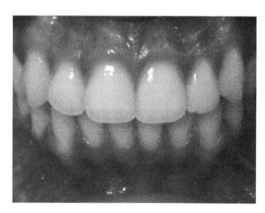

FIGURE 1   A majority of the judges correctly identified this person as female.

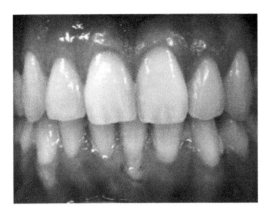

FIGURE 2 A majority of the judges correctly identified this person as male.

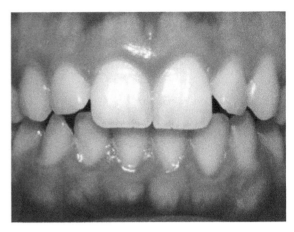

FIGURE 3 Example of a photograph of a male patient that was judged incorrectly as female.

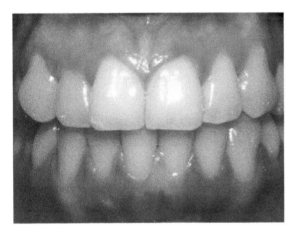

FIGURE 4 Example of a photograph of a female patient that was judged incorrectly as male.

The main criteria used for the layman group for gender determination were

- For women: small, aligned, delicate teeth; small dental arches; and high levels of oral hygiene.
- For men: large, broad, and overlapping teeth; mis-aligned, serrated teeth with diastemas; yellow hues; large dental arches; and normal levels of oral hygiene.

DISCUSSION

The factors of gender, personality, and age were reported by Frush and Fisher.[13,16] Regarding gender, they stated that rounded contours of incisal angles produced spherical effects of maxillary central and lateral incisors. They classified these characteristics as feminine. Straight angles, which produced cube-like effects in teeth, were classified as consistent with the male gender. In the present study, factors related to anatomical contours and alignment of teeth did not appear to be isolated determinants for correct gender identification.

Judges did not receive information regarding identifying characteristics relative to the determination of gender prior to the evaluations. This enabled all judges to use their perceptions of esthetics. It may be concluded that, in this study, professionals used their knowledge and/or perceptions that they received as part of their life experiences and/or training; this is consistent with the observations of Hyde et al.[2]

In a study by McCord et al,[1] patients, dental students, and prosthodontists attempted to determine the gender and age of patients from photos of complete dentures. They reported that this was not a reliable method to identify gender and age. Hyde et al[2] reported that specialists, when asked to distinguish gender from plaster casts prepared from natural dentitions of men and women, could not differentiate between casts according to gender; however, they considered that casts reproduced the shapes, contours, and angulations of the teeth, but anatomical features such as hue, chroma, and value and the texture of gingival tissues could not be determined. In a study reported by Wolfart et al,[4] black and white intraoral photographs were used specifically avoid identifying the coloration of teeth and gingival tissues. The authors of the present study, in contrast to the above-mentioned studies, used color photographs. It should be noted that all of the above studies drew similar conclusions to those in this study: judges, whether professionals, patients, or laymen, were not able to identify gender in a statistically significant manner. These results are also consistent with reports published by Burchett and Christensen,[15] Sellen et al,[3] and Berksun et al[9]

The judges were asked about their evaluation criteria, something not done in the studies mentioned above. The answers confirmed that the professionals made their decisions based on the "dentogenic" esthetic concepts. Only two photographs in the present study were correctly identified by more than 90% of the evaluators; three of the 40 photographs were erroneously identified by more than 85% of the evaluators. Thus, it may be assumed that criteria used by professionals are not based on gender differences. In fact, there may be no discernible differences in tooth morphology related to gender. The "dentogenic theory" could therefore not be confirmed.

Regardless of whether the decision of the judges was correct, an analysis of the selection of each evaluator in the two phases was carried out. The rate of agreement varied between 52.5% and 82.5%. These results were close to those obtained by Wolfart et al[4] who observed variations between 54% and 77%. In this study, the intraobserver agreement was not statistically significant for any evaluator. In the study by Wolfart et al[4] 8 of 10 dentists showed statistically significant results. It can thus be observed that, in this study, none of the evaluators, despite having in mind certain criteria to differentiate gender, failed to replicate the second phase responses to the first phase. Thus, besides gender difference criteria not being evidence based, judges still applied the principles to the task at hand.

Factors influencing identification were length, position, and proportion of teeth, and the results of oral hygiene practices of the subjects. This latter factor, according to the observations of this study, was a criterion frequently used by layman judges, who had no anatomical references. In relation to the factors that influenced dentists, these were probably influenced by doctrines and theories widely discussed in dental schools, and are frequently mentioned in publications.[11–14,16,17] This may explain why some photographs with characteristics typical of one gender, according to the literature, were identified, in high percentages, correctly or incorrectly.

CONCLUSIONS

In this study, the photographs of male patients were correctly selected 58.8% of time; females were correctly identified 57.6%. It was not possible to correctly identify gender exclusively from intraoral photographs (anterior teeth). Dentists should be careful to create dental restorations consistent with patients' individual needs, whether the patient is male or female.

REFERENCES

1. McCord JF, Burke T, Roberts C, et al: Perceptions of aesthetics: a two-centre study of denture wearers and denture providers. *Aust Dent J* 1994;39:365–367.

2. Hyde TP, McCord F, Macfarlane T, et al: Gender aesthetics in the natural dentition. *Eur J Prosthodont Rest Dent* 1999;7:27–30.

3. Sellen PN, Jagger DC, Harisson A: An assessment of the ability of dental undergraduates to choose artificial teeth which are appropriate for the age and sex of the denture wearer: a pilot study. *J Oral Rehabil* 2001;28:958–961.

4. Wolfart S, Menzel H, Kern M: Inability to relate tooth forms to face shape and gender. *Eur J Oral Sci* 2004;112:471–476.

5. Goldstein RE: Attitudes and problems faced by both patients and dentists in esthetic dentistry today: an AAED membership survey. *J Esthet Restor Dent* 2007;19:164–170.

6. Jørnung J, Fardal Ø: Perceptions of patients' smiles: a comparison of patients' and dentists' opinions. *J Am Dent Assoc* 2007;138:1544–1553.

7. Adams TC, Pang PK: Lasers in aesthetic dentistry. *Dent Clin N Am* 2004;48:833–860.

8. Anderson KM, Rolf GB, McKinney T, et al: Tooth shape preferences in an esthetics smile. *Am J Orthod Dentofacial Orthop* 2005;128:458–465.

9. Berksun S, Hasanreisoglu U, Gökdeniz B: Computer-based evaluation of gender identification and morphologic classification of tooth face and arch forms. *J Prosthet Dent* 2002;88:578–584.

10. Morley J: The role of cosmetic dentistry in restoring a youthful appearance. *J Am Dent Assoc* 1999;130:1166–1172.

11. Rufenacht CR: *Principles of Esthetic Integration.* Chicago, Quintessence, 2003, pp. 205–241.

12. Williams JL: The esthetic and anatomical basis of dental prosthesis. *Dent Cosmos* 1911;53:1–26.

13. Frush JP, Fisher RD: Introduction to dentogenic restorations. *J Prosthet Dent* 1955;5:586–595.

14. Waliszewski M: Restoring dentate appearance: a literature review for modern complete denture esthetics. *J Prosthet Dent* 2005;93:386–394.

15. Burchett PJ Jr., Christensen LC: Estimating age and sex by using color, form, and alignment of anterior teeth. *J Prosthet Dent* 1988;59:175–179.

16. Frush JP, Fisher RD: How dentogenics restorations interpret the sex factor. *J Prosthet Dent* 1956;6:160–172.

17. Jameson WS: Dynesthetic and dentogenic concept revisited. *J Esthet Restor Dent* 2002;14:139–148.

28

GUIDELINES FOR MAXILLARY INCISAL EDGE POSITION—A PILOT STUDY: THE KEY IS THE CANINE

CARL E. MISCH, DDS, MDS
Clinical Professor and Director, Oral Implantology, Temple University, Philadelphia, PA

Keywords
Esthetics; maxillary complete dentures; maxillary implant overdentures; maxillary implant fixed prostheses

Correspondence
Dr. Carl E. Misch, Misch International Implant Institute, 16231 W. Fourteen Mile Rd., Beverly Hills, MI 48025.
E-mail: Info@misch.com

Accepted August 22, 2006

Published in *Journal of Prosthodontics* 2008; Vol. 17, pp. 130–4

doi: 10.1111/j.1532-849X.2007.00259.x

ABSTRACT

Purpose: The purpose of this pilot study was to evaluate the relationship between the vertical position of the maxillary central incisal edge and the maxillary canine relative to the maxillary lip line in repose of dentate patients. This may be beneficial for clinicians in establishing guidelines for the rehabilitation of edentulous patients.

Materials and Methods: One hundred and four Caucasian dentate patients (59 men and 45 women) between the ages of 30 and 59 years were evaluated. A millimeter ruler was used to measure the maxillary right central incisor edge and the maxillary right canine tip to the maxillary lip in repose. Data were collected in reference to sex and age.

Results: For the female group, average central incisor exposure in relation to the relaxed maxillary lip line was 3.8 mm, and the range of exposure was −1 to +8 mm. In the 30- to 39-year olds (17 patients), the average was 4.1 mm with a range of 0 to 8 mm. The average in the 40- to 49-year-old group (16 patients) was 2.8 mm with a range of −1 to +6 mm. In 50- to 59-year olds (12 patients), the average was 1.8 mm with a range of −1 to +5 mm. In the male group, the average central incisor exposure was 2.5 mm, and the range was −3 to +7 mm. The average for the 30- to 39-year-old group (20 patients) was 3.2 mm with a range of 0 to 7 mm. For the 40- to 49-year group (18 patients), the average was 2.4 mm and for 50 to 61 years (21 patients), it was 1.4 mm with a range of −3 to +5 mm in both latter age groups. The canine position for the female group average exposure was 0 mm, with a range of −2 to +2 mm. For the 30- to 39-year old group, average exposure was 1 mm with a range of −1 to +2 mm. The 40- to 49-year-old group exposed an average of 0.4 mm with a range of −1 to +2 mm. For the 50- to 59-year old group, canine exposure was −0.5 mm with a range of −2 to +1 mm. The male average canine exposure was −0.5 mm, and the range was −3 to +2 mm. For the 30- to 39-year old group, the average was 0.9 mm with a range of −1 to +2 mm. The 40- to 49-year-old group exposed an average of 0.2 mm, with a range of −1 to +2 mm. For the 50- to 59-year old group, average was −0.9 mm with a range of −2 to +1 mm.

Conclusions: There was a large range of maxillary central incisal exposure in relation to the maxillary lip line. The average dimension of central incisor exposure represented less than 30% of the subjects in the study and could not be used predictably to assess incisal edge position. The range of canine exposure was narrower. The average dimensions of canine exposure to the lip were within 1 mm for both men and women in all age groups. Further studies are needed to confirm these preliminary results. The average dimensions for the different sex and age groups related to canine exposure represented a greater proportion of the subjects. Therefore, it is suggested that the average canine exposure dimension can be used clinically to assess anterior incisor edge position when restoring edentulous patients.

The ideal goal for a restorative dentist is to return a patient to normal contour, comfort, function, esthetics, speech, and health of the stomatognathic system. The anterior teeth play an important role in esthetics, phonetics, and incision of food. When restoring or replacing these teeth, esthetics is often a primary focus.

When a patient is missing all of the maxillary anterior dentition, the restorative dentist should attempt to position the teeth in a fashion similar to the arrangement of ideal dentate patients of similar age, gender, race, and facial structures.[1] Phonetics and/or the vertical position of the maxillary central incisors with the lip in repose may be evaluated with this goal in mind.

Various authors have used phonetic guidelines to establish the vertical maxillary incisal edge position in the fabrication of maxillary dentures.[2–4] For example, Payne used phonetics to determine the position of the maxillary anterior teeth using the sounds "S," "Z," and "C."[3] He reported that if the vertical positions of the teeth were too low, the teeth would "click" together. Boucher observed that the vertical positions of the maxillary anterior teeth were determined by phonetics, especially with labiodental sounds.[1] He noted that the maxillary central and lateral incisors touched the lower lip during pronunciation of the letters "F" and "V." He also noted that when the maxillary lip was at rest, the incisal edges of the maxillary teeth were usually visible.

Several authors have reported that the vertical positions of the central incisors were primarily determined by their relationship with the lip in repose (say "emma" and relax) regardless of age or sex.[7–10] As a general rule, these authors observed that the occlusal aspect of maxillary occlusal rims (maxillary central incisors) should extend approximately 1 to 2 mm below the lip in repose. Speech ("F" sounds) was then used to modify this vertical position. A survey of the maxillary lip in repose relative to the maxillary central incisor position of dentate patients was performed by Vig and Brundo.[11] They evaluated the maxillary central incisor position of dentate patients related to sex, race, lip length, and age. The average amount of central incisor exposure with the lip in repose was 1.91 mm for men and 3.4 mm for women. Relative to race, Caucasians averaged 2.43 mm, blacks 1.57 mm, and Asians 1.86 mm. People with a short upper lip (10 to 15 mm) exposed 3.92 mm, whereas people with 31 to 35 mm length lips exposed an average of 0.25 mm. Relative to age, averages were 3.31 mm for patients less than 29 years, 1.58 mm for 30 to 39 years, 0.95 mm for 40 to 49 years, 0.46 mm for 50 to 59 years, and 0.04 mm for above 60 years of age.[11]

The measurements of Vig and Brundo for central incisor exposure were averages, and did not report the number of patients, the method of evaluation, or the range of incisal edge exposure in dentate patients. When an average dimension is used to determine maxillary central incisor position without consideration of the extent of the range, the average may be inaccurate.

Frush and Fisher stated that the "smiling line" helped determine the vertical position of the maxillary teeth in complete dentures.[12] They observed that the central incisors were longer than the other maxillary teeth, and the curvature of the maxillary teeth followed the curve of the upper border of the lower lip during smiling. Using their guidelines, the locations of the maxillary anterior teeth were suggested to just barely reach the lower lip during smiling.

Misch stated that the vertical position of the maxillary anterior teeth and the lip in repose should be determined by the maxillary canine position, rather than the central incisal position.[13] He noted the range of exposure of the central incisors was greater than the range of exposure of canines. Many authors have noted that maxillary central incisors' incisal edges were longer than the cusp tips of the canines compared in the horizontal plane.[1,4,7–10] Therefore, once the vertical position of the canine tips have been identified, the central incisal position can be established; however, no range or average dimension of the maxillary anterior teeth exposure was reported by Misch, relative to the lip in repose.

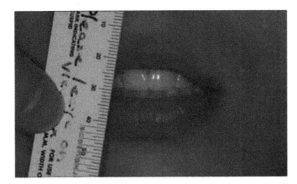

FIGURE 1 The vertical exposure of the maxillary central incisal edge in relationship to the lip in repose was measured in 104 patients (59 men and 45 women). This 32-year-old female patient exposes 5 mm of the central incisor in the midline.

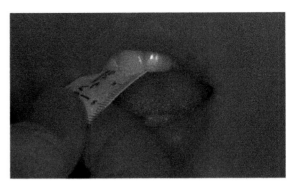

FIGURE 2 The vertical position of the maxillary canine in relationship to the lip in repose was also measured in these same 104 patients. This 32-year-old female patient exposes −1 mm of canine with the lip in repose.

The purpose of this study was to evaluate the position of the incisal edges of maxillary central incisors and maxillary canines in relationship to the maxillary lip in repose in Caucasian dentate patients.

MATERIALS AND METHODS

Fifty-nine male and 45 female (30 to 59 years) Caucasian adults were enrolled from a private practice. All 104 subjects had at least first molar occlusions. Patients were excluded if they had a history of plastic surgery to the lips or orthodontics used to modify the anterior incisal edge positions. Also excluded from this study were any subjects with moderate to severe wear of the maxillary anterior teeth.

Measurements were made by the same examiner with the patients seated upright in a chair with their heads

unsupported. Each patient was asked to say "emma" and relax his/her face and lower jaw. A millimeter ruler was used to measure and record the vertical distance (in mm increments) from the most inferior position of the maxillary vermillion border of the lip in repose to the maxillary right central incisor edge (Fig 1). A similar procedure was used to measure the position of the maxillary right canine tip to the maxillary lip in repose position (Fig 2). There was no accounting for incisal tooth wear, orthodontic skeletal position, or lip length. The data from these adults were separated by age and sex. Age brackets used for the study consisted of three groups: 30 to 39, 40 to 49, and 50 to 59 years old.

RESULTS

In the female group, the overall average central incisor exposure was 3.8 mm, and the overall range of exposure was −1 to +8 mm (Fig 3). In the 30- to 39-year-old group (17 patients), the average was 4.1 mm with a range of 0 to 8 mm (Fig 4). The average central incisor tooth exposure in the 40- to 49-year-old group (16 patients) was 2.8 mm with a range of −1 to +6 mm. In the 50- to 59-year-old group

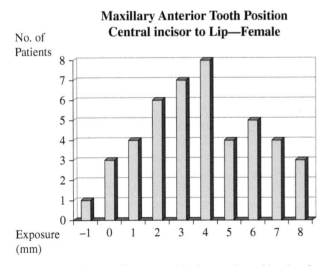

Maxillary Anterior Tooth Position Central incisor to Lip—Female

No. of Patients

Exposure (mm)

FIGURE 3 The maxillary central incisor tooth position in relationship to the maxillary anterior lip in repose was evaluated in 45 women between the ages of 30 and 59 years. Less than 20% of the female population was similar to the average.

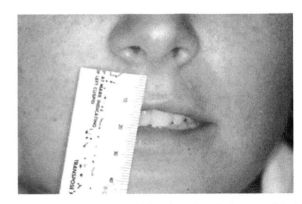

FIGURE 4 This 30-year-old female patient had a central incisor exposure of 6 mm, and her canine exposure was 1 mm.

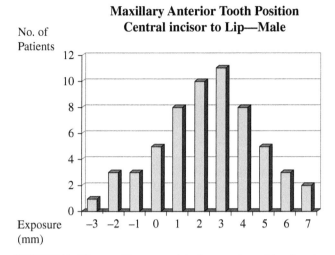

FIGURE 5 The maxillary central incisor tooth position in relationship to the maxillary anterior lip in repose was evaluated in 59 men between the ages of 30 and 59 years. Sixty-five percent of the subjects were not similar to the average.

(12 patients), the average was 1.8 mm with a range of −1 to +5 mm.

In the male group, the overall average central incisor exposure with the lip in repose was 2.5 mm and the range was −3 to +7 mm (Fig 5). In the male 30- to 39-year-old group (20 patients), the average was 3.2 mm with a range of 0 to 7 mm. In the 40 to 49-year-old group (18 patients), average was 2.4 mm and in the 50 to 59-year-old group (21 patients), the average was 1.4 mm with a range of −3 to +5 mm in both latter age groups.

In the same 104 dentate patients, the right maxillary canine incisal edge exposure with the lip at rest was measured. The overall female average exposure was 0 mm; the range was −2

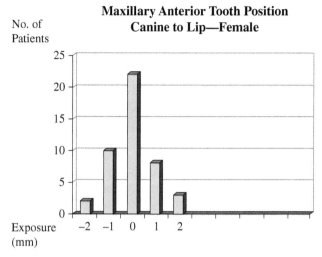

FIGURE 6 The maxillary canine lip exposure was evaluated in relation to the maxillary lip in repose in the same female group as in Figure 3. Almost 50% represented the average, and only five subjects were more than 1 mm from the average.

to +2 mm (Fig 6). For the 30- to 39-year old, average exposure was 1 mm; range was −1 to +2 mm (Fig 4). For the 40- to 49-year-old group average exposure was 0.4 mm; range was −1 to +2 mm. For the 50- to 59-year old, average exposure was −0.5 mm; range was −2 to +1 mm.

The male average position of the canine in relation to the lip in repose was −0.5 mm: range was −3 to +2 mm (Fig 7). The 30- to 39-year-old subjects' average was 0.9 mm; range was −1 to +2 mm. The 40- to 49-year-old group exposed an average of 0.2 mm canine incisal edge; range was −1 to +2 mm. For the 50- to 59-year old average exposure of the canine was −0.9 mm; range was −2 to +1 mm. The average values for canine exposure were within 1 mm for both male and female subjects.

DISCUSSION

The determination of the vertical position of the maxillary anterior teeth is an important criterion in patients missing these teeth. One of the goals in prosthetics is to replace these teeth in positions similar to dentate patients of the same gender, age, race, and facial structures. Hence, a clinical study of the averages and ranges of these elements in dentate patients was needed to record these values.

The amount of maxillary central teeth exposure with the lip in repose is a highly variable position and is dependent on many factors. One central incisor to lip in repose average position is not specific enough to use in edentulous patients of various ages. In fact, because the range in this study was so large and the sample size so small, only 20% of the patients under 40 years exhibited an average exposure.

The use of averages with a narrower range (3 to 4 mm in the canine position) may be more predictable than using averages with a wider range (6 to 8 mm in the central incisor

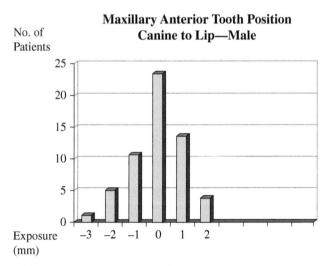

FIGURE 7 The maxillary canine exposure was evaluated in relation to the maxillary lip in repose in the same male group as in Figure 5. Sixty of the subjects were similar to the average, and only 10 subjects were more than 1 mm from the average.

position). As reported in this study, the canine tip position was usually −1 to +1 mm longer than the maxillary lip in repose at the ages of 30 to 59 years. In this report, it was also observed that the canine position varied less with age or sex, compared to central incisor positions. In other words, the canine position in relation to the maxillary lip at 35 years is more similar to its position at 55 years of age than the central incisor positions at these ages. Therefore, this study suggests that, for Caucasians between the ages of 30 and 59 years, the canine tip has a more consistent position to the resting maxillary lip position than the maxillary central incisor edge. Exposure of maxillary incisors was 1 to 2 mm longer than the canines in reference to a horizontal plane. Therefore, the vertical position of the maxillary central incisal edge may be positioned after the canine tip position is determined.

A potential flaw in the design of this study was measuring the amount of tooth display with a handheld ruler, because the examiner might distort the lip/tooth relationship. The limitations of the study include the number of patients in each age group, the clinical method to evaluate the canine lip/tooth position, and the fact that only one investigator made the measurements. It should be noted that when the canine was above the lip in repose, it was necessary to slightly distort it to make the measurement. As a result, photographs or other passive measurements would not allow assessment of the tooth position. This report also limited its evaluation to subjects with little to no wear of the anterior teeth. The limited sample size and method to assess the canine versus the central tooth position suggests further studies are necessary before a broad generalization of the results.

The consequences of incorrectly positioning the maxillary central incisors in relation to the maxillary lip line include both obvious esthetic consequences and other more subtle problems, including improper plane of occlusion, occlusal vertical dimension, occlusal scheme during mandibular excursions, and moment forces placed on anterior teeth, dentures and/or implants. For example, when the central incisor exposure is insufficient (too apical), the canine may also be apically positioned. This may result in an incorrect position of the maxillary teeth. The anterior point of the plane of occlusion for an edentulous patient is determined by the incisal edge position, whether it is parallel to Camper's Plane or one-half the length of the retromolar pad.[4,5] A consequence of improper central incisor edge position may be that the entire vertical position of the maxillary occlusal plane may be affected.

CONCLUSION

For patients in this pilot study, the range of exposure of maxillary central incisors was wide, and the use of an average dimension as a guide may not be accurate in clinical practice.

This study also found that the relationship in the exposure of the cusp tips of maxillary canines to the maxillary lip in repose position exhibited a narrow range. The average dimensions for maxillary canines relative to age and sex were closer to the extremes of the range. In this patient population, the canine position relative to the maxillary lip appeared to be a more predictable determinant for establishing the vertical position of the maxillary anterior teeth. In this study, the maxillary canine position to lip in repose had an average dimension within 1 mm of the upper lip, regardless of sex or age. Hence, it is suggested that this relationship may be used as one of the determinants of anterior tooth position in edentulous, Caucasian patients. Additional studies are mandated to further verify this clinical observation.

REFERENCES

1. Boucher CO: Arrangement of teeth. in Boucher CO (ed): *Swenson's Complete Dentures*, (ed 6). St. Louis, MO, Mosby, 1970, pp. 155–210.

2. Pound E: Esthetic dentures and their phonetic value. *J Prosthet Dent* 1951;1:98–111.

3. Payne SH: Contouring and positioning, in Moss SJ (ed): *Esthetics*. New York, NY, Medicine, 1973, pp. 50–54.

4. Zarb GA, Bolender CL, Hickey JC, et al: Creating facial and functional harmony with anterior teeth, in Zarb GA (ed): *Boucher's Prosthodontic Treatment for Edentulous Patients*, (ed 10). St. Louis, MO, Mosby, 1990, pp. 382–424.

5. Tallgren A: The reduction in face height of edentulous and partially edentulous subjects during long-term denture wear: a longitudinal roentgenographic cephalometric study. *Acta Odontol Scand* 1966;24:195–239.

6. Gruber A, Solar P, Ulm C: Maxillomandibular anatomy and patterns of resorption during atrophy, in Watzek G (ed): *Endosseous Implants: Scientific and Clinical Aspects*. Chicago, IL, Quintessence, 1996, pp. 29–62.

7. Heartwell CM: Tooth arrangement, in Heartwell CM (ed): *Syllabus of Complete Dentures*. Philadelphia, PA, Lea and Febiger, 1968, pp. 261–276.

8. Sharry JJ: Anterior tooth selection, in Sherry JJ (ed): *Complete Denture Prosthodontics*, (ed 3). New York, NY, McGraw-Hill, 1974, p. 234.

9. Ellinger CW, Rayson JH, Terry JM, et al: Arrangement of anterior teeth, in Ellinger CW (ed): *Synopsis of Complete Dentures*. Philadelphia, PA, Lea and Febiger, 1975, p. 163.

10. Landa SL: Anterior tooth selection and guidelines for complete denture esthetics, in Winkler S (ed): *Essentials of Complete Denture Prosthodontics*. Philadelphia, PA, Saunders, 1979, pp. 282–300.

11. Vig RG, Brundo GC: The kinetics of anterior tooth display. *J Prosthet Dent* 1978;39:502–504.

12. Frush JP, Fisher RD: How dentogenics interprets the personality factor. *J Prosthet Dent* 1965;67:441–449.

13. Misch CE: Partial and complete edentulous maxilla implant treatment plans, in Misch CE (ed): *Dental Implant Prosthetics*. St. Louis, MO, Elsevier/Mosby, 2005, pp. 295–300.

29

NASAL WIDTH AS A GUIDE FOR THE SELECTION OF MAXILLARY COMPLETE DENTURE ANTERIOR TEETH IN FOUR RACIAL GROUPS

FABIANA MANSUR VARJÃO, DDS, MSC, PHD[1] AND SERGIO SUALDINI NOGUEIRA, DDS, MSC, PHD[2]

[1]Private Practice, Former Graduate Student
[2]Associate Professor

Keywords

Complete denture; dental esthetics; artificial teeth; race

Correspondence

Fabiana Mansur Varjão, DDS, MSc, PhD, Av. 22 de Agosto, 318, ap. 23, Araraquara-SP-Brazil, CEP 14810-125.
E-mail: fabianamansur@uol.com.br

From the Department of Dental Materials and Prosthodontics, São Paulo State University, Araraquara Dental School, Araraquara, São Paulo, Brazil.

Accepted June 23, 2005

Published in *Journal of Prosthodontics* 2006; Vol. 15, pp. 353–8

doi: 10.1111/j.1532-849X.2006.00134.x

ABSTRACT

Purpose: Selecting artificial teeth for edentulous patients is difficult when pre-extraction records are not available. Various guidelines have been suggested for determining the width of the maxillary anterior denture teeth. This study was undertaken to evaluate the use of the nasal width as a guide for the selection of proper width maxillary anterior denture teeth in four racial groups of the Brazilian population.

Materials and Methods: One hundred and sixty subjects (40 Whites, 40 Mulattos, 40 Blacks, and 40 Asians) were selected. Using a sliding caliper, the nasal width and the intercanine distance were measured. The Pearson product-moment correlation coefficient was used to determine the relationship between the above measurements. A prediction was made of the percentage of subjects of the White, Mulatto, Black, and Asian populations in which the selection error due to the clinical application of the method of the nasal width would be within 0 to 2 mm, within 2 to 4 mm, and greater than 4 mm.

Results: The four racial groups showed a weak correlation between the intercanine distance and the nasal width. In 39.7% of the White, 55.7% of the Mulatto, 81.9% of the Black, and 48.2% of the Asian populations, errors greater than 4 mm would be present with the use of the nasal width.

Conclusions: The correlation found between the intercanine distance and the nasal width was not high enough to be used as a predictive factor. The relationship between natural tooth width and artificial tooth width as predicted by the nasal width showed that the nasal width method is not accurate for all the studied groups.

Selecting and arranging artificial teeth for edentulous patients is difficult when pre-extraction records are not available. Errors at this stage can often result in patient rejection of otherwise well-constructed, comfortable, and efficient dentures.[1–5] In an effort to solve this problem, various guidelines have been suggested for determining the width of the maxillary anterior teeth.

One of the available methods that can aid in the selection of the width of anterior teeth is the use of the nasal width, the so-called "nasal index."[2,6] In this technique, it has been suggested[7] that the projection of perpendicular lines downward from the alae of the nose to the buccal surface of the upper occlusal rim may be used to determine the position of the tips of the artificial canines. To select the correct size of the six anterior artificial teeth, the distance between the canine marks projected to the buccal surface of the maxillary occlusal rim is measured around the curve of the rim with a flexible ruler.[2,5,3] Since tooth mold charts for anterior teeth give dimensions from the distal of one canine to another, 8 to 10 mm should be added to this value to obtain the distance between the distal surface of the canines.[8]

Previous studies attempted to determine the nasal width dimension and its relation to the intercanine distance.[1–5,9,10] Most of them have shown no significant relationships between these two measurements.[1,2,4,5,8] However, most of the studies regarding the selection of complete denture teeth were conducted in Caucasian population samples,[1,3–5,11,12] and the findings have been extrapolated to other ethnic groups. In 1992, Johnson[13] pointed out that the prosthodontic literature seems to pertain only to the Caucasian race with little noted about other races. Furthermore, the author reported that the knowledge of racial norms for facial appearance might aid practitioners, since the treatment given would then be in harmony with the facial appearance for patients of different races.

The Brazilian society consists of a diverse mix of races, with some of the ethnic groups remaining racially homogenous while others have mixed with other races. The purpose of this article is to evaluate the use of the nasal width as a guide for the selection of proper width maxillary anterior denture teeth in four racial groups of the Brazilian population.

MATERIALS AND METHODS

The research plan was prepared in accordance with guidelines appropriate to research involving human subjects, as set down in Resolution 196/96 of the National Health Council and approved by the Research Ethics Committee of São Paulo State University.

One hundred and sixty Brazilian subjects (40 Whites, 40 Mulattos, 40 Blacks, and 40 Asians—Japanese and Chinese) of mixed sex and age (ranging from 18 to 33 years) were selected for this study. The subjects met the following criteria: (1) they had all natural permanent maxillary teeth with no history of orthodontic treatment or extraction, (2) the canines and incisors were in good alignment without drifting or attrition in more than one third of incisal edge of the canines, and (3) they had no congenital or surgical facial defects.

Before any procedures, all subjects received detailed information about the research and were then asked to sign a Free and Clarified Consent Form.

The external width of the alae of the nose was measured at the widest point using a digital sliding caliper (Mitutoyo Sul Americana Ltda., São Paulo, Brazil). Artificial stone casts of the maxillary arches (Rock Plus, Polidental Ind. e Com Ltda, São Paulo, Brazil) were made from irreversible hydrocolloid (Jeltrate, Dentsply Ind. e Com. Ltda., Petropolis, Brazil) impressions made in perforated stock trays. The maxillary intercanine distance was measured from the stone cast using the sliding caliper. Each measurement was made in a straight line from canine cusp tip to canine cusp tip on three occasions. The original cusp tip was considered to have been at the intersection of a line drawn with graphite along the mesial and distal cutting edge and a line along the buccal and lingual long axis of the tooth.

Each measurement was made on three separate occasions. The average of the three measurements was used. The same examiner carried out all procedures, performed all measurements, and recorded all information.

Analysis of variance was used to determine whether the nasal width and the intercanine distance were different in relation to race. To compare different means, the Tukey test ($p < 0.05$) was used. The Pearson product-moment correlation coefficient was used to determine the relationship between the intercanine distance and the nasal width in the four racial groups studied.

The selection error due to the application of the method of the nasal width was also determined, in millimeters. First, the curve distance between the cusp tips of the canines (IcD) was measured. For that, dental floss was placed at the greatest facial curvature of the maxillary arch, sectioned with a blade

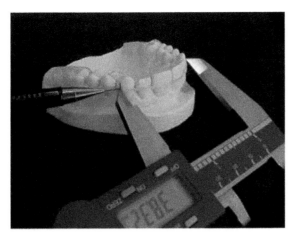

FIGURE 1 Sliding caliper positioned on the dental floss and mark made with graphite.

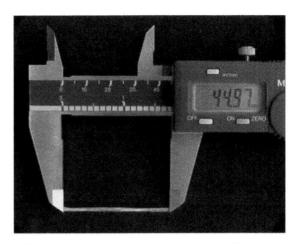

FIGURE 3 Dental floss measured with the sliding caliper.

at the location of the cusp tips of the canines, and then measured with the sliding caliper. Dental floss was also placed at the greatest curvature of the maxillary arch and fixed with adhesive tape. The sliding caliper was opened to the value obtained for the nasal width. The sliding caliper was positioned on the dental floss, and two marks were made with graphite, one each side (Fig 1). The floss was sectioned in the marks' locations (Fig 2) and measured with the sliding caliper (Fig 3). The value obtained for this measurement corresponded to the intercanine distance predicted by the nasal width (IcD′). Each measurement was made three times on three separate occasions. The selection error was defined as the difference between the width of the artificial teeth estimated by the nasal width and the real width of the natural teeth (IcD′ minus IcD).

In addition, a prediction was made of the percentage of subjects of the White, Black, Mulatto, and Asian populations (using a 95% confidence interval) in which this error would be within 0 to 2 mm, within 2 to 4 mm, and greater than 4 mm.

RESULTS

The mean values of the intercanine distance and of the nasal width of the four racial groups and the result of the Tukey test are presented in Table 1. For the nasal width, the Black group was significantly different from the White, Mulatto, and Asian groups. Between the Mulatto and Asian groups, there was no significant difference. For the intercanine distance, the Black group was significantly different from the White, Mulatto, and Asian groups. The Mulatto group was not statistically different from the White and Asian groups.

Pearson correlation analysis showed a weak correlation between the intercanine distance and the nasal width in the four studied racial groups. It was not high enough to be used as a predictive factor. The following coefficients (r) were obtained: White = 0.238, Mulatto = 0.436, Black = 0.286, and Asian = 0.089. The correlation between the two measurements in the four races is shown in Figures 4 to 7. The dotted lines present the linear regression line for the values. In the White, Black, and Mulatto groups, although the coefficients were all weak, there was little tendency for

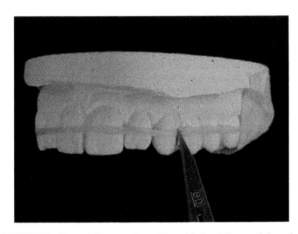

FIGURE 2 Dental floss sectioned by a blade at the mark location.

TABLE 1 Values for the Nasal Width and the Intercanine Distance

Measurements	Statistic (mm)	White	Mulatto	Black	Asian
NW*	Minimum	30.07	30.40	34.39	30.68
	Maximum	40.57	45.29	53.80	43.07
	Mean	35.28[a]	36.89[b]	42.39[c]	37.27[b]
	SD	2.62	2.99	3.40	2.88
ID*	Minimum	29.01	28.67	30.67	29.95
	Maximum	39.26	39.19	39.97	38.75
	Mean	33.55[a]	34.31[ab]	36.03[c]	34.83[b]
	SD	2.30	2.49	2.07	1.77

Same superscript letters indicate that the Tukey test showed no significant difference ($p < 0.05$). NW = nasal width; ID = intercanine distance.
*p Value = 0.0000.

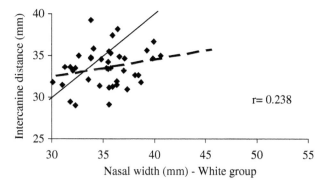

FIGURE 4 Correlation between the nasal width and the intercanine distance for the White group.

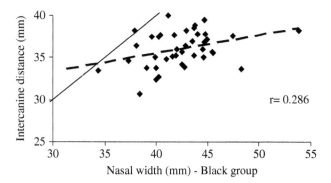

FIGURE 6 Correlation between the nasal width and the intercanine distance for the Black group.

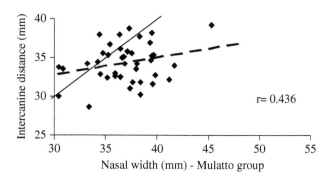

FIGURE 5 Correlation between the nasal width and the intercanine distance for the Mulatto group.

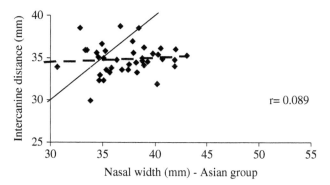

FIGURE 7 Correlation between the nasal width and the intercanine distance for the Asian group.

the variables to increase linearly in the same way. The full lines indicate the position of the points in the diagram if there was equality between the variables.

Table 2 contains the information regarding the selection errors due to the use of nasal width for the selection of the six anterior teeth width. In all racial groups studied, the use of the nasal width would lead, in general, to the selection of wider artificial teeth.

DISCUSSION

The mean nasal width dimensions were 35.28 mm for the White group, 36.89 mm for the Mulatto group, 42.39 mm for the Black group, and 37.27 mm for the Asian group. The White value is in agreement with the studies of Mavroskoufis & Ritchie (35.3 mm);[3] Scandrett et al (34.4 mm);[4] and Smith (33.5 mm).[5] However, Latta et al,[14] studying White

TABLE 2   Selection Errors Due to the Use of the Nasal Width for the Selection of the Six Anterior Teeth Width

Information	Race			
	White	Mulatto	Black	Asian
Error statistics (mm)				
Largest error for wider teeth	8.75	14.67	27.29	14.65
Largest error for narrower teeth	−8.25*	−9.24	−3.77	−9.08
Mean	0.17	2.39	9.85	1.73
SD	4.72	6.34	7.23	5.41
Prediction of errors %				
Within 0 to 2 mm	32.8%	23.1%	8.8%	27.4%
Within 2 to 4 mm	27.5%	21.2%	9.3%	24.3%
Higher than 4 mm	39.7%	55.7%	81.9%	48.2%

*The minus sign (—) demonstrates the selection of narrower teeth.

edentulous patients, found a value of 40 mm. Other studies did not include races in their respective patient populations, although they found values for the nasal width close to those of the results of this study. Puri et al[10] found 37.13 mm for men and 33.05 mm for women, and Hoffman et al[1] found 34.28 mm.

In the Black group, the mean nasal width was statistically different from the White and Mulatto mean values. Latta et al,[14] studying Black edentulous patients, found a different value (47 mm), although this value lies between the minimum and maximum values found in this study.

The nasal width values obtained by Keng,[2] studying Chinese patients, were close to those of the results of this study: 39.60 mm for men and 36.41 mm for women.

For the intercanine distance, the White group presented a mean value of 33.55 mm, while the Mulatto group presented 34.31 mm, the Black group presented 36.03 mm, and the Asian group presented 34.83 mm. The White value was in agreement with the studies of Smith (33.2 mm);[5] Mavroskoufis & Ritchie (34.3 mm);[3] Hoffman et al (35.35 mm);[1] and Puri et al (36.5 mm for men and 33.67 mm for women).[10]

With respect to the intercanine distance of the Black group, the mean value obtained was statistically higher than the mean values of the White and Mulatto groups. One of the factors that may influence this distance is the width of the teeth. The studies of Grave,[15] Lavelle,[16] and Mack[17] demonstrated that Black subjects have wider teeth than other races, which may explain the greater intercanine distance found in the Black group.

In the Asian group, the intercanine distance obtained was in agreement with the values found in Keng's study (35.60 mm for men and 34.96 mm for women).[2]

The correlation coefficient (r) found in the White group (0.238) is in disagreement with those found by Smith (0.37)[5] and Hoffman et al (0.413).[1] Scandrett et al[4] obtained a coefficient of 0.366, although they determined the correlation between the nasal width and the curve distance between the distal of the canines, and not the straight distance between the tips of the canines.

The mean selection error due to the application of the method of the nasal width was calculated by subtracting the value obtained for the curve intercanine distance predicted by the nasal width from the value obtained for the real curve distance between the tips of the canines. Thus, the positive mean values (Table 2) indicate that the use of this method would lead to the selection of wider artificial teeth for all the racial groups.

The prediction of the percentage of subjects of each race in which the selection error would be within 0 to 2 mm, within 2 to 4 mm, and greater than 4 mm showed that errors greater than 4 mm would be present in 39.7% of Whites, 55.7% of Mulattos, 81.9% of Blacks, and 48.2% of Asians (Table 2). Since the method of the nasal width determines the position of the cusp tips of the canines, the addition of 8 to 10 mm is necessary to obtain the distance between the distal surface of the canines.[8] This addition could introduce an additional error.

The results of this study suggest that the method of the nasal width is not accurate for all the racial groups studied, rendering the worst result for the Black group; however, this method may aid in an initial selection of the width of the artificial anterior teeth for the White group, although other variables are needed to predict the width of the maxillary anterior teeth, such as the patient's physical size, jaw ridge size, and esthetic sensitivity.

CONCLUSIONS

From the results of this study, the following conclusions were drawn:

For all the studied racial groups, the measurements of the nasal widths showed a weak correlation with the intercanine distance, not high enough to be used as a predictive factor.

The relationship between natural teeth width and artificial teeth width as predicted by the nasal width showed that the nasal width method is not accurate for all the studied groups and would lead, in general, to the selection of wider artificial teeth.

REFERENCES

1. Hoffman W Jr, Bomberg TJ, Hatch RA: Interalar width as a guide in denture tooth selection. *J Prosthet Dent* 1986;55: 219–221.

2. Keng SB: Nasal width dimensions and anterior teeth in prosthodontics. *AnnAcad Med Singapore* 1986;15:311–314.

3. Mavroskoufis F. Ritchie GM: Nasal width and incisive papilla as guides for the selection and arrangement of maxillary anterior teeth. *J Prosthet Dent* 1981;45:592–597.

4. Scandrett FR, Kerber PE, Umrigar ZR: A clinical evaluation of techniques to determine the combined width of the maxillary anterior teeth and the maxillary central incisor. *J Prosthet Dent* 1982;48:15–22.

5. Smith BJ: The value of the nose width as an esthetic guide in prosthodontics. *J Prosthet Dent* 1975;34:562–573.

6. Lee JH: The appearance of artificial dentures. *Aust Dent J* 1964;9:304–308.

7. Scott JE: The Scott system of precision articulation in three-dimensional occlusion. *J Prosthet Dent* 1952;2:362–380.

8. McCord JF, Grant AA: Registration: stage III—selection of teeth. *Br Dent J* 2000;188:660–666.

9. al-el-Sheikh HM, al-Athel MS: The relationship of interalar width, interpupillary width and maxillary anterior teeth width in Saudi population. *Odontostomatol Trop* 1998;21:7–10.

10. Puri M, Bhalla LR, Khanna VK: Relationship of intercanine distance with the distance between the alae of the nose. *J Indian Dent Assoc* 1972;44:46–50.

11. Grove HF, Christensen LV: Relationship of the maxillary canines to the incisive papilla. *J Prosthet Dent* 1989;61: 51–53.

12. Lieb ND, Silverman SI, Garfinkel L: An analysis of soft tissue contours of the lips in relation to the maxillary cuspids. *J Prosthet Dent* 1967;18:292–303.

13. Johnson PF: Racial norms: esthetic and prosthodontic implications. *J Prosthet Dent* 1992;67:502–508.

14. Latta GH Jr, Weaver JR, Conkin JE: The relationship between the width of the mouth, bizygomaticwidth, and the interpupillary distance in edentulous patients. *J Prosthet Dent* 1991;65:250–254.

15. Grave AM: The frequency of various molds in a sample of natural and artificial dentitions. *J Prosthet Dent* 1987;57: 195–197.

16. Lavelle CL: Maxillary and mandibular tooth size in different racial groups and in different occlusal categories. *Am JOrthod* 1972;61:29–37.

17. Mack PJ: Maxillaryarch and central incisordimensions in a Nigerian and British population sample. *J Dent* 1981;9:67–70.

30

QUALITATIVE AND QUANTITATIVE GUIDES TO THE SELECTION AND ARRANGEMENT OF THE MAXILLARY ANTERIOR TEETH

DOUGLAS A. HOCK, DDS, MS
Private practice, Ypsilanti, MI

Keywords
Qualitative/quantitative guides; maxillary anterior teeth

Correspondence
Address reprint requests to Douglas A. Hock, DDS, MS, 3075 W Clark Rd, Suite 409, Ypsilanti, MI 48197.

Published in *Journal of Prosthodontics* 1992; Vol. 1, Issue 2, pp. 106–11

doi: 1059-941X/92/0102-0007$5.00/0

ABSTRACT

A literature review of the selection of the maxillary anterior teeth is presented. Although several different qualitative guidelines are cited, the best method for the selection of the maxillary anterior teeth is the use of pre-extraction records or old photographs. Numerous qualitative and quantitative guidelines are cited in the literature for the proper placement of the maxillary anterior teeth. Through careful and proper construction of the maxillary wax occlusal rim. these factors may be recorded and relayed to the dental laboratory technician.

The field of complete denture prosthetics has approached new thresholds with the development of dental implants for implant-supported dentures. At times, from a clinical perspective, it seems that concepts of denture esthetics are being overshadowed by mechanistic concerns for denture stability and function. Patients, however, are most concerned about the appearance of their prosthetic treatment.[1,2] The question comes back to, "How do we select the anterior teeth?" and, "How do we determine the proper esthetic arrangement of the anterior teeth?" It seems that these two very basic requirements are often lost in a sea of technological advances and philosophical changes of emphasis during the course of prosthodontic treatment. Therefore, the purpose of this article is to examine, through the use of the literature, qualitative as well as quantitative guides to the selection and arrangement of the maxillary anterior teeth.

ANTERIOR TOOTH SELECTION

Leon Williams is generally given credit for the development of the "Law of Harmony," which states that basic tooth forms of square, ovoid, tapering, and the combination of these forms will match the outline of the patient's face.[3] Berry, however, wrote in 1906 (a decade earlier) that the inverted outline of the face will correspond to the appropriate tooth form.[4] House strongly endorsed the efforts of Williams because it was believed that Williams' work gave a sound, scientific foundation for the selection of artificial teeth.[5] Before the efforts of Williams and Berry, denture tooth selection was based upon the "Tempermental Theory," which ascribed tooth form characteristics to basic personality types. A "billious" individual would be expected to have short, broad, tapering incisor teeth, whereas a "sanguineous" individual would possess long, thin, and narrow teeth.

Wright was one of the first to disagree with Williams' theory. Based on clinical observations of patients with natural teeth, he noted that in one third of the patients he studied that face and tooth form did not match.[6] It was pointed out that these individuals did not present with "incongruous" faces. It was believed that this was caused by the fact that from a standpoint of casual, conversational esthetics it is difficult to detect discrepancies of tooth and facial form because teeth are relatively small when compared to the face. He further noted that the arrangement of the teeth, irrespective of the outline form, is in an alignment that harmonizes with the facial contours. Wright should be given credit for saying that when selecting artificial teeth, photographs, old models, or pre-extraction records should be used when available.

As time went on, researchers began to question Williams' Law of Harmony. Mavroskoufis et al examined the face shape and photographs of the central incisors of 70 dental students. They discovered that in only 5.7% of the students did the facial outline and tooth forms coincide. Another 25.6% were similar, but not identical. A rather striking 68.7% of the students showed no correlation between facial and tooth outline forms.[7]

Brodbelt et al studied 81 subjects with normal, healthy maxillary anterior dentitions. They made studies by plotting 21 points along the outlines of the face and the corresponding maxillary central incisors. They determined that no truly tapering faces existed and no square faces had square teeth. In addition, it was found that the majority of the faces were ovoid, and 87% of these had ovoid teeth.[8] Seluk et al found that with respect to patient preference, there are significant differences between facial form and tooth molds when the patients were asked to choose between three sets of dentures with square, tapering and ovoid tooth forms. They also noted that any given tooth mold may appear square, tapering, or ovoid depending on how the gingival contours are waxed.[9]

French, while disagreeing with the Law of Harmony, favored interproximal wear as well as incisal wear for older patients.[10] In the 1950s, Frush and Fisher in a series of articles introduced the concept that they called dentogenics. According to the authors, dentogenic is the description of a denture "which is eminently suited for the given wearer, which adds to a person's charm, character, dignity or beauty." It was believed that it is necessary to convey age, sex, and personality in complete dentures. With respect to age, it was believed that the older the individual, the darker the teeth. Older teeth have greater incisal and interproximal wear. With increasing age, greater rounding of the interdental papillae and festooning of the free gingival margin takes place. A discussion of what constitutes male and female characteristics was presented. As interpreted by the authors, when one thinks of feminine characteristics, one thinks of roundness, smoothness, and softness. Therefore, it was believed that the incisal edges should be rounded or curved. Masculine characteristics, it was believed, are cuboidal, hard, muscular, and vigorous. Following these interpretations, the incisal edges of a man's denture tooth should be squared. The position of the maxillary anterior teeth with respect to one another may also be sex specific. Rotating the lateral incisor, making the distolabial line angle prominent, creates an illusion of harshness. Tucking the cuspids distally was considered feminine, while making them prominent was considered to be masculine. The authors furthered stated that the teeth and their arrangement should coincide with the patient's personality. They believed that vigorous teeth should be used with vigorous patients.[11–13]

Roberts supported Frush and Fisher by stating that modifications should be made to the shape of selected denture teeth to account for the patient's age and sex.[14] Although much credit should be given to Frush and Fisher for their ideas about the importance of age and sex, personality factors should not enter into tooth selection. To ascribe tooth forms and their arrangement based upon perceived personality factors is akin to the Tempermental Theory, which was debunked earlier in this century. The perceived personality of a patient in a dental office may be quite different from that observed in a less formal atmosphere where the patient may not be under such close scrutiny and, perhaps, not under as much stress.

Esposito noted that the replacement teeth of complete dentures tend to be too small.[15] Vig observed that using replacement teeth that are too small contributes to what he describes as the undesireable "denture look."[16] McArthur examined study casts of three different groups of patients. In the group of young patients, the average mesiodistal width of the maxillary central incisor was 8.87 mm. In adults, because of proximal wear, the average incisor width was 8.67 mm. In denture patients, the average mesiodistal width of the maxillary central incisor was found to be only 8.36 mm. Because of the relatively small difference, it was believed that the perception that denture teeth are too small may be caused by the results of decreased vertical dimension, inadequate lip support, and lack of natural effects or characterization.[17]

AUTHOR'S VIEWPOINT: TOOTH SELECTION

Patient input is of tantamount importance when the selection of denture teeth is to be made. One cannot overlook the significance of patient satisfaction and of what the patient perceives as being correct and esthetic. The patient should believe that he or she has a share in the responsibility of determining what their finished prosthesis will look like. This is not to say that the patient should be allowed to capriciously take over the tooth selection process. The patient should be educated about the parameters with which their case presents. For example, if a clinician is faced with the task of selecting teeth for a very tall, large-boned male with very large edentulous arches, the suggestion might be made that a large tooth mold should be used. The patient may agree and the selection process may be further narrowed to a particular mold. The patient may disagree, saying that he originally had very small teeth with considerable spacing.

Old photographs or pre-extraction records not only provide a wealth of information regarding the patient's pre-edentulous state, but also provide a focal point for discussion. The patient may voice approval or express concerns with the appearance of his or her previous natural dentition. If the patient's previous natural dentition is deemed to be unesthetic, appropriate changes should be made. Under these circumstances the patient will always wish to look better.

The patient's input can put the clinician on the right path to the correct selection of anterior teeth. The patient's age and sex should be taken into consideration. Maxillomandibular relations may influence the tooth selection process. There are times when a shorter tooth must be selected to provide the correct amount of incisor display because a very large or prominent alveolar process may be present. The tooth selection process should follow the recording of the maxillomandibular relations on occlusal wax rims.

MAXILLARY ANTERIOR TOOTH PLACEMENT

House spoke of a need to move away from mechanical approaches to denture construction in favor of esthetic and natural considerations. In his article he made a great deal of use of dried skull specimens to illustrate how teeth occur in nature.[5] Pound eschewed mechanical methods of denture construction in preference of a natural approach. He stated "To reproduce or imitate nature should be our aim." It was believed that the anterior and posterior teeth should be replaced in the same natural position relative to the lips, cheeks, and tongue. He acknowledged that as the edentulous

ridges resorb, the correct placement of the teeth will become more off-center with respect to the edentulous ridges.[18] In support of his predecessors, Boucher stated "The only correct position of a tooth is the one in which it was placed by Nature." He added, "Perhaps dental schools should no longer teach the ideal tooth arrangement. Instead, they might place greater emphasis upon the relations of natural teeth to the alveolar ridges from which the teeth erupt."[19] In a later publication, Boucher illustrates how the maxillary anterior alveolus protrudes at an angle from the rest of the face. This profile should be duplicated with the labial flange of a complete denture.[20] Vig described what he termed "the denture look" as being that typical facial appearance common to most denture wearers. He asserted that placing the teeth too close to the ridges is the greatest contributor to "the denture look."[16] Lombardi furthered this assessment by stating that the principle failure in denture esthetics is not setting the teeth in a dynamic way with the face. Too often, he observed, the maxillary anterior teeth are set too high up and too far back.[21] Curtis et al noted that immediate dentures are usually the most esthetic because esthetic perception is enhanced if the replacement teeth are placed in relatively the same position as the former healthy, natural teeth.[1] While agreeing with the problems encountered with correct maxillary anterior tooth placement, Sharry points out that as a general rule, the labial surface of the mandibular incisors should not be set out beyond the plane perpendicular to the mucolabial fold.[22]

Any discussion of correct maxillary anterior tooth placement should not be undertaken unless morphological changes that take place under denture bases are first understood. Tallgren, in a series of articles, researched changes that occur in the bone of denture wearers. By using serial roentgenographs, she examined patients that wore dentures for 7 years. She found a mean reduction in vertical height of 8.5 mm caused by the loss of alveolar bone. She did not find any changes in the basal bone, or the gonial angle of the mandible, or cranial base and upper face.[23,24] Later, in a study covering 25 years of denture wearing, she found continued and marked vertical reduction in the residual ridges whereby the mandibular residual ridge resorbed at a rate four times greater than that of the maxilla.[25] Atwood found that the rate of residual ridge reduction averaged 0.5 mm per year. The rate of reduction was 0.1 mm per year for the anterior maxilla and 0.4 mm per year for the anterior mandible.[26] Bergman and Carlsson, in a long-term study of denture wearers, found that after 21 years of denture wearing the occlusal vertical dimension was found to be too low in two thirds of the patients.[27] Watt and Likeman studied maxillary postextraction changes over a period of 2½ years. The only stable area was found to be 1 cm palatal to the original position of the natural teeth. They observed that bone loss occurs labially and buccally as well as vertically, ranging from 3.5 mm in the central incisor and premolar area to 4 to 5 mm in the molar region. The incisive papilla was found to move anteriorly 1.6 mm and superiorly 2.3 mm.[28] Maritato and Douglas, in an effort to find stable anatomical landmarks, determined that the subspinale (point A) is not subject to change. Because the alveolar process in a dentate state angles labially from point A, it was concluded that the border of the labial flange can be used to help create the labial contour of the wax occlusal rim. It should also follow that the border of the labial flange of the maxillary denture should be thin.[29]

Harper was the first to describe the incisive papilla as a guide in denture prosthetics in determining the labial extent of the central incisors. He cautioned against the use of the incisive papilla to determine the midline of the replacement teeth, noting that in one half of the patients observed, the maxilla lies off-center with respect to the midline of the face.[30] Schiffman studied 507 maxillary casts of dentate patients. An imaginary line passing through the tips of the cuspids was found to be within 1 mm of passing through the center of the incisive papilla in 92.1% of all the casts.[31] Ehrlich and Gazit produced findings that supported Schiffman's. In a study of 430 dentate casts of patients with Angle's Class I malocclusion, they also found that the average distance from the posterior edge of the incisive papilla to the labial surface of the right central incisor was 12.31 mm, with a range from 12 to 13 mm.[32] Grove and Becker agreed with the use of the posterior border of the incisive papilla because it is closest to the stable, unchanging area of the palate. Their findings were in agreement with those of Ehrlich and Gazit. Two groups of dentate and denture patients were studied. They found the labial surface of the central incisor of maxillary dentures to be almost 2 mm closer to the posterior border of the incisive papilla, indicating that denture teeth are set too far posterior.[33]

Hoffman et al found that the nasal interalar width could be used as a guide for determining the width of the maxillary anterior teeth. On average, the intercuspid tip width was found to be 3% greater than the interalar width. It was believed that this finding could be used as a guide in fabricating the maxillary occlusal wax rim.[34]

Esposito noted that the vertical placement of the maxillary anterior teeth should allow for light incisor contact with the lower lip with the pronunciation of f and v sounds.[15] Vig and Brando examined the amount of incisor display with the lips at rest. Men tended to show 1.91 mm and women 3.4 mm of the maxillary incisors. It was further noted that with increasing age, there is a decrease in the exposure of the maxillary incisors and an increase in the display of the mandibular incisors.[35] Tjan et al examined the smiles in photographs of 454 dental and hygiene students. In 10.57% a high-lip-line smile was observed, showing the total cervicoincisal length and a continuous band of gingiva. In 68.94% an average smile was observed, with 75% to 100% of the cervicoincisal length of the maxillary incisors exposed. In 20.48% a low smile with less than 75% of the length of the incisor teeth showing was observed.[36] Araki and Araki found that the

head angulation may have an influence on the maxillary lip posture, and concluded that maxillomandibular relations should be recorded with the patient in a comfortable, upright posture.[37]

AUTHOR'S VIEWPOINT: MAXILLARY ANTERIOR TOOTH ARRANGEMENT

The first step in determining the correct placement of the maxillary anterior teeth is the fabrication of the wax occlusal rims. It is from the wax occlusal rims that the laboratory technician determines the placement of the anterior teeth. When done correctly, the wax occlusal rims inserted into the patient's mouth should properly support the lips at the proper vertical dimension of occlusion.

Using point A (subspinale) and the incisive papilla as anatomical guides, the maxillary wax occlusal rim should be constructed with a convex anterior profile. One should envision the labial surface of the anatomical crown and root of the maxillary central incisor as coinciding with the anterior profile of the rim (Figs 1 and 2). The labial extent of the rim should be approximately 12 mm from the posterior border of the incisive papilla. The edge of the labial flange should be kept relatively thin. The approximate placement of the maxillary cuspids should be envisioned. The tips of the cuspids should form an imaginary line roughly passing through the center of the incisive papilla.

When the maxillary baseplate is inserted into the mouth, the upper lip should appear unstrained and relaxed. With the lips lightly parted, depending upon the age of the patient, approximately 2 mm of the rim should be exposed. When the patient speaks, the wax rim should be visible. Observe the patient's smile. If considerable vertical height of the wax rim is visible, ask the patient if they had a tendency to show their "gum line" when they smiled with their natural teeth. This may be another opportunity for the use of old photographs. The edge of the wax rim should lightly touch the lower lip with f and v sounds.

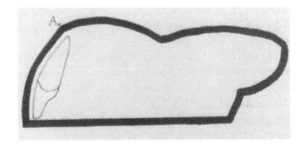

FIGURE 1 A schematic depiction of a maxillary interocclusal rim. The A point is the subspinale, from which the anterior profile of the wax rim curves outward. Note how the labial surface of a maxillary central incisor coincides with this profile.

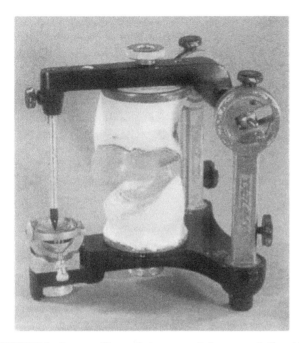

FIGURE 2 Intermaxillary relations recorded on a semiadjustable articulator. Note the outward curved anterior profile of the wax occlusal rim.

The quantitative measurements used in determining the placement of the maxillary anterior teeth should be used only as approximate guides and not as hard-and-fast boundaries. If the maxillary wax occlusal rim does not fall within the numerical guidelines given in this article, the rim should not necessarily be discarded. It should be re-examined for correctness.

REFERENCES

1. Curtis TA, Shaw EL, Curtis DA: The influence of removable prosthodontic procedures and concepts on the esthetics of complete dentures. *J Prosthet Dent* 1987;57:315–323.
2. Goldstein RE: Study of need for esthetics in dentistry'. *J Prosthet Dent* 1969;21:589–598.
3. Williams JL: *A New Classification of Natural and Artificial Teeth.* New York, NY, The Dentist's Supply Go, 1917, pp 1–76.
4. Berry FH: Is the theory of temperament the foundation to the study of prosthetic art? *Dentist's Mag* 1906;1:405–413.
5. House MM: Art-A fundamental in denture prosthesis. *J Am Dent Assoc* 1937;24:406–422.
6. Wright WH: Selection and arrangement of artificial teeth for complete dentures. *J Am Dent Assoc* 1936;23:2291–2307.
7. Mavroskoufis F, Ritchie GM: The face form as a guide for the selection of maxillary central incisors. *J Prosthet Dent* 1980;43:501–505.
8. Brodbelt RHW, Walker GF, Nelson D, et al: Comparison of face with tooth form. *J Prosthet Dent* 1984;52:588–592.
9. Scluk LW, Brodbelt RHW, Walker GF: A biometric comparison of face shape with denture tooth form. *J Oral Rchabil* 1987;14:139–145.
10. French FA: The selection and arrangement of the anterior teeth in prosthetic dentures. *J Prosthet Dent* 1951;1:587–593.
11. Frush JP, Fisher RD: Introduction to dentogenic restorations. *J Prosthet Dent* 1955;5:586–595.
12. Frush JP, Fisher RD: How dentogenic restorations interpret the sex factor. *J Prosthet Dent* 1956;6:160–172.
13. Frush JP, Fisher RD: The age factor in dentogenics. *J Prosthet Dent* 1957;7:5–13.
14. Roberts AL: Present-day concepts in complete denture service. *J Prosthet Dent* 1959;9:900–913.
15. Esposito TJ: Esthetics for denture patients. *J Prosthet Dent* 1980;44:608–615.
16. Vig RG: The denture look. *J Prosthet Dent* 1961;11:9–15.
17. McArthur DR: Are anterior replacement teeth too small? *J Prosthet Dent* 1987;57:462–465.
18. Pound EO: Lost-Fine arts in the fallacy of the ridges. *J Prosthet Dent* 1954;4:6–16.
19. Boucher CO: The current status of prosthodontics. *J Prosthet Dent* 1960;10:411–425.
20. Boucher CO: *Swenson's Complete Dentures (ed 6).* St Louis, MO, Mosby, 1970, pp 155–166.
21. Lombardi RE: The principles of visual perception and their clinical application to denture esthetics. *J Prosthet Dent* 1973;29:358–382.
22. Sharry JJ: *Complete Denture Prosthodontics (ed 2).* New York, NY, McGraw-Hill, 1968, pp 235–237.
23. Tallgren A: The reduction in face height of edentulous and partially edentulous subjects during long-term denture wear. *Acta Odontol Scand* 1966;24:195–239.
24. Tallgren A: The effect of denture wearing on facial morphology. *Acta Odontol Scand* 1967;25:563–592.
25. Tallgren A: The continuing reduction of the residual alveolar ridges in complete denture wearers: A mixed longitudinal study covering 25 years. *J Prosthet Dent* 1972;27:120–132.
26. Atwood DA, Coy WA: Clinical, cephalometric, and densitometric study of reduction of residual ridges. *J Prosthet Dent* 1971;26:280–295.
27. Bergman B, Carlsson GE: Clinical long-term study of complete denture wearers. *J Prosthet Dent* 1985;53:56–61.
28. Watt DM, Likeman PR: Morphological changes in the denture bearing area following the extraction of maxillary teeth. *Br Dent J* 1974;136:225–235.
29. Maritato FR, Douglas JR: A positive guide to anterior tooth placement. *J Prosthet Dent* 1964;14:848–853.
30. Harper RN: The incisive papilla. *J Dent Res* 1948;27:661–668.
31. Schiffman P: Relation of the maxillary canine to the incisive papilla. *J Prosthet Dent* 1964;14:469–472.

32. Ehrlich J, Gazit E: Relationship of the maxillary central incisors and canines to the incisive papilla. *J Oral Rehabil* 1975;2: 309–312.

33. Grove AMH, Becker RJ: Evaluation of the incisive papilla as a guide to anterior tooth position. *J Prosthet Dent* 1987;57: 712–714.

34. Hoffman W, Bomberg TJ, Hatch RA: Interalar width as a guide in denture tooth selection. *J Prosthet Dent* 1986;55:219–221.

35. Vig RG, Brando GC: The kinetics of anterior tooth display. *J Prosthet Dent* 1978;39:502–504.

36. Tjan AHL, Miller GD, The JGP: Some esthetic factors in a smile. *J Prosthet Dent* 1978;39:502–504.

37. Araki NG, Araki CT: Head angulation and variations in the maxillomandibular relationship. Part II: The effects on facial contour and lip support. *J Prosthet Dent* 1987;58: 218–221.

INDEX

A

abutment teeth, 173
  preset of, 175
acquired or congenital maxillofacial defects, 27
acrylic prosthetic denture teeth, 6
acrylic teeth, 152
acrylic varnish, 124
adaptol, 181
  border-molded custom tray, 182
adjunctive diagnostic procedures, 53–54
adjunctive diagnostic techniques, 52–53
Aggregatibacter actinomycetemcomitans, 60, 89, 90, 92, 93, 95, 96
aging, 9, 33, 44, 49, 58, 67, 84, 129, 172, 207, 243
albumin, 68, 70, 71
alcohol, 49
aligned artificial tooth (1SA) system, 153
  digital design, 153
alternative medicines, 135
Alzheimer's Disease, 43
amphotericin B, 107, 108, 131, 136, 138–140, 142, 144
Angle's Class I malocclusion, 264
ANOVA design, 212
anterior tooth, 246
  and dentogenic theory, 249
  factors influencing identification, 249
  factors of gender, personality, and age, 248
  female patient, 248
  Kappa values, 247
  law of facial harmony, 246
  layman group for gender determination, 248
  male patient, 248
  natural dentition, 246

photographic evaluation, 247–248
  reliability/validity, 247
anthropometric assessment, 67, 68
antibacterial agents, 58
antifungal agent, 60, 131, 135, 144, 146
antifungal agents, 12, 60, 131, 135, 146
  combination therapy of, 135
antifungal therapy, 81, 99, 107, 108, 135, 140, 142
antimicrobial treatment, 81, 108
antiseptic agent, 129
AOP. *see* artificial occlusal plane (AOP)
artificial canines, 256
artificial food, chewed
  mean weight and standard deviation (SD) of, 208
  period granulation, 209
artificial occlusal plane (AOP), 195, 197
  Camper's I, II, and III, 195, 196
  dentate group, 195
artificial teeth, 24, 153, 160, 174, 196, 197, 207, 256–259, 262
aspiration pneumonia (AP), 6, 41
  risk factors, 81
autopolymerizing resin, 222

B

Bacillus subtilis, 131
bacterial endocarditis, 6, 60
bacterial species, in healthy patients, 6
barium sulfate creamy mix, 195
bilateral balanced occlusion
  buccal view of, 222
  fully, 222
  lingual view, 222
biochemical assessment, 67, 68

Journal of Prosthodontics on Complete and Removable Dentures, First Edition. Edited by Jonathan P. Wiens, Jennifer Wiens Priebe, and Donald A. Curtis.
© 2018 American College of Prosthodontists. Published 2018 by John Wiley & Sons, Inc.